THE AVOIDABLE CAUSES OF DISEASE,

INSANITY AND DEFORMITY.

BY

JOHN ELLIS, M.D.

PROFESSOR OF THE PRINCIPLES AND PRACTICE OF MEDICINE IN THE WESTERN MEDICAL COLLEGE OF CLEVELAND, OHIO; AUTHOR OF "MARRIAGE AND ITS VIOLATIONS."

A BOOK FOR THE PEOPLE AS WELL AS FOR THE PROFESSION.

"The Prevention of Disease is more important than its Cure."

NEW YORK:

PUBLISHED BY THE AUTHOR,

ROOM 20 COOPER INSTITUTE.

1860.

[S. & A. HOYT, Printers, etc.]

CONTENTS.

PREFACE.

CHAPTER I.

CHAPTER II.

CHAPTER III.

CHAPTER IV.

CHAPTER V.

PREFACE.

For many years, while engaged in the practice of medicine, the author of this volume has been more and more impressed with the idea that the causes of the suffering, diseases, and premature deaths, which we witness around us on every hand, lie nearer our own doors than the transgression of the fair mother of our race; and that the men and women of to-day are, at least, equally as reprehensible for existing suffering, as those who have gone before them, and often much more so. In fact, he feels satisfied that by far the greatest portion of all the suffering, disease, deformity, and premature deaths which occur, are the direct result of either the violation of, or the want of compliance with the laws of our being; calamities, which, were the requisite knowledge possessed by the community, can and should be avoided. The physician, while he confines himself to the treatment and cure of diseases and deformity, does nothing but plaster over the evils of humanity. He is at best but a simple scavenger—useful, it is granted, in a low degree—so long as he confines himself entirely to the removal of the effects, or symptoms and diseases, which are the result of causes still operative. Every true lover of humanity, in the medical profession, has before him a nobler calling, and he neglects the great duty of his life if he fails to point out to the community the causes of the ills which he is called upon to treat; and if he does not, by his own example, strive to induce others to shun them, he is unworthy of that noble calling.

Whatever may be the value of this volume, it is not the mushroom production of a night, but it is the result of years of careful observation and reflection, and has been written after having carefully read many volumes bearing upon the subjects discussed in it. It has been the aim of the author to furnish the reader with the greatest amount of useful information possible in a small compass; and as far as practicable, to give the why and wherefore, in language which all can understand. He has endeavored to point out distinctly the causes of diseases, and to show the reader how to avoid them, and how to ward diseases off, at their commencement, by obedience to the laws of health and life: but for their proper treatment, when they are fully developed, the reader is referred to his physician.

Several of the chapters contained in this volume were first prepared as lectures, and delivered in Detroit, Cleveland, and other places. They afterwards appeared in a series of articles in different periodicals. Six of the chapters are now for the first time in print. The portions heretofore published have been carefully revised, and have received much additional matter, the result of further observation, reflection and reading.

The first part of the chapter on Education, when it appeared in the *Detroit Tribune*, attracted so much attention that it was published in a pamphlet form, by some of the friends of education in Detroit, and twenty-seven hundred copies were circulated gratuitously. The pamphlet had for its title, "The Physical Degeneracy of the American People: showing that an Imperfect System of Education, and abuse and neglect of Children, are among the Chief Causes of this Degeneracy." So firm was the conviction in the mind of the author at the time of writing, that our American people are degenerating, that he only devoted about two pages to a superficial view of the evidences that such a change is taking place, as he did not for a moment suppose that any one would seriously call it in question. In this he was mistaken, as several periodicals in noticing this pamphlet, earnestly denied there being any such degeneracy. It is not the aim of the author, in this volume, to advocate either side of this question, for he does not feel prepared to do justice to the subject; and furthermore, he loves his native land and his countrymen, and nothing would give him greater pleasure than to find after a thorough examination of the subject, and comparison of Americans with the races from which they have sprung, that he has been mistaken in supposing that the American people are degenerating. He hopes to have an opportunity, after the census of 1860, to thoroughly examine all the evidence upon both sides of this question, in the light of statistics, physiology and pathology; and to lay the result, whatever it may be, before the public. In the mean time he has thought that it might not be either uninteresting or unprofitable to the reader, to have placed before him what has already been written upon both sides of the question, although it may be, as it certainly is, superficial and unsatisfactory. The portion of the pamphlet referring to this subject will first be inserted, then will follow a notice of the same from the New York *Evening Post*, which embodies the substance of all which the author has seen upon that side; after which will follow a copy of a reply which was forwarded to the *Evening Post*, with some slight alterations made to prevent unnecessary repetition, and remedy defects.

[For the Detroit Tribune.]

PHYSICAL DEGENERACY OF AMERICANS.

"Mr. Editor:—I noticed in your paper of April 1st, an article on this subject. If it is true, that the people of the United States are physically deteriorating, it would seem that the subject should command the serious attention of every patriot and philanthropist, to say nothing of the Christian portion of the community. With what force the subject appeals to the latter, will be evident if we bear in mind that men and races of men do not deteriorate, physically, without a cause. If it is true, that, while we are justly pitying the poor benighted heathen nations on earth, and are spending our money and the lives of philanthropic men, to send them knowledge, we are ourselves being slowly and surely destroyed as a race, through a lack of knowledge of the physical laws of our being, or still worse, wilfully violating known laws, how much more do we need the active labors of efficient missionaries at home.

"That the people of the United States are deteriorating, is in accordance with the testimony of travelers who have been among the nations of Europe, from which ours has sprung; and its truth can be very easily confirmed by comparing our citizens with the foreign emigrants who flock to our shores. We shall find the emigrant more robust, hardy, and firmly built; and that this is not simply an external appearance, will be manifest if we carefully compare the different structures of the body. Even if we descend from the most delicate, to the very bones: Compare the teeth, if you please, of foreigners, with the teeth of Americans, and you will find the most surprising deterioration in the latter. Toothache, decayed teeth, and toothless gums, are far more common; nor is this all, for even the very jaws themselves will be found more perfectly developed in foreigners than in Americans; the former having, usually, thirty-two teeth and room for them in the jaws; but the latter, in a far greater number of cases, are compelled to lose four teeth, one on each side of each jaw, or to have them crowded and deformed. Here, then, we see that the most solid structures of the body are degenerating; and how much more manifestly the more delicate structures are deteriorating, may be seen in the delicate and slender form of the body, attenuated face, and expression of the countenance. It is not necessary that a man or a race of men should be large in order to be well built and healthy. Why do we have all this deterioration of our race in the United States? We are told by some that it is the effect of the climate. If this were true, there would be little or no prospect of its being remedied; but I shall endeavor to prove that it is not true—that the Lord has not permitted one race of people to be swept off from this broad continent and another to take its place, and yet the latter not capable of taking the place of the former residents. I think that it can be easily shown, that there are actual evils of life, voluntarily indulged in, (notwithstanding all the lights of science and the gospel,) either one of which is doing more—yes, many times more—towards destroying our American people, than all the effects of climate. I have no hesitation in asserting, that climate has comparatively very little to do with causing the delicate, deformed, nervous, dyspeptic and consumptive race of men and women we see around us. Abundant evidence of the truth of this is to be found in the very simple fact, that our females do not enjoy as good health, and are not proportionally as hardy and robust as our males, showing conclusively that the causes are more active among them than among the males; and yet climate affects both alike. Again, pass over into Canada, beyond immediate contact with our people, and we shall find that the writer in the '*Atlantic Monthly*' states the truth, when he says, that 'certainly no one can visit Canada without being struck with the spectacle of a more athletic race than our own. On every side one sees rosy female faces and noble manly forms,' even in the latitude of Detroit, central New York, and New England.

"Is there anything in the atmosphere of our republic, which is inconsistent with symmetry of form, substantial structures and physical health? If there is we had better forthwith change our form of government. But no! the causes of this degeneracy are to be found deep within the human soul; in the perversion of God-given faculties, and the resulting vanity, sensualism and miserly selfishness of the day, which ultimate themselves in the neglect and ill-treatment of our children, and in the violation of physical laws, and consequent deformity and disease.

"With your leave, Mr. Editor, I propose to point out, with a gentle hand, some of the causes of this physical degeneracy, in a series of articles for your paper; and if, without much ceremony, I may chance to expose some of the cancerous ulcers of our present social fabric, you will pardon me, as I shall have but one end in view, and that will be to expose them in the light of reason, that the proper remedies may be the more effectually pressed home to the consciences of our citizens, that our race may be saved from dwindling away; our men saved from destruction by dissipation, which is so fearfully prevalent among the young; our ladies from spinal distortion and irritation, neuralgia, hysteria, and female diseases; and that our children may be saved from an untimely grave. As the violation of natural laws commences at the cradle—or even before our children are born, but I forbear—I propose to review some of the shortcomings of our present system of education."

In noticing the pamphlet from which the above is taken, the New York *Evening Post* says:

"It has been popular for a long time to represent the inhabitants of this country as undergoing physical degeneration. Educational, medical, and other journals, print essays, showing how the decay may be arrested. The introduction of athletic games, archery, and other exercises into school discipline, are constantly recommended by 'progressive educators.' A physician of Detroit has published a pamphlet, setting forth that our imperfect system of education is one of the principal causes of the physical degeneracy of our people. This is probably not unjust; our teachers not only instruct too much and educate too little, but confine their efforts to the intellect, to the neglect of the body. Such a state of things so far as it exists should receive attention.

"But it may be doubted whether this great degeneracy really exists. We will not deny that there is a margin for improvement; but is it not quite probable that our people, even now, are making upward progress? Is the average duration of life shortening? It may be that we have fewer old men and old women, but a larger proportion of children attain maturity than formerly. Statistics indicate that the ratio of mortality is actually on the decrease. It must be admitted then that our people possess a larger aggregate of vitality, though perhaps exhibiting fewer 'remarkable instances of longevity.' The French nation has lost two inches and more in average stature within fifty years, while the Americans are taller than their European progenitors. It is argued that we have less fat upon our muscles, and that we exhibit signs of over-taxed energies. The rapidity with which we make our way in the world shows the possession of high vital stamina; while large accumulations of fat are only proof that there is an inactivity of the vital functions. Lean men will generally endure severer privation, and they are more ready for physical and mental exertion than the fleshy. The dread which Cæsar entertained of Cassius is the tribute paid to the men who really perform most of the work of the world.

"It is true that Americans 'study much,' and that severe mental labor taxes the energies. But few persons die from this cause, for the most laborious students the world over have been the longest livers. Only when bad habits have existed, or other duties to the mind have been neglected, has much study resulted in deterioration of the health. They are mistaken who imagine that mental development involves physical degeneracy. Without intellectual cultivation the liability is far greater. Thus in our prisons, the labor, though forced, is less severe than that of farmers and mechanics, merchants and editors; and very often the apartments are better ventilated than our residences and school-houses. Yet convicts are of a lower type of health than people outside pursuing similar employments.

"In unfavorable localities, particularly in cities densely populated, there exist many counterbalancing circumstances. There is not that equal distribution of labor which is necessary to develop the highest physical power. Fashions of dress are often pernicious; so are residences, public buildings and workshops, when badly constructed or located in unhealthy places. But there evils may be obviated, and such examples are not illustrative of the general principle.

"The immigrants added to our own population do not appear to equal our own people in vital power. Epidemics are more fatal among them, more of them die in early life, and they are less able to do manual labor. At the plough and hoe, the axe and carpenter's plane, in the haying and harvest field, Americans will achieve more in a given time than they. The Arab and Tartar are not our equals in power of endurance. Even the Indian possesses a smaller stock of vitality, and fails when required to perform stated labor.

"The energy of our people is due to the high cultivation of their faculties. So far from being in a state of decadence, they are yet in early manhood, with an eventful future before them. Luxuries that kings could not afford, five centuries ago, are now enjoyed by our common laborers. The comforts of life in profusion are in our grasp. We have much to learn yet, but our attainments already achieved are neither small nor unimportant; and not among the least of these is the enhancement of our stock of vital power."—N. Y. Eve. Post.

Soon after the publication of the above the following reply was written by the author, and forwarded to the *Evening Post.*

"MR. EDITOR:—A late number of your paper contains a notice of a pamphlet, composed of the first ten of a series of articles I am writing for the Detroit *Daily Tribune.* The pamphlet was published by some of the friends of education, for gratuitous circulation in Detroit. In your notice you call in question the position assumed in this work—that the American people are physically deteriorating—and intimate that they are actually progressing, and you have given certain reasons why you suppose this to be true.

"Upon the supposition that neither of us have any motive for writing upon this subject, except the welfare of our race, I have good reason to hope that you will cheerfully permit me, through your columns, to call in question your positions. If you are right, no harm will result to your readers. If I am correct, and can show that the people of the United States are degenerating, good may result, by inducing our citizens to examine into the causes of such degeneracy, and to put them away.

"That there is nothing in the climate to prevent the highest and most perfect development and health of the human body, when the laws of physical development and preservation are heeded, we have abundant evidence; for no finer specimens of men can be found in any part of the world, than can be found in almost any part of the United States; so that, if we are, as a race, physically degenerating, there is no need of it, and it should be checked by a speedy reformation of bad habits; and such a reformation becomes a duty, which we owe, not only to ourselves, but also to our country, and to the future of our race. That there are causes enough operative among us to destroy any race, must be manifest to every intelligent and careful observer. Causes always have and always will produce their effects. With a knowledge of how our children are fed, housed, dressed and educated; of the habits and fashions of our ladies; of what we eat and drink, at our meals, and of the various poisonous substances which are so generally used, any one, possessing a reasonable amount of knowledge of the laws of physical development and preservation, would be able to say with certainty, without even looking around him, that we are degenerating. I am not among those who 'imagine that mental development involves physical degeneracy.' No mistake could be greater, or more pernicious. It is only when such development is one-sided,—the intellect educated, and the body neglected—that this results. It is true that 'the most laborious students the world over, have been the longest livers,' when they have inherited good physical constitutions, and have lived according to the laws of health. The highest intellectual development, of which the individual is capable, is only attainable in a well developed and healthy body, which alone can withstand prolonged mental application.

"Is the fact that emigrants, subjected to a change of air, water and food, cannot withstand the diseases of our climate as well as our own people, and that more of them die young, any evidence that they do not equal us in 'vital power?' If so, we must figure very low in vitality, when compared with the Mexicans; for where are the young men, who, but a few years ago, enlisted for the Mexican War? What proportion of them ever returned, and how many of those brave soldiers are alive to-day? Is the fact that the emigrant, Arab and Indian, cannot endure an amount of physical labor for which their muscles have not been trained, and to which they are not accustomed, equal to Americans, any evidence that they possess less vitality than the latter? Could our farmers, untrained, excel the Indian in the race? or the Arab in endurance on horseback? The question is asked: 'Is the average duration of life shortening' with us? The admitted fact that we have fewer aged persons than in days past, is sure evidence, it seems to me, that our vitality is being impaired, and our race becoming degenerated. If it could be proved by statistics that fewer children die, owing, perhaps, to greater care and improved medical treatment, and thereby, the average duration of human life has been increasing, it would be no positive evidence that we are not on the decline; for some diseases, like the small pox, which were formerly very fatal, destroy but comparatively few to-day; and many diseases, which manifest unmistakably a loss of vital power, such as the consumption, dyspepsia, insanity, nervous and female diseases, are rarely manifested during childhood, even when there is a strong hereditary predisposition. Is not the increasing prevalence of such chronic and constitutional diseases, far better evidence of decadence, than deaths from acute diseases, war, starvation, and accidents, even although the latter may carry off a larger proportion of a community while young? Then, again, many of the habits and fashions which are doing so much towards destroying our race now, were comparatively inoperative, except, perhaps, in our cities, thirty or fifty years ago. Young men used less tobacco then than now; children, especially girls, were not so recklessly deprived, then, of the necessaries of life—sunlight, air, active exercise and labor—as in our day. Those monstrosities of the Press, the fashion-plates of our popular periodicals, containing most miserable caricatures of the female form, represented as model forms, had not then reached the fireside of the farmer, and mechanic, to destroy their daughters. A pale, bloodless skin, and delicate body, were not regarded as essential to beauty, and cultivated, by carefully excluding by the aid of blinds and curtains, the life-giving light of the 'god of day.' Active, useful labor was honorable among the young ladies who were to be the mothers of the present generation, and the spinning-wheel and loom were heard in almost every farm-house. To such mothers, comparatively well formed and industrious, do we owe much, for the physical strength and mental force of the present adult generation. What is the prospect for the future? Statistics have not had time to tell their story; one or two generations more must pass away first.

"But has the careful observer no signs by which he can judge whether we, as a people, are physically progressing or retrogressing? Surely he must have. I have already alluded to the increase of chronic and constitutional diseases among us. It is certainly true that an excess of fat is no evidence of an excess of vital power, but rather the reverse; and the same is true of premature wrinkles. Nor is the fact that men are very tall, any evidence of superior health and vital power; or that they are short, any evidence that they are lacking in these respects. But we find positive evidence of degeneracy in the thin sharp faces of Americans; not thin from the absence of fat only, but from the absence of bone, for we find the bones of the face not as well developed as in foreigners. Every dentist can testify that the teeth of the Americans are far more liable to decay early, from being less perfectly developed, than the teeth of foreigners; yet the teeth and jaws are among the most substantial structures of the body. Narrow chests, round shoulders, and slender bodies, denote a lack of vital force. It must be manifest, to every observer, that the causes of this degeneracy are much more active among the female portion of our population, than among the male; for the American women are not so healthy, and robust, when compared with the women of other nations as they should be, for with us they hold no comparison in either of these respects, or capacity for endurance, to the men. Can any one say that the females of our country are not physically degenerating? Miss Catherine Beecher truly says:

"An English mother at thirty, or thirty-five, is in the full bloom of womanhood; as fresh and healthy as her daughters. But where are our American mothers who can reach this period unfaded and unworn? Mary Lamb writes to Miss Wordsworth, (both ladies being over fifty years of age:) 'You say you can walk fifteen miles with ease; that is exactly my stint, and more fatigues me." How many young ladies have we who could walk fifteen miles, or even five? How many healthy ladies, beneath the age of thirty or forty, with well developed chests and waists, can be found in our land? Comparatively very few. Is it possible for our delicate, pale-faced, small waisted women to become the mothers of healthy children? Never! The pale, delicate faces, and slender bodies of the children of such parents, which we witness around us on every hand, answer most emphatically, never!—that if the mothers of our land are degenerated, their children will inherit imperfect organizations, and the coming generation will be found wanting in physical development. Is it true that we as a nation have enhanced our stock of vital power? It certainly does not appear to be true; but we have our nervous excitability, activity and energy, and if we only had corresponding physical development, our nation would soon outstrip all others. Our soldiers possessed the energy to astonish the natives, and even the world on the plains of Mexico, but their frail physical bodies could not withstand such excessive draughts upon their vitality, and a fearful mortality, from the diseases of the climate was the result. Dr. Kane accomplished wonders in his Arctic voyages; and had he possessed physical capacity equal to his mental energy, he might have lived to have yet carried his explorations, perchance, to the very Pole, instead of resting from his labors with 'our nation's honored dead.' How many of our young mothers do we witness, who have the mental energy, soon exhausting their feeble vital powers in the care of their children, and thus leave them to the care of strangers? It is impossible to do justice to this subject in the short space of a newspaper article, yet if the reader will but seek with ordinary diligence, he will find an abundance of evidence that the citizens of this great republic are physically in their decline, and that nothing but a speedy reformation of bad habits, especially so far as our children and ladies are concerned, can open to us, as a nation, a glorious and 'eventful future.'"

DETROIT, Aug. 30, 1858.

As has already been stated, the object of this volume is neither to advocate nor defend the views contained above, still the author can but intimate that it will not be for the good of our nation and race for our citizens to allow their eyes to be blinded as to the probable destiny of the American people, if danger actually exists, and that duty would seem to require that we should not permit the voice of warning, which has been raised by so many observers, to pass unheeded.

Although it may not be very flattering to the vanity of young America to be compelled to believe that we are physically in our decadence, and that there is reason to fear that a fate similar to that of the Spanish race in Mexico, is to be our fate; still it will be best for us to look the truth in the face, and take timely warning, if actual danger exists; for all history shows that if a nation physically declines, it cannot long maintain its physical or even mental supremacy. If there is no cause for alarm, no harm will result from an examination of the subject, and the anxiety felt by many sincere lovers of our country will, perhaps, thus be quieted.

But surely, without raising the question whether our countrymen are degenerating or not, when we look around us and see the amount of disease and suffering, and the number of premature deaths, or deaths which occur before old age, we may well begin to enquire into the causes which produce such fearful effects, and especially when we bear in mind that the effects of these causes cease not with this life, but follow us to eternity. The rum-drinker's and the tobacco or opium-user's appetite, is not simply an appetite of the material body, but it is a craving of the spirit for unnatural excitement, and it is well known that the use of these substances excite the passions, and render reformation and regeneration difficult, if not impossible, so long as their use is continued. The infatuation of the love of approbation, when it leads its victims to violate conscience, and to continue in known injurious practices, is not less injurious to physical and spiritual life than natural drunkenness.

Can any subject be more important to the sincere Christian at this day than the subjects discussed in this volume? A man must know before he can do, he must see evil before he can put it away; and nowhere can he see his own evils as distinctly as in his external acts; and he must cease to do evil, before he can cease to think and will evil. That there are fearful evils running riot over our land, which are even threatening the physical destruction of the American people, is certain, and have we not reason to fear that a large portion of the nominal members of our Churches, are being overwhelmed by the flood, instead of seeking the ark of safety? To bring those evils to light, will be the aim of the author in this volume.

It is high time that those who profess to be Christians, should awake to the importance of ultimating that which they profess in life, even in their external lives.

As the natural world is the ultimate or basis of the spiritual world, so man's natural body is the ultimate of his spirit, and it is through his natural body that he acts in this world. A man may, as to his intellect, be raised into angelic knowledge, so as to behold in their beauty and adaptation to the wants of man, the truths of God's Word, and yet if that knowledge be not ultimated in the external acts of his daily life, or if he is not engaged in the effort to ultimate it, his religion is like a house without a foundation, or a house built upon the sand, and will be swept away by the rains and floods, or the sophistries of the natural man. "Cease to do evil and learn to do well," are the commands of the Lord; but before we can do well, we must cease to do evil; cease to do evil in our external acts, as well as cease to think and will evil. The author would by no means undervalue the importance of spiritual truth, and the spiritual or higher degree of man's being, for he well knows that no reformation of man's external life will be permanent, unless it arises from an earnest desire to shun evils as sins against God; and to do right because it is right, and in accordance with the Divine commands. Here lies the great difficulty with the moral reforms of the day; they have no true spiritual foundation, they are earth-born and crumble back to earth. They may have palliated for a season, the various evils they were intended to correct, but we find a reaction following. We behold, for instance, even in our fair land, the dark form of intemperance arising, and spreading devastation and ruin in its train; and where are the eloquent advocates of the temperance reform, whose voices were heard in thunder tones but a few years ago? If echo alone answered where, it would be a relief, but, alas! of not a few it may be said, their banners are furled, and they are rushing on in mad haste, as if to catch up with time lost in the cause of temperance, on their march to the drunkard's grave. Why do we see all this backsliding in this worthy cause? Simply because the motives which prompted the reformation were too frequently natural, and not spiritual; therefore temporary and not eternal. Man's evils may be restrained from going forth into act, by counteracting evil affections. The miser is often restrained, by the love of money, from an indulgence which will require the sacrifice of his treasure, but a change of circumstances, or an increase of wealth, may remove this restraint. Love of approbation, often restrains men from gratifying in external act, their evil desires; but a change of location or of society, may remove this restraint. How many men have lived virtuous and temperate lives, in external act, among their old neighbors and friends, but after being lured, by the love of gold, to the shores of the Pacific, have become vicious and dissipated. Fear of the loss of health, may restrain men while symptoms of disease are present, but a return of health removes this restraint, at least for a season; or the man counts the cost between the unlawful gratification, and the suffering from the disease which results, and chooses the gratification. A fear of death, it would seem, should restrain men, if any selfish consideration can deter them permanently, from evil actions. But how often has the author heard, even young persons, declare that they would rather live ten years in the gratification of their perverted appetites, than to restrain their appetites, and live as we should live, fifteen years. In all these selfish and natural motives for reform, there is no spiritual life; man is his own center, and the gratification of his selfish desires, his chief delight; and his evils can never be permanently removed until he comes to act from higher motives.

We are born naturally into the love of self and the world, but the Lord declares that we must be born again, or we cannot enter the Kingdom of Heaven. The Lord must become the center, and we must acknowledge him as such; and we must open our hearts to the reception of His love, and our understandings to the perception of the Divine precepts of His Word, and permit the new life to flow forth into our external acts. Love to the Lord and to our neighbor, must take the place of love of self and the world; then the motives which prompt our acts will be spiritual and eternal. If we eat and drink it will not be simply to gratify our appetite, or taste, and the inquiry will be, not what will taste the best, and give the most present gratification, but what aritcles of food, and quantity of them, will be the most conducive to health; for in order that we may keep the Lord's commands, and overcome our evils, and do good to others, a healthy body is very important. So in regard to our clothing, the important question will be, not what is the most beautiful and dazzling to the eyes of others, but what will be the most healthy and useful, and after this, the most appropriate, having in view our being able to perform uses to our fellow-men. So in regard to the acquisition of wealth; it is right and proper to labor to feed and clothe ourselves and families comfortably, and to make reasonable provision for old age and sickness, and also to acquire it to be able to perform more efficiently, acts of usefulness to others, but never for the sake of being called rich, or for the sake of unnecessary sensual gratifications.

If we would direct our steps to a world of peace and joy, whether we eat or drink, or whatever we do, we must do all to the honor and glory of God; and we honor Him when we keep His commands; when we shun our own evil acts, thoughts and desires, as sins against Him, and engage in a life of active usefulness, at the same time humbly acknowledging that all goodness and truth are from the Lord; that it is He who worketh in us, to will and to do of His own good pleasure. Then will the appetites and passions of the natural man be under subjection to the spiritual man. Love of the Lord, and a desire to live in obedience to His commands, and love of the neighbor, and a desire to do good to all, will become the ruling loves, to which all the sensual and natural appetites must bow and be brought under subjection. Use then, will be the great end in all sensual and worldly gratifications, and pursuits, and man's reformation will be prompted by heavenly affections, having in view, not the vain baubles and selfish pleasures of earth, but the life which is to come, a heaven of truth and love above the fleeting things of earth.

How far above is such a life to the life of self-love, which seeks instead of the welfare and prosperity of our neighbors, to rule over them, to outshine them in wealth, apparel and gaudy display; and which is jealous and envious when others excel, or which seeks its chief delight in the gratification of the sensual appetites, without regard to use; and even indulges knowingly in the use of substances which are known to be injurious to the health, and destructive to the moral nature, or which will, without hesitation, to gratify vanity, follow fashions which are known to be injurious to the health, and even destructive to life.

When self-love, and love of the world, are the ruling loves, we shall look in vain for any genuine reformation of the passions and appetites, for self-gratification is the chief object desired, and it is the same with the various passions, and appetites of the individual man, as it is with a society of such men, they can only be restrained by each other, but not radically reformed. In order for a genuine and permanent reformation, man must be regenerated, or born again. The old man, or self-love, with his deeds, must be put off, and the new man, or love to the Lord and neighbor, put on. The great object of our lives will then be, to do right, to do good, and to live right, taking no thought so far as the sensual or selfish gratification is concerned, as to what we shall eat or drink, or wherewithal we shall be clothed, knowing full well that our Heavenly Father permits the highest delight to flow from living in true order, or in accordance with His laws.

It is right and proper that we desire and strive so to conduct ourselves as to win the approbation of all good men; of all whose good opinion can be gained by doing right; but the motive which should prompt us in our efforts, should not be our own gratification, it should be to enable us to do more good to others, and to do right because it is right, not for the sake of applause or flattery. But when we seek to obtain the applause of others by doing wrong, or by following fashions which are injurious and destructive to health or life, especially when we do this knowingly, therefore in violation of conscience, we destroy both soul and body in the fire of worldly love.

Against fashions and habits, which are harmless, the author proposes to wage no war, although, in regard to the former, he feels free to say, that if we would consult the wisdom which is displayed in all the works of our Creator, variety would take the place of slavish uniformity.

AVOIDABLE CAUSES OF DISEASE.

CHAPTER I.

DISEASES FROM A SPIRITUAL OR MENTAL ORIGIN, OR FROM THE PERVERSION OF THE PASSIONS AND FACULTIES OF THE SOUL.

WE may denominate the harmonious action of all the organs, faculties and functions, of both body and mind, or spirit, as a state of health; and any change of structure, or variation of function, as a state of either disease or deformity. Disease is an effect of a preceding or co-existing cause, which may still be operative, and require to be removed before any permanent cure can be effected. Before we can either remove or avoid the causes of diseases we must understand them.

But before we are prepared correctly to understand our subject it is necessary for us to have some knowledge of man who is the subject of disease; and as we are about to consider, in this chapter, the origin of diseases from the perverted passions and faculties of the human spirit, it is necessary for us to have a distinct idea as to man's spiritual nature.

Believing, with St. Paul, that "There is a natural body, and there is a spiritual body," I have an abundance of evidence to satisfy me, that the latter is far more real and substantial than the former, for man's natural body is but an effect. If we would seek causes we must seek them in the world of causes; matter in itself is dead.

Go with me gentle reader, to yonder forest; the trees which were once living and towered in all their majesty toward the heavens, now lie prostrated by the woodman's ax, and lifeless; no more shall they be clad in living green, their glory has departed.

Go with me to yonder dark shaft, from which the laborious miner raises from the bowels of the earth the copper and iron ore, and you will behold the materials from which the steam engine, and cars, are built—an almost shapeless stick of wood in one case, and a mass of minerals in the other. Tell me if they are the cause of the beautiful steam engine which you see flying over the iron rail at the rate of thirty, or forty miles an hour? Or are they simply the materials from which it is formed?

Go and examine the anatomy of the engine, study its physiology, or the functions of the various parts; behold the evidence of design in every part and piece, and then tell me if you find the cause of its existence in it, or that it was the cause of itself; or, again, that it is a part of its own cause. No! you exclaim, the cause is not in it; it is not the cause of itself, and it constitutes no integral part of the cause. Then, if the cause which has produced the engine is neither the matter of which the engine is built, nor included in it, where shall we seek its cause? Shall we seek it in matter, or in the material world? No; for matter, it is evident, in itself is dead: we will seek the cause in the mind of the architect who has fashioned it; for it is but a manifestation of his thoughts, and the thought existed before the external form.

We have now traced the cause of the engine to the thoughts of the builder, but are we sure that we have reached the real cause? Let us see: what is the cause of the thoughts which have given life to this beautiful machine? Are they their own cause, or are they but an effect of a certain affection, or love, which desires the accomplishment of a certain end or object; which may perchance be to save labor, horse-flesh, time, or, to make money? Then we see that even the thought is but an instrumental cause in the formation of the engine; the real cause is love, the love of accomplishing a certain end. Love is the very life of man, and we read that even "God is love," and His wisdom is but a manifestation of His love, as our thoughts are but a manifestation of our love, or loves. Then all the works of man which we behold are but manifestations of his affections, through the instrumentality of his understanding.

Let us turn from the comparatively dead works of man, which are but surface works, to the nobler works of God, which are infilled with life to every fibre. Let us read the thoughts of the great Architect in all the works of Creation which we behold around us; in the substantial earth upon which we stand, the blade, the leaf, and full grown plant and tree, of the vegetable kingdom; in the worm that crawls at our feet, the insect that flies at our approach, the animals which acknowledge the supremacy of man; in the fowls of the air, and the fishes of the sea. All these manifest thought and design, far more than the works of man, and could only have had their origin from an intelligent personal being. We behold springing forth from the earth the tiny vegetable, but warmed by the solar rays, and moistened by the rains and dews of the natural heavens, it grows, blossoms, and bears fruit for the sustenance of the animal kingdom. We behold then, even in the creation of the mineral kingdom, an end, or object, for which it was created; for without the mineral kingdom vegetables could not have been created: but the great end or object of the creation of this beautiful universe is not to be found in the vegetable kingdom, for creation rests not there, but this kingdom is but instrumental for the development of higher orders of life, or the animal kingdom. From the lowest forms of animal life we shall need to ascend step by step, until we arrive at the creation of man, before we reach the crowning act of creative energy. Comparative anatomy teaches us that in man is to be found the various forms of the animal kingdom beneath him.

Throughout the entire works of Creation, we are able to read the design of the Almighty, and clearly to see that the creation of man was the end in view.

Revelation teaches us that man, differing from all the rest of the animal kingdom, was created in the image and likeness of God his creator. We find man more perfect in organization than any animal; and, although without the strength or bulk of many animals, yet able to subject them all to his dominion. We find him endowed with mental faculties immeasurably above the brute creation. He alone possesses the power of reasoning, reflecting or thinking. He alone is endowed with conscience and freedom of will. Yet man, although capable of loving, reasoning and executing, or clothing his thoughts in words and external forms, is not his own creator, any more than the steam engine is its own creator. He is not the creature of chance, or unintelligent nature, for we behold in his beautiful and erect form, the surprising adaptation of parts, and wonderful delicacy of structure, far more evidence of thought and design, than can be found in all the works of man, or even in creation beneath him. We find that he possesses in a finite degree, those faculties which are manifested in the works of the infinite Creator—love and wisdom. But man does not possess life in and of himself, nor does he possess love or wisdom of himself, he is simply an organ receptive of the life which is ever flowing in from the giver of life. Even his body does not live of itself, but is only sustained in being, by the constant reception of materials from the external world, or by food and drink, which is for a time made alive by the indwelling spirit or soul. The spiritual world then is the world of causes. Man is at one and the same time an inhabitant of two worlds; his external body is an inhabitant of the natural world, and his spiritual body (composed apparently of affections, intellectual and perceptive faculties) which gives life to the natural body, is an inhabitant of the spiritual world. Even man's external acts and works, have their origin in his spirit, for affections and thoughts are spiritual, and not material; and when the artist forms the image of a man, or animal, from granite, or a machine from iron and wood, it is but an embodiment of a spiritual form or thought.

If all the works of man have a spiritual origin, and are but the clothing of spiritual forms, or thoughts, how much more must the works of God have a spiritual origin; for they are the clothing of the Divine thoughts, in matter, which give life to all the organized forms of the vegetable and animal kingdoms.

Man's material body then is but the clothing of his spirit or soul, and must correspond to it in every particular. It follows that there cannot be an organ, member or fibre in the body, which possesses life, which does not derive that life from the spirit. The spirit being the real man, is of course in the form of man, or of the body.

We read that God created man upright, but that man has sought out many inventions. That he was created free from evil and free from disease. Even aside from revelation, I cannot for a moment suppose, that the first man was created the sinful and diseased being we behold in the men of this day.

Not a few believe that our race has always been progressing, from the time of the very first creation of man on earth. But that man has degenerated upon the earth, it seems to me, must be manifest to all who are capable of reflecting, if they are not blinded by the theories of progress, so prevalent among those who worship nature instead of God.

It is known that vast cities and mighty nations have passed away, that arts once possessed were lost for many centuries, some of which have not yet been re-discovered. The relics of past greatness are being discovered on every hand. "The languages of savage nations, however," says a recent writer, "show this corruption of a noble primitive tool still better; for they point backwards into the dim past, to a time of perhaps even greater perfection of speech than Latin or Greek. Alexander von Humboldt, the man best fitted to speak with weight upon this subject, describes the American races as singularly remarkable for the degradation of their faculties from an original standard whence they have fallen; while he says that their languages resemble the relics of some great ruin or mighty devastation. In their study, the scholar wanders among the fallen columns and overgrown ruins of a once noble temple of human words; the relics of desolation, not the first, crude, undeveloped germs of language yet to be. Niebuhr also, the historian,—and higher authority could hardly be quoted,— insists strongly, that the languages of savage nations are only the poor fragments of a once glorious instrument of thought; and declares that language, as well as history, points backward to a lost civilization and a golden age."

It seems impossible to avoid the conclusion that our race has fallen from the state of purity and innocence which existed, when man stood forth in the garden of Eden, the image and likeness of his Creator. To me nothing is more irrational than the supposition that man has not fallen, but that he has always been progressing.

Man is not a creature of chance or blind nature, for we behold even in his fallen state, abundant traces of the handy workmanship of an intelligent, all wise and merciful Creator; and to suppose that man, when he came from the hands of such a being, and was pronounced by him "very good," was the poor, miserable, sinful being we behold him to-day—spiritually with his affections perverted, and his intellectual horizon full of every variety of unclean thoughts—is to suppose that God is directly the author of evil, or that a good tree can bring forth evil fruit. I ask the reader if it is possible that man could have been created the poor, diseased, broken down object we see him now; even his body, full of hereditary tendency to the development of scrofula, cancer, consumption and insanity, which are so common, to say nothing of the specimens of puny and delicate organization which we so generally witness around us? Is it possible that the time has never been, when the inhabitants of our earth were in the possession of better physical organizations than they are now?

How few strictly healthy men can be found in our land. Can you find one entirely free from disease, free from pain and suffering, from the cradle to the grave, whose lamp of physical life goes out gently like the setting of the summer's sun, or the closing of the eyes of the innocent babe in quiet slumber? Such would be the life of a truly healthy man, and such the *only natural* death. But alas! how far from this is the sad reality we witness around us in the present life of man. Behold the innocent babe suffering and dying in its mother's arms, perchance amid contortions and convulsions terrible to witness. Behold the prattling child, the playful boy or girl, the youth, the middle-aged and the old, stricken down by disease and cut off by a premature death; tell me, if the first men on earth, when God breathed into man the breath of life, and he became a living soul, were so created that necessarily nearly one-half of the children born into the world died before they were ten years old, as at present? Enlightened reason rebels against such a conclusion, and sustains revelation when it teaches that man has fallen. That our race from a primitive state of innocence, peace and physical health, has degenerated until the darkness of night has shut out from man's spiritual perceptions, the bright rays of the Sun of Heaven; until selfishness, violence, vice, and sensualism have sapped even the physical constitutions of the inhabitants of our earth. Evil is not undeveloped good, but the opposite of good, or a perversion of good; nor is falsehood undeveloped truth, but the opposite of truth. Nor are disease and suffering undeveloped health, and happiness; for they hold the same relation to health that evil and falsehood do to goodness and truth; and all progressive increase of disease and suffering, tends towards the destruction of the life of the natural body, in the same manner that an increase of evil and falsehood tends to destroy spiritual and heavenly life in man; for disease and suffering hold the same relation to evil and falsehood that effect does to cause. If man was free from sin he would understand more fully the physical laws by which he is surrounded; and what is even more essential, he would be willing to live in accordance with them; for even the brute creation—the horse, the ox, and sheep, cull the life-giving grass from the same field where grows the poisonous plant, and even the young lamb will rarely touch the deadly laurel, except when driven to it to prevent starvation, when the green grass and other vegetation are covered with snow. The animals in the world, when unperverted by man, live in the order of their creation. But man, standing at the head of the animal kingdom, endowed with freedom, and reason to guide him, is found both physically and mentally, or spiritually perverted, and he is constantly suffering, both physically and spiritually, from the consequences, or penalties which follow the violation of natural and spiritual laws. This fact, of itself, should be satisfactory evidence that man is responsible for his acts, and that he is not simply the child of circumstances, therefore irresponsible for his doings.

Revelation teaches that God is not the author of evil, and if not the author of evil, of course not the author of diseases which are but the effects of evil. God is the author of life; evils which cause diseases tend to destroy the life of the body, through the instrumentality of such diseases.

If evil is the cause of disease, it becomes important for us to inquire what constitutes evil, and from whence is its origin, if not from God. Without the aid of revelation it might be difficult for us to answer this question; but the truth, when once revealed, can be seen in the light of reason.

I have said man is endowed with freedom of will, without which he would not be man, and of course not responsible for his acts, any more than beasts. Does any one question that man is responsible for his acts? How otherwise can we account for the present fallen state of our race? Every youth has a clear perception that he has freedom of will; external circumstances may often prevent him from carrying out his designs, but he can harbor them, and have the will to do in spite of circumstances. The dealing of man with man, and our entire system of government, are founded upon the assumption that man has such freedom, and is therefore responsible to society for his acts, so long as he is a sane man. In fact, upon this very point, in a great measure, turns the question of man's sanity or insanity. The insane man has not, for the time being, such freedom, and therefore we do not hold him responsible for his acts. So clear is our perception that we are free to will to do right or wrong, that it is next to impossible for us not to manifest our instinctive faith in free will in our external acts. The light of perception flows into man from the Lord, the Sun of Heaven, and the very moment we close our eyes to that light, and call it in question, that moment we plunge into mental darkness on that subject. Therefore, if we call in question our mental freedom, after having perceived that we have freedom of will, and by the unaided light of our understandings attempt to reason about it, we may confirm ourselves in almost any absurdity upon this question, and it will appear to us as truth. We perceive, for instance, that we live in a real and material world; now we may call in question this light of perception, and begin to reason about it, and we may readily confirm ourselves in the opinion that there is no real world, that we are only living in an ideal world, and not a few have done this very thing. The light of perception is above the light of man's understanding, and if we desire to understand and analyze man's perceptions, we must make the attempt in their own light; for the light from the Lord to the perceptions, is to the spirit of man what the light of the natural sun is to man's natural vision, and we can no more understand these matters of perception, when we call in question, or deny their existence, than we can understand and analyze the light of the natural sun when we close our natural eyes, call in question the existence of the sun's light, and sit down by a coal fire to reason about the solar rays. Every child, for instance, born into the world, understands by instinct or perception how to draw his nourishment from his mother's breast; but you feed that child a few times with a spoon, and his instinctive knowledge is lost or gone, and you will find it very difficult, and in some cases almost impossible to teach him to nurse.

Man has conscience to restrain him when he knowingly inclines to do wrong, which the brute creation has not; but conscience does not teach him what is right or wrong, Revelation teaches him this; and the right is summed up in the two great commandments, "Thou shalt love the Lord thy God with all thy heart, and with all thy soul, and with all thy strength, and with all thy mind, and thy neighbor as thyself." These commandments together with an acknowledgment that all goodness and truth are from the Lord, constitute the tree of life in the midst of the garden; and when man partakes of its fruit, it gives life and health to both soul and body. To live in accordance with the commands of the Lord is the great end and aim of life. The Lord is the center, and a firm reliance on the Divine Providence gives peace, contentment, and quiet; and an earnest desire to do good to all, leads to unity, and harmony among men. No selfish or angry passions bear sway, and even the sensual appetites are under subjection to reason; use, is then the great object in all sensual indulgence. If a man eats and drinks, it will not be to gratify his appetite, but to give strength and substance; and, of course, such food, and such only, as will build up a healthy body, will be selected and used. So of the other sensual appetites, use alone will govern their indulgence. So in regard to dress, use alone must govern, and not vanity.

When man thus lived he was free from diseases, because he was free from their causes; and when man shall return again to the "tree of life, which (we read) bears twelve manner of fruits, and yielded her fruit every month: and the leaves of the tree were for the healing of the nations," diseases will vanish with their causes—the evils of the human heart. But man we read, and we see evidence of its truth all around and even within ourselves, chose to abuse his freedom and to eat of "The tree of knowledge of good and evil," of which he was commanded not to eat. Or, in other words, instead of acknowledging that all life and all goodness and truth are from the Lord, and striving to live according to the Divine laws, both spiritually and naturally, he began to persuade himself that he had life and goodness and truth in himself, and came to love himself, and the sensual gratifications of earth, more than he loved his Creator. Here was the origin of evil, and a fruitful tree, this "tree of the knowledge of good and evil" has proved to be. When man came to love himself supremely, and the gratification of his selfish desires above his neighbor, self became the end and aim of his life, the center around which he revolved. Then his interest was at war with the interest of every other man, and an endless strife for the mastery, for the acquisition of power, reputation, wealth, display, and the sensual things of earth, has been the result ever since. Anger, hatred, revenge, love of dominion and money, have desolated our earth, with fire and the sword; flourishing nations have been overthrown, cities have been destroyed, and fruitful fields have been desolated, until briers and brambles, useless, and even poisonous weeds, and pestilential marshes, flourish where gardens once furnished sustenance for man. Pestilence and famine have followed in the wake of these infernal gratifications—the inevitable and natural result. Vanity, or perverted love of approbation, has led to the adoption of fashions and habits, which are destructive to life and health. The perversion of amativeness, from its legitimate use, to selfish gratification, has filled our world with licentiousness, and impotency syphilis and gonorrhœa, constitute no inconsiderable share of the diseases which the physician is called to treat. These are the legitimate effects of vice.

Disregarding the legitimate use for which he should eat and drink, that is, that he shall eat and drink to build up a healthy body, or to live, man has perverted this department of his being, or has come to live to eat and drink, and to make such gratifications one of the chief objects of his life; and not satisfied with plain, wholesome, nourishing food, he seeks out those substances which stimulate his perverted passions. As a result, gluttony and drunkenness cover the land, and degrade man, the noblest work of God, beneath the brute; for he sacrifices to gratify his unhallowed cravings, his freedom, and becomes an abject slave to his appetite; his rationality, and becomes a fool, and even his instincts, and thereby sinks beneath the brute, at least for the time being. A large share of the diseases, which the physician is called to treat, have their origin in the perversion of the appetites by which man's body is nourished and sustained. We see then, that directly or indirectly, diseases are but an effect of the evils in the heart of man; and these evils are a perversion of God given faculties and appetites; not always with the individual suffering, for diseases are sometimes transmitted from parents to offspring; and a tendency to similar diseases, to those which have afflicted parents, is generally transmitted. The child has thus to suffer physical consequences which result from the evils of his parents. So the child inherits a tendency to the predominant spiritual evils of his parents, but this inheritance is not his fault, and he only becomes evil when he voluntarily does evil, or that which he knows to be wrong himself. If the hereditary inclination to do evil is so strong, that the child or man cannot avoid acting it out, or doing evil, and therefore he is not in freedom to do or not to do, he is insane and not responsible for his acts.

It may be asked why man was created with the ability to do evil, as well as good. To which we may reply, simply because if he had not been so created he would not have been man, with the capacity of thinking and reasoning, and then of acting out his thoughts, or not, as in freedom he may choose. Deprive man of freedom of will, and he would be compelled to act out his impulses, as are the brutes; and like them could only be restrained through fear; now he is able to sit in judgment on his impulses, and to reason about them, and restrain them if need be. With freedom of will he possesses an endless capacity for improvement; and, although born into the world more ignorant than the brute creation, he is raised immeasurably above it in capacity for development.

But to strive to justify the order of creation is unnecessary, as practical men we have to do with the world as it is. The fact that revelation teaches us a true life, which will lead us to unity and peace, to happiness and health, and, although men are able to see that this is true, and yet do not lead such a life, is positive evidence that they have freedom of will, even to do evil when they know what is good. The implantation of conscience in the human soul would have been an act of cruelty, and entirely superfluous, if man had not been endowed with freedom of will. The mental suffering which follows doing wrong is farther evidence, for in no other way can its existence be reconciled with the wisdom and goodness of God; and the consciousness which every man has of such freedom is an unanswerable argument in favor of its existence. Man by sophistical reasoning may persuade himself that white is black, and black white, but truth is eternal notwithstanding.

I have already intimated that the causes of disease, although spiritual, may be divided into two great classes. The one internal—the perverted affections of the human soul, acting directly on the body, causing unnatural excitement or depression, or perverted action in the organism,—the other external, or poisonous substances, miasms, or mechanical agents, acting directly on the *organism*, either internally or externally. When man, to gratify his perverted affections or appetites, voluntarily and knowingly cultivates or indulges in deleterious habits or practices, or brings himself under the influence of external causes of disease, the real cause of the disease, it will be seen, is spiritual, or his perverted affections, and the external agents are but instrumental causes. But where he is brought, either ignorantly or unavoidably, under the influence of external causes of disease, the cause of the disease which follows would seem to be external, still, even this may be but an appearance, for, have we not reason to think that, the entire amimal, vegetable, and even mineral kingdoms, derive all the life they possess, from the spiritual world—from spiritual influx? And that all substances derive their character from the quality of the influx which has given them form, and individual life? The actual ultimate constituents of which different substances are composed, which are capable of causing very different effects when taken into the stomach, are sometimes so nearly alike that the chemist can detect no difference, except from sight, smell, touch, taste, and effects.

If, as perhaps enlightened reason may yet teach, all chemical and mechanical changes or effects, are but the ultimation of spiritual causes, it will be seen that all the causes of disease are spiritual.

It is questionable whether matter alone possesses the ability to manifest activity, life, or intellect, unaided by spiritual influx. We can perhaps more distinctly see the truth of this position by an examination of our own senses. Does the eye see? No, for in cases of mental abstraction, or where our thoughts are intently engaged upon other subjects, or objects, how often are the rays of light reflected from the printed page directly upon the retina, without our seeing distinctly a single word, or letter, or perhaps even knowing that a book is before us. Who has not passed his own door, or failed to recognize his most intimate friends in the street, not because they were not within the angle of vision, but because his affections and thoughts were directed elsewhere? But let a desire arise to possess the treasures of the printed page, or to see the loved ones at home, or to recognize an expected friend, and every word will be distinctly seen, every door noticed, and every face carefully scrutinized. Then it is not the eye which sees; nor is it the brain, for the rays of light, reflected from objects, may strike the retina just as distinctly, and the impression may be carried to the brain just as perfectly, when we do not recognize the objects, as when we see every thing, plainly. So we are compelled to admit that it is not the eye that sees, but the spirit, or soul within the body, which sees through the eye. And the same is true of all the other senses. The vibrations of the air strike the auditory membrane just as distinctly during sleep as when awake, and yet a severe thunder storm will not arouse many individuals. I have spent weeks within a few rods of one of the largest bells in Detroit, without even scarcely recognizing its regular ringing, not from the lack of ears, but because my affections and thoughts did not flow into the ear to hear. I have, perhaps, never been awakened a dozen times by thunder in my life, and yet my door bell rarely ceases ringing for the first time, during the night, however sound asleep I may be, before I am on my feet. Separate the spirit from the body or any part of it, and sensation, circulation, and nutrition, cease; decomposition follows, and it returns to its native elements. When once the soul is fairly or fully separated from the body, however perfect the organization may be, we can get no manifestations of life from the latter.

The internal or spiritual causes of disease require at our hands a more extended notice. Nor do they have that place in medical works which their importance demands, although it is true that with some physicans, and some of our medical works, far more importance is attached to mental symptoms in selecting remedies, than with others; and yet, even such, hardly begin to realize the importance of an inquiry in regard to the mental causes, and symptoms of diseases.

Mental emotions, which are but manifestations of the affections, or loves, cause diseases by producing undue excitement or depression, or perverted action in the organism. Phrenology teaches that the intellectual and perceptive faculties, the moral sentiments, and the passions, are manifested through different portions of the brain; and that we can judge with some degree of certainty as to the comparative natural strength of the different faculties by the external development, or form of the head. The natural is not the cause of the spiritual, but the latter clothes itself with a body of matter, as with a garment, through which it manifests itself in this world. Not only the head but the whole body manifests the character, or comparative strength of man's intellectual faculties, and affections; for, as I have already said, we have every reason to think that man's affections and intellectual faculties compose the very substance and form of his spiritual body, or soul; and the latter lives in, and gives life to every part of the natural body. For this reason we are by no means confined to the form of the head in making up our mind in regard to a man's mental capacity, but we all judge almost intuitively from the form and expression of the face; and had not man the ability to play the hypocrite, we should be able to read character far more accurately in the pliant structures of the face than in the more unyielding form of the head. Nor are we confined to the head and face alone, for we can see a manifestation of the quality of man's spirit in the form of the body, and extremities, even to his finger and toe nails: also in the tone of his voice, in his gait, and his handwriting. Man can hardly prevent his passions being manifested in the tones of his voice; and very impressible persons, it is said, can judge in regard to a writer's state and character, by simply placing a piece of paper upon which he has written, to their foreheads. While at a hat store not long since, I noticed that the measures of two heads by the conformateur were almost exactly alike, both as to shape and size, and a very striking similarity exists in the handwriting of the two gentlemen. This would doubtless often be found to be the case where the handwriting is natural and not changed by art.

As the harmonious action of all the parts and organs of the body constitutes physical health, so the freedom from undue excitement or depression of the mental faculties, at the same time that there is a manifestation of mental strength and power, denotes spiritual health.

Man's spirit requires food and drink as well as his body; truths or knowledges, for the intellect, and love or affection, for the affections; both are necessary, as both water and bread are necessary for the body. Water satisfies man's natural thirst, knowledges his spiritual thirst. Water is the medium in and through which substantial food is carried to the structures of the body, to nourish it, so truths, or knowledges, are the medium, if you please, through which correct and true principles and affections reach man's spiritual structures. Life from man's spirit flows into the body and makes alive the nutritious substances which are received from the food, and moulds them into vital structures. So life from the Father of our spirits flows in and moulds the spiritual food we eat, or good affections we cultivate, into our spiritual body, and it becomes a part of us. After the days of childhood are over, we voluntarily select, eat and drink such food and drink as we please, of which to build up our bodies. So we voluntarily seek such knowledges, and cultivate such affections as we desire, for the sustenance of our spirits.

As man's body may be surfeited by eating and drinking too much good food and drink, more than the digestive organs can digest, or than the different structures can assimilate, so that the secreting organs become diseased, and the body becomes an unwieldy mass of fat, instead of being adapted for use; or, in other instances, as the undigested food irritates the stomach and bowels, thereby causing disease, so likewise man's spiritual organism may be surfeited with even healthy spiritual food, and drink; for he may acquire knowledges faster than he can carry them into life, or even has any desire to do it, and when he fails to live according to the truths he possesses they are worse than useless. The noblest affections of the human heart, veneration for the Supreme Being, benevolence, and conscientiousness, when incessantly fed and excited by long continued religious observances, exciting appeals, and example, may become so far surfeited, as to render the man a recluse, enthusiast, or a monomaniac. To man is given reason, and through his understanding he should watch over his affections, and thereby avoid enthusiastic excitement; for such excitement, even in a right direction, is mental disease. Excessive joy may cause mental alienation, disease of the organism, or death. Intense and long continued mental application to religious subjects, not unfrequently causes disease of the brain, and nervous systems, and also mental derangement. As man may supply nourishment of a poisonous quality for the sustenance of his body, so he may spiritual nourishment of like quality for his soul; and he does this when he voluntarily seeks false teachings, and is influenced by bad example to do wrong; to break the Divine command; also when he ceases to rely upon the Divine Providence, forgets to be cheerful and contented, and to look forward with hope, but suffers from unnecessary fears, anxiety for the future, unavailing grief, disappointed hope, and a murmuring and discontented spirit.

Love is spiritual heat, and truth spiritual light. The temperature of man's body depends much upon the state of his affections; when they are warm and alive, they flow into or excite the natural body to activity; the heart beats with increased force, the respiratory organs are more active; more air, and consequently more oxygen is received into the lungs; oxydation of combustible materials throughout the body is more rapid, and the result is that the heat of the body is increased. All this will ensue although there is not a voluntary muscle moved. But the brain and nerves of voluntary motion partake of the increased excitement of the involuntary system, and there is an increased inclination to voluntary action, even although such action is restrained, by the will.

Man's affections when perverted to evil ends, and allowed to flow out into act unrestrained, are a fruitful source of disease. Unnatural mental excitement causes unnatural excitement and consequently disease of the body. Anger causes excitement of the brain, which may result in apoplexy, paralysis, congestion, convulsions and even insanity. It excites the heart to unnatural activity, which may result in dilatation, or other form of cardiac disease; it may cause hemorrhage from the lungs, also derangements of the functions of the liver, kidneys, and bowels; and disease of these organs can often be traced to this cause. Anger may cause inflammatory fever, or develop other fibrile diseases, when there is a predisposition to them latent in the system. A desire for revenge may so far take possession of the human soul, as to be a cause of disease of the brain, and insanity; and, although perhaps more slow in its effects, it may disturb the functions of the vital organs to the extent of causing disease and death. Avarice, or the unrestrained love of money, when unduly excited by sudden prospects of wealth, or by its actual acquisition, may cause excitement and disease of the brain, resulting in sudden death or insanity. It may also affect the functions of the heart, lungs, and other organs as seriously as anger. Perverted love of approbation, or vanity, may be attended with similar results, and so of all the other perverted passions. Lasciviousness, or perverted amativeness, is a frequent cause of nocturnal emissions, spermatorrhœa, leucorrhœa, and impotence.

The diseases which result from the direct excitement of the passions, are, as a general rule, congestive or inflammatory; or diseases of nervous excitement;—debility or depression of course may follow the undue excitement, in such as in other cases.

There is another class of spiritual causes of disease which is perhaps, even more potent than the one we have been considering. I allude to the depressing mental emotions. Love, or man's affections, as we have seen, constitute the very life of man; and with every man there is a ruling affection, which is predominant, to which all the other affections are, to a greater or less degree, tributary and subordinate. The ruling affection may be good and heavenly—love to the Lord, neighborly love, or love of obeying the truth; or, it may be evil—the love of self, the love of ruling over others, the love of approbation, or the love of wealth. A blow which results in a wound of man's ruling love, or even one of the prominent subordinate affections, spends its force, not alone on man's spirit, for it depresses all the functions of the body, sometimes to the extent of causing sudden death. In the latter case the eye grows dim, the ear dull of hearing, the blood forsakes the surface, respiration ceases, the heart ceases to beat, and the body is dead, and all from a wound received by man's spirit. If man is in true order, or has his ruling love centered out of himself, and he is seeking, not so much his own happiness, as the happiness of others, he is comparatively safe. If death snatches beloved friends from his very hearth, he feels an assurance that what is his own loss, is their gain, and however severe the parting, consolation will come. If disappointed in love, by the refusal of one of the opposite sex to join hands and hearts as partners for life, he is aware that her welfare, which he has at heart, requires that her hand should only be given with her heart, and he rejoices in seeing her happy, perhaps, in the arms of a rival suitor. The loss of wealth, of power, place, public favor, and even of earthly friends, or of his good name, does not reach his heart, or his ruling love, and his trust in the Divine Providence sustains him in the hour of trial.

Not so with the man who has made some selfish object the chief aim of his life. If money is his god, take from him his wealth and you strike a blow at the very heart of his spirit, and if his earthly tenement survives the shock, instead of being reconciled to his loss, he, perchance, murmurs against the Almighty, or permits his spirit to burn with feelings of revenge towards his fellow-man. The same is the case with all the other selfish passions, when encountering losses and disappointed hopes, or expectations. Such mental blows often depress man's spirit even when the life of the body is not immediately endangered, and slowly impair the functions of important organs, causing debility and disease, if not directly, at least indirectly, by rendering the organism more susceptible to the influence of the external causes of disease. Fear and apprehension, render the system far more susceptible to the action of epidemic and miasmatic poisons; and protracted grief predisposes to, if it does not actually cause dyspepsia, jaundice, neuralgia, hypochondriasis, phthisis pulmonalis or consumption, and many other diseases.

CHAPTER II.

NATURAL CAUSES OF DISEASE.—A GENERAL VIEW.

THE causes of disease have been divided, by medical writers into predisposing, exciting and proximate causes. But as the proximate cause as represented by writers, is but the pathological condition, or the change of structure which is the immediate cause of the symptoms, it is but a part of the disease itself, and, of course, it cannot be classed with the causes of disease, as it is only a cause of the symptoms. I shall then discard the term, "proximate cause," in our present inquiry.

We have only to consider the predisposing and exciting causes of disease. The co-operation of both the predisposing and exciting causes, is generally required to produce disease. The entire community are exposed to a sudden change of atmospheric temperature; one is attacked with a cold in the head, another with pneumonia, or pleurisy, another with diarrhœa, another with acute rheumatism, and still another with an inflammatory fever, and by far the largest number escape entirely, without any disease; and yet all are exposed to the same cause, but each of the different individuals attacked, were predisposed to a different disease from the others, which manifested itself as soon as the exciting cause was applied; while the majority had no predisposition, and the exciting cause was harmless without a predisposition to some particular disease; and the predisposition was insufficient until the exciting cause was applied.

But the predisposing cause may be sufficiently strong, to develop disease without, or with but a very slight exciting cause; thus a person with a very weak stomach will have indigestion, however careful he may be in his diet, and does not need any exciting cause to develop it. So likewise an exciting cause may be strong enough to produce disease when no predisposition to such disease exists. Thus a large dose of ipecac will cause nausea and vomiting without a predisposition, but a small dose will require a predisposition before it will produce these effects.

The spirit which lives in and gives life to the natural body, which preserves from decomposition the nutritious materials which are needed to build up and sustain the different structures, and withdraws them from the circulation at the very point where they are needed, which presides over the development of childhood, and youth, and fixes bounds for the full development of manhood, and permits the physical body to gradually decline as old age approaches, until wrinkles, wasted structures, and helplessness take the place of the growing roundness and activity of childhood, and the firmness and energy of adult age, alike watches over the organism to preserve it from the harm of noxious agents. It is no more on the alert to build up the organism from the nutritious materials in the blood, than it is to get rid of those which are pernicious. The latter are allowed to escape through the organs of secretion, often with a great increase of the secretion, which may be natural or depraved, aside from the presence of the noxious substances. Improper food is often ejected by vomiting, or passes off by stool. The system is generally relieved from the bad effects which would result from the suppression of perspiration, during a change from warm weather to cold, by the kidneys taking on a vicarious action, thereby increasing the flow of urine, and thus relieving the system from an excessive accumulation of fluid in the blood vessels. So when one of the organs of secretion, as the liver for instance, becomes diseased so as not to be able to perform its duty in the removal of effete or worn out particles, the kidneys and even the skin strive to aid by taking on a vicarious action, and bilious matter appears in the urine, and even sometimes in the perspiration, and thus is the organism often in a measure protected from harm.

I have already alluded to the fact that the predisposing as well as the exciting cause of disease, is often to be found in the spirit or soul of man; in excessive and prolonged intellectual application, or, more frequently, in undue excitement, or depression, or perversion of the affections. Grief, fear, despondency, disappointed ambition, avarice, and love, are among the most frequent predisposing causes of disease.

Predisposition to disease may depend upon deficiency of power to resist the influence of exciting causes, rather than on the existence of anything positive, but sometimes it depends on something positively wrong in the organism; this may be hereditary or acquired.

An exciting cause of disease sometimes acts simply as a predisposing cause, and may require the action of a second exciting cause to develop the disease, as in the following instance: all who reside in a miasmatic district, are under the influence of the cause which produces intermittent and remittent fevers; where the system is not able to ward off the influence of the poison, or in other words, such individuals as have a strong predisposition to such fevers are attacked; whereas many others who have not such a predisposition may escape entirely, although the poison has entered the systems of all alike. Now let those who have escaped be exposed to any cause which shall depress the vital powers, such as excessive fatigue, depressing mental emotions, or profuse evacuations, and they will be very likely then to begin soon to show the effects of the poison.

PREDISPOSING CAUSES OF DISEASE.

I will hastily call the attention of the reader to a few of the chief predisposing causes of disease.

The power of resisting disease depends in a great measure on constitutional strength, vigor and health. Exceptions to this may exist in cases of particular idiosyncrasies, where there is an unusual susceptibility to be affected by certain noxious causes, which is not in keeping with the general strength of constitution, and health.

Debilitating causes of predisposition are, perhaps, the most numerous of any, especially such as enfeeble the circulation and the digestive organs. Among these may be mentioned:

1. Imperfect nourishment, whether from want of capacity in the digestive organs, or from defect in the quantity or quality of the food. This produces a liability to low forms of fever, and epidemic diseases. Pestilence usually follows in the wake of famine. There is an increased liability to contract infectious, or epidemic diseases, even while temporarily fasting, and this is a serious objection to the custom of fasting during the prevalence of epidemics.

2. Confinement in impure air. Even an abundance of good food, and every other comfort will not compensate for the lack of pure air, as is manifestly to be seen in the pallid and cachectic complexion, and delicate structures of the inhabitants of crowded cities, factories, prisons and mines, or even those confined in splendid houses or palaces. The deprivation from the light of the sun, under such circumstances, is perhaps quite as fruitful a source of mischief, as the impure air. The inhabitants of such localities are far more liable to contract disease, particularly those of the nutritive and nervous systems, than those who enjoy the free air and light of the country. But I shall call the attention of the reader to the importance of pure air, light, and exercise, and to the sufferings which result from a deficiency of these requisites for physical development, in another chapter.

3. Excessive exertion of mind or body, especially without sufficient sleep, is a frequent predisposing cause of disease. Although exercise is all important for the preservation of health, still when it exceeds what the strength can bear, especially when deprived of an opportunity to recruit during sleep, the system is exhausted, and nervous excitability takes the place of strength, and there is an increased susceptibility to the action of exciting causes of disease.

4. Long continued heat, from a residence in a warm climate, especially with those who are not accustomed to a hot climate, predisposes to attacks of functional, and organic diseases of the liver, also to dysentery, and cholera morbus, and even cholera. Overheated rooms and excessive clothing also predispose to disease, by their relaxing and weakening influence; especially to diseases of the nutritive and nervous functions.

5. Long continued cold when its influence is not counteracted by muscular exertion, or artificial protection by the means of shelter, clothing and fires, predisposes to epidemic disease; generally of a typhoid character. Cold, when moderately or temporarily applied to the body, is invigorating, if reaction follows, but if it is long continued or excessive, its sedative and debilitating effects are pernicious. Malignant and low forms of fever most frequently prevail toward the close of severe winters, and among the poor who have not been properly protected against the inclemency of the season.

6. Excessive and repeated evacuations either of blood, or of some secretion from it, are frequent predisposing causes of disease. The continued loss of blood by various hemorrhages predisposes to attacks of local congestion, spinal irritation, and various diseases which result from an anæmic or bloodless state of the system. Excessive venereal indulgences induce extreme debility, and premature decay, and predispose the body and mind to various diseases. Leucorrhœa, uterine ulcerations, and hysteria in the female, can frequently be traced to this, as an exciting cause; and the debility which results in both sexes, renders individuals who are addicted to such excessive indulgences, far more liable to be attacked by any prevailing disease than others. Few causes more strongly predispose to disease by weakening the vital powers, than solitary vice; and, in this sensual age of the world, this pernicious practice is fearfully prevalent among the young, of both sexes; although, beyond all question, far more prevalent among males than females. Extensive inquiries have satisfied me, that few young men reach the age of twenty years, without having been at some period addicted to this practice, and it is not uncommon among small boys long before they reach the age of puberty, even as young as five or six years; of course at this age there is no seminal discharge, but the effect is scarcely less pernicious upon the mental and physical health of the young child, than upon that of the young man. But this whole subject will receive the attention its importance demands in another work.

7. The habitual use of intoxicating drinks, the use of tobacco

and opium, abuse of digestive organs in eating, and the fashions and bad habits of the ladies, are all predisposing causes of disease; but, as the consideration of these causes is very important, from the fact that they are causes which may and should be avoided, I shall call the attention of the reader to them in separate chapters.

8. Previous debilitating diseases, and especially, the treatment which is sometimes resorted to for their cure, predispose to disease. During convalescence from severe diseases, even under any treatment, the body is weak, and the functions of the different organs are but just resuming their balance, and have less power of resistance than during robust health, and the former or some other disease, may be very readily produced by improper food, exposure to cold, over exertion, or excitement. The heroic antiphlogistic treatment, which was formerly more used than at present, for the cure of acute diseases, by reducing the quantity of the vital fluid below even the standard of the existing disease, predisposes to the same, or some other acute disease, as soon as the blood vessels become over-distended, as they are very likely to become, after such reduction from depletion, when the recuperative energies of the system have had a few months of uninterrupted activity. For this reason it is far more common for a second attack of pleurisy, or pneumonia, to occur in patients treated by excessive blood-letting, and other evacuents, than in those treated by milder measures.

9. The use of certain remedies leaves a predisposition to disease. Patients who have been once salivated by mercury, are very liable to have ptyalism again from the slightest cause; and such patients are very subject to rheumatism from the slightest exposure, and this predisposition often lasts for many years. The use of cathartics renders the intestines liable to inflammation and irritation from exposure to cold, or from errors of diet; they also predispose to constipation. A proclivity to disease is frequently caused by the previous existence of the same disease; thus a child who has once had the croup, or convulsions, or a person who has had the cholera, hysteria, rheumatism, or gout, is more liable to an attack of the same disease, than one who has never

had the disease. There is doubtless some change in the structures involved which keeps up the predisposition, or it may perhaps depend in some cases simply upon functional derangement. Certain structural diseases, such as tubercles and cancerous affections, manifest a very strong predisposition to return, when the organism has once been invaded by them. This doubtless depends on errors in the processes by which the body is nourished, or on those by which it is cleansed from worn out or improper substances.

10. Organic disease, existing in an important organ, frequently predisposes to disease; thus, disease of the heart causes a tendency to hemorrhage from the lungs, and apoplexy, on the occasion of violent physical exertion. Disease of the kidneys and liver predispose to hypertrophy or enlargement of the heart.

11. A predisposition to disease is often hereditary, or born with the individual, and inherited from one or both parents. It is well known that epilepsy, asthma, insanity, scrofula, cancer, gout, hemorrhages, blindness and deafness, occur more frequently in some families than in others, depending on individual peculiarities transmitted from parents to offspring. All the children of the same parents do not inherit this predisposition alike, any more than they do the same form of features. One child may resemble the father in temperament, form of body, and mental peculiarities, more than he does the mother, whereas another may bear the greatest resemblance to the mother; and, so far as my observation extends, the strength of the hereditary tendency to disease, is in a great measure in keeping with such resemblance.

The fact that an hereditary disease, or rather predisposition to disease, is not manifested in the child, is no evidence that it may or will not be in the grandchild, for the latter often much more closely resembles the grandparent, than does his own child. Individual peculiarities, both physical and mental, often manifest themselves in the great, and even great great grandchildren. It then certainly would not be strange if a proclivity to disease should skip, or jump over, one or two generations, and yet manifest itself in succeeding generations. Observation shows that such is very frequently the case, and that where parents may have escaped, the grandchildren often manifestly inherit the tendency, and all this without any change of habits to manifest that it is acquired. But, in connexion with this view, we should ever bear in mind that the child is just as capable of developing a tendency to disease, and even to disease of the same character, by the violation of the laws of health, as was the parent and grandparent, and not permit ourselves to indulge in the delusion that the consequences of our own evils, in the form of diseases, or a tendency to disease, are the result of the sins of our ancestors.

12. Temperament is often connected with peculiarities of constitution which predispose to particular diseases. Individuals of predominant sanguine temperament, in which the arterial system is active, and red blood abundant, are more liable than others, to active congestion, inflammation and active hemorrhage. Those of the bilious temperament are liable to melancholy, derangements of the liver, and digestive organs. Those of the phlegmatic or lymphatic temperament, in whom there is a deficiency of red blood, and of vascular action, and tone, are liable to dropsy, leucorrhœa, and other watery fluxes; while those of the nervous temperament are predisposed to hysteria, spasms, neuralgic and nervous pains.

13. Age is classed by writers among the predisposing causes of disease; and, whether correctly so classed or not, it is certain that there exists a proclivity to diseases corresponding to the changes which the animal frame undergoes at different periods of life. In early infancy the skin is very susceptible to the action of the air, and to cold, and is very liable to erythematous redness, and to various eruptive diseases. The alimentary canal is very susceptible of disorder, and consequently colic, vomiting, and diarrhœa, are not uncommon.

During childhood, or the period from early infancy to puberty, those functions which administer to growth are most active; hence there is a predisposition to derangements of the stomach and bowels; and, as owing to the activity of the nutritive functions, the blood is rich in fibrine and albuminous matter, and red globules, there is an increased liability to inflammation and to membranous effusions, such as occur in croup. The brain and nervous system, excited by the novelties of the external world, become rapidly developed, and are liable to various diseases, such as different forms of convulsions, inflammation and hydrocephalus. The process of teething adds an irritation which increases the tendency to diseases of the head, bowels, and lungs.

Puberty brings with it, especially in the female sex, an increased susceptibility to disease. A new function is to be established, which has its nervous as well as its vascular relations; which is liable to be retarded, or deranged after its development, by many causes, and thus a predisposition may be given to many diseases, affecting the circulation, the nervous system, and the secreting organs.

The termination of growth, when nourishment ceases to be appropriated for the development of the body, is another critical period; and there is often a predisposition to fullness, hemorrhage and inflammation in the robust, and in the cachectic, to morbid depositions, especially of the tuberculous kind.

From the cessation of growth, to the beginning of old age, in men, there is perhaps less predisposition to disease than with women, and less than at most other periods of life. But, with women, there is often a predisposition to various diseases in connexion with the generative functions. Pregnancy predisposes to vascular fullness, and local determination of blood, owing often to mechanical obstruction by pressure, to the flow of blood through the large blood-vessels of the abdomen, giving rise to palpitation of the heart, ringing in the ears, headache, and even convulsions, swelling of the lower extremities, etc. The sympathy which exists between the uterus and stomach predisposes to various derangements of the latter organ, such as nausea, vomiting and heart-burn.

Parturition, or confinement, predisposes to inflammation of the uterus and its appendages; and to irritation and inflammation of the mammæ or breasts, before the secretion of milk is fully established. Lactation predisposes to anæma, nursing sore mouth, diarrhœa, and various other diseases, especially of the nervous system. At the final cessation of the menses, or turn of life as this period is called, there is a disposition or tendency to various diseases connected with vascular plethora, or fulness, such as morbid growths, of various kinds, particularly in the uterus, ovaries or mammæ. The approach of old age brings with it an increased tendency to various diseases. The gradual wasting of the structures and body, which attends old age, is not necessarily attended with disease, any more than its growth in youth; but the bad habits of youth, and adult age, when they are not sufficient to affect the health seriously, or destroy life during the vigor of manhood, are sufficient to gradually affect the organism, when its power of resistance grows less, as old age approaches, and thus a predisposition to disease is established, when none is inherited; and few, if any, die from old age free from disease. There is a predisposition to induration and ossification, or change to bone, of the valves of the heart, and of the arteries, also to obstruction of the most delicate blood vessels, or capillary circulation, which often cause hypertrophy of the heart, and serious derangements in the circulation. If the heart acts with increased energy, in such cases, there is often a tendency to apoplexy, palsy, hemorrhages, asthma, and diseases of the urinary organs; whereas if the heart's action is weak there will be imperfect circulation, and tendency to venous congestions, dropsical effusions, varicose or enlarged veins, disordered secretions, and general failure of all the functions which depend on a supply of arterial blood.

The attention of the reader has now been hastily called to a general view of the chief predisposing causes of disease, both to the avoidable, and to such as cannot be avoided; for it is important to have a general idea of the latter, although very little time has been, or will be, devoted to their consideration. By knowingly violating the laws of our being, and thus lessening our power of resistance, we render ourselves far more liable to be affected by the unavoidable causes of disease. After taking a hasty general view of the exciting causes of disease, I shall commence a more careful consideration of specific causes, especially of such as can be avoided, as it is to the consideration of the latter that this work is chiefly devoted.

A truly healthy man should neither be diseased nor have any predisposition to disease; and all the predisposing causes of disease which we have been considering, with few exceptions, are but the effect of the spiritual causes we have considered in the first chapter, or else of the violation either intentionally, or unintentionally, knowingly or ignorantly of physical laws.

EXCITING CAUSES OF DISEASE.

Some of the exciting causes of disease, such as poisons, and strong irritants, may be so powerful as to produce disease without any predisposition, but where the agents are less energetic, the effects, or even whether there shall be any effect at all, will depend very much on predisposition; and, as has already been intimated, when disease does follow the action of an exciting cause, its character, and even location, will depend much on predisposition.

Exciting causes have rightly been divided into Cognizable, or those mental and physical agents of whose existence we can take cognizance independently of their operation in producing disease, and Non-cognizable, or those causes which elude our senses; and we only infer their existence from their morbific or disease creating effects. Thus we know nothing of malaria, and infection, except from the diseases which they cause.

The following are the Cognizable Agents enumerated; Mechanical, Chemical, Ingesta, Bodily exertion, Mental Emotions, Suppressed or defective evacuation, Excessive evacuation, Temperature and changes.

The Non-cognizable Agents are; Endemic, Epidemic, and Infectious—poisons. I shall call attention hastily to these different classes of agents or causes of disease, in the order in which they have been named, with the exception of those which I shall leave for a special chapter.

1. The Mechanical causes act, either by injuring the structures, or by impeding or deranging the functions of the body. Those which act by cutting, tearing, pinching, striking, bruising, and straining, produce effects or lesions which come within the province of surgery; but there are many other mechanical causes which give rise to diseases which come within the jurisdiction of the physician for treatment. Tight stocks and neckcloths, by

impeding the flow of blood from the head, may cause congestion of the brain or apoplexy. I shall call attention to tight dressing, or lacing, in a separate chapter. Indigestion may be caused by sitting in a bad position after a meal. Pressure caused by gravitation, by the weight of the body, on a part or parts, from long continuance in one position, whether standing, sitting, or lying, by partially obstructing innervation and circulation, may produce paralysis, and swelling of the lower parts, or of those beyond the seat of the pressure; and, if long continued, may cause inflammation and sloughing of the parts pressed upon, and death.

A stone in the bladder or urinary passages, or in the gall duct, may stop the flow of urine, or bile, or cause irritation of the parts with severe suffering. The digestive organs may be irritated by the presence of indigestible substances, swallowed accidentally, or taken in food, such as pins, needles, cherry stones, and the like. The respiratory organs may be irritated by the inhalation of dust, or of fine particles of metal or stone, as happens with stone-cutters, and needle-grinders. Then the products of disease, and morbid growths, often press mechanically upon surrounding parts, as in empyema and hydrothorax or suppuration and dropsy of the chest, or in the case of polypus, or enlarged glands. Then mechanical injuries may cause inflammation and fever, when there are no external wounds; inflammation of the brain and hydrocephalus may result from even slight concussion or jarring of the brain.

2. The chemical causes of disease are such agents as tend to decompose the tissues, or structures of the body, or irritate and disorder the functions, by their affinities. Acids, alkalies, and many salts, whether applied in a liquid form or inhaled in the form of gas, or vapor, are chemical irritants. The strong acids, caustic alkalies, corrosive sublimate, and other metallic salts, are chemical poisons, and act by their powerful chemical affinities. When food, for any cause, is not digested in the stomach and bowels, it becomes subject to chemical, instead of vital laws, and rapidly ferments and putrifies, which cause eructations of gas, and sour liquid from the stomach, and unnatural discharges from the bowels; and these chemical processes may give rise to irrita-

tion of the mucous membrane, spasms of the muscular coat of the stomach and bowels, gastralgia, colic and various other diseases.

3. Violent bodily exertion may be a cause of disease, especially with those not accustomed to such exertion; the circulation is increased, the heart is excited to inordinate action, is over distended, and its functions, or even its structure and that of the great vascular trunks, may be impaired in consequence. The brain is liable to be congested, and we may have, from this cause, giddiness, ringing in the ears, deafness, defective vision, convulsions, palsy and even apoplexy. The lungs are liable to suffer from the blood being returned to them faster than they can arterialize or purify it, and thus causing congestion; hence may ensue cough, dyspepsia, and hemorrhage and even inflammation. Hemorrhage from the nose, stomach, bowels, and urinary organs, has been caused by violent exercise; also derangements of the liver, stomach, bowels and other organs. The excessive exercise of the vocal organs may cause hemorrhage from them, or other forms of disease. Bodily exertion may cause a predisposition to disease by its exhausting effect, or it may even cause syncope and death; short of this, it may simply cause debility, or derangement of the functions of different organs. A low or typhoid form of fever is said sometimes to follow prolonged fatigue.

The effects of mental emotions have already been considered.

4. The retention, diminution, or suppression of secretions and evacuations, either natural, or simply habitual, frequently causes disease. Feculent matter retained in the intestines is a bugbear to most patients, and to some physicians and writers, but in reality it is attended with far less danger than the measures frequently adopted for its removal; still injury may sometimes result when the bowels are neglected.

Retention of urine may cause irritation, inflammation, ulceration, and even rupture of the bladder; and its suppression will cause deterioration of the blood, disease and death. Retention or suppression of the menses is a fruitful cause of disease. Long continued looseness of the bowels, or hemorrhages, such as from piles, if suddenly checked, especially by the use of astringents, may cause fullness of the blood vessels and disease. Also the sudden healing up of old ulcers, or of cutaneous eruptions, especially when this result is caused by external applications, is a fruitful cause of disease.' The following are among the diseases which most frequently result from such suppressions, viz.: various inflammations, congestion of the brain, apoplexy, epilepsy, hysteria, chorea, asthma, dyspepsia, mania, &c.

5. The excessive loss of blood, or of secretions from the blood, may cause fainting, and general debility, palpitation of the heart, and convulsions.

6. Extremes of heat and cold, or sudden transitions from hot to cold, or from cold to hot, are among the most frequent causes of diseases. Heat above 160 degrees coagulates the albumen of the blood, and thus obstructs the blood vessels, and destroys the vitality of the parts. Cold below 32 degrees freezes the water of the fluids, and destroys the vitality of the parts; whether from the stoppage of the circulation, or from the injury to the tissues from the expansion of the ice, is not known. Heat, when insufficient to cause destruction of parts, is directly stimulant. When applied to the whole body, it causes feverish excitement, when applied to a part, it excites its functions. The fever, fulness and throbbing, caused by heat, are relieved in a measure by the profuse perspiration which usually follows. Solar or artificial heat to the head may cause severe headache, congestion of the brain, and even apoplexy. Heat to the spine may cause sickness of the stomach, fainting, and even convulsions. The local application of heat may cause inflammation of the eyes or skin, or of other parts.

Cold is directly sedative; it contracts the tissues and the blood vessels, and renders the skin pale and shrunk; it tends to depress the vital powers when extreme, and causes dullness and torpor, both physical and mental. Such is its direct action, but its indirect action is very different; for there is in the living organism a disposition to react against the effects of depressing agents, and so long as the application of cold is not so extreme, or long continued, as to prevent reaction, or as to cause excessive reaction, it is a useful tonic and gives vigor, activity and strength to the organism. But it not unfrequently excites a reaction which results in congestion, irritation and inflammation, especially when the reaction is sudden. Such are the effects of cold on the parts to which it is applied, but this is not the most common mode in which it excites disease. A person is exposed to a draught of cold air, gets his feet wet, or is exposed when not properly clad; he afterwards becomes diseased, but not in the feet or part exposed, but in some internal part. He gets inflammation of the lungs, rheumatism, looseness of the bowels, or sore throat, or cold in the head, or any other disease to which he is predisposed.

Non-cognizable agents. As little or nothing is known in regard to this class of causes, except from their effects, or from the diseases which they cause, it is hardly necessary to devote more space to their consideration than is necessary to name them, and make a few practical suggestions for their avoidance.

Endemic causes, are such as exist and cause disease in particular localities; as the cause of ague in marshy districts, or goitre in certain localities.

Epidemic causes, are such as spread over large sections and affect many persons at the same time; scarlatina and cholera result from such causes. Infectious and contagous causes, are such as are developed by those already suffering.

Intermittent, and remittent, fevers.—These fevers are supposed to be caused by a peculiar exhalation, which results from the decomposition of vegetable substances, denominated marsh miasm. This miasm, if it exists, has never been detected, and is only known by its effects; we may therefore dismiss this term and consider the diseases which result. Intermittent and remittent fevers are contracted in the neighborhood of marshes, swamps, mill-dams, rivers, and low lands, where vegetable matter is undergoing decomposition, during the hot weather of summer. These fevers do not often prevail beyond the 56th degree of latitude, as the summers do not seem to be long enough to generate in sufficient force the poison which causes them. Large cities although located in districts where they prevail, are generally comparatively exempt; so that however prevalent they may be in the immediate vicinity, or even the outskirts of a city, very few cases occur in the densely peopled portions. Low timbered lands are often quite healthy when first settled, until somewhat extensive clearings are made, and the surface and soil exposed to the sun. The side of a marsh, or bank of a stream, or mill-dam, in the direction of the ordinary winds, is often more sickly than the opposite. The evening, night and morning air, is more injurious than the air during the day, for the poison is dissipated with the fog and dew by the heat and light of the sun, but retained near the earth by the damp air of night.

To avoid these fevers, persons who live in miasmatic districts should, during the hot weather of summer, and until frosts come, remain within their houses during the evening, night, and until some hours after sunrise, and carefully exclude the night air. The light and heat of the sun and the air, should be freely admitted during the middle of the day to purify the house. Those residing in cities, in such districts, should avoid visiting the outskirts, or suburbs, of such cities during the evening and early morning. Those who reside in healthy districts, should never, if they can well avoid it, visit miasmatic sections of country between the first or middle of July, and the occurrence of severe frosts in the fall.

In regard to the miasm which is supposed to cause typhoid and typhus fevers, even less is known as to its cause, and the circumstances under which it is generated, than is known in regard to marsh miasm. These fevers are more prevalent and malignant in crowded, ill-ventilated and filthy localities and apartments, and yet they are by no means confined to such situations, but not unfrequently occur under quite the opposite circumstances. In regard to the Cholera, nothing is known as to its cause. It is an epidemic disease, spreading from Asia over Europe and America. It, like typhoid and typhus fevers, is more apt to occur among the residents of crowded streets, alleys, ill-ventilated and filthy apartments, and especially the intemperate; but it may attack those differently situated, and even the temperate.

To prevent typhoid and typhus fevers and the cholera; abstain entirely, and habitually, from the use of alcoholic and fermented drinks; be temperate in eating and drinking; seek proper and cheerful amusements, especially in the open air; be industrious, but avoid excessive labor; banish fear by a firm reliance on the Divine Providence; admit freely the light of the sun, and fresh air into every room of the house; remove all decaying vegetables from the cellar, drain off all stagnant water around or under the house; see that filth, animal and vegetable matters, are not allowed to accumulate and decompose about sinks, penstocks, drains, or doorsteps; and pay proper attention to personal cleanliness.

Measles and hooping-cough arise from an exposure to a specific poison generated by those already suffering from the same complaint. As these diseases are as light during childhood as during any period of life, and every one is almost sure to have them, sooner or later, it is hardly best to strive to avoid them.

Scarlet fever frequently occurs epidemically, and is to a limited extent a contagious disease. It rarely attacks adults, and for this reason it is desirable to avoid it during childhood if possible. Children may have it without exposure to those suffering from the disease, but are more likely to have it after exposure.

To prevent scarlet fever, children suffering from it should be separated from the healthy when practicable, not only during the fever, but also for at least three weeks after its termination, as it is the opinion of some writers, which from observation I think is correct, that the disease is as likely to be communicated during desquamation, or the separation of the scarf-skin, as during the fever; and it is also important to confine patients to an even temperature within doors, for at least three weeks after the termination of the fever, to prevent troublesome sequelæ, or after diseases, from exposure, as well as to avoid exposing others. Belladonna, in very small doses, first introduced by Dr. Hahnemann, has been recommended by many writers, both homœopathic and allopathic, as a preventive. So far as concerns preventing the disease after exposure, it has not answered my expectations, when I have used it, but it has seemed to lessen its severity as a general rule.

The smallpox. This is a contagious disease, and very few, in however good health, will fail to take it if exposed.

Vaccination is the great preventive measure, as is well known, but it is not so generally understood as it should be, that re-vaccination is indispensable in order to prevent the disease with any degree of certainty. A child who has been vaccinated within the first year of life, by the time he is eight or ten years old, if exposed, will be very liable to have at least varioloid. If vaccinated before puberty an individual is very liable to have the disease during manhood if exposed. A child, where there is the least possibility of exposure, should be vaccinated within the first year, re-vaccinated when seven or eight years old, and again when eighteen or twenty years of age. A person who has been vaccinated during adult life for the first time, should be re-vaccinated after a few years; but it is not generally necessary to re-vaccinate more than once, or at most twice, during adult life, as the effects of vaccination do not wear off as readily or rapidly as during childhood and youth. Re-vaccination after an interval of several years, with good matter, is a very sure preventive of small-pox, perhaps quite as sure as having the disease itself. If proper care is used in selecting matter from healthy subjects no harm results from vaccination or re-vaccination. That troublesome and dangerous diseases are sometimes communicated in this manner is certain, but with proper care there is no need of it. If matter is selected from a child, it is not only important to know that the child is to all appearance healthy, but it is about equally important to be satisfied that the parents of the child are free from all hereditary or acquired predisposition to chronic or other troublesome diseases. Vaccine matter should only be selected from the arms of the healthy children of healthy parents.

CHAPTER III.

USE AND ABUSE OF THE DIGESTIVE ORGANS.

ALTHOUGH man's natural body is but the clothing of his soul or spirit, and depends upon the indwelling spirit for its form and life, still the changes which are constantly taking place within the organism will be found to be, at least in a great measure, in accordance with the laws of the natural world. Within the last few years Physiology and animal Chemistry have been rapidly revealing the hitherto hidden processes which are constantly going on within, in the building up, sustaining and wasting of our earthly tenements.

To study the laws of our being is clearly a duty, and to conform to them should be a pleasure; for obedience to law is true order, and leads to health, life and happiness. In the first place, the attention of the reader will be called to the proper use of the digestive organs, and afterwards, more especially, to the abuse to which they are subjected at this day, and also to the consequences which follow.

The digestive organs in the animal kingdom answer to the roots of trees and plants in the vegetable kingdom, and the lungs to the leaves of the trees; but trees are attached to the earth, and draw their nourishment from the earth, as well as from the air; but men, and all the higher order of animals, have no such attachment to the earth; and yet they require to be sustained by something more than air. To meet this want, men and animals are furnished with digestive organs. It is only by the reception of new material, which goes to supply the place of worn-out particles that man's body is sustained. Few persons are aware of the rapidity of the change; but of the urgency of the demand, every one may soon become conscious by withholding supplies. Without air man can live but a few minutes, and without water and food, but a few days. We may form some idea of the rapidity of the change which is constantly taking place in the tissues of the body, by witnessing the rapid emaciation which follows when food is withheld. The actual materials of which the entire soft parts of the body are formed to-day, will have disappeared in a few weeks or months, and new substances will have taken the place of the old; and within a few years even the particles of which the very bones are formed, will have, in a great measure, given way to new material. Then we see that, so far as the material body is concerned, man has no identity. The real man, and that which sustains the apparent identity of the body, must necessarily be the spirit, or "living soul" within the body.

An adult man requires to be fed with more than a ton weight of material in a single year; and, of course, should waste the same quantity; if he does not, he grows larger; if he wastes more than he receives, he grows thin. The child receives more than he loses, the old man loses more than he receives; but the middle aged are sustained in a state of equilibrium between the two.

From the army and navy diet-scales of England and France, it is inferred that about two and one-half pounds, avoirdupois, dry, or comparatively dry food, per day, are required for a man in active life—of this about three-quarters vegetable and the rest animal. At the end of an entire year this amounts to over nine hundred pounds; of water, or some substitute for pure water, in the form of a solvent or fluid, it is estimated that about fifteen hundred pounds per annum are required, and about eight hundred pounds of oxygen; making in all over three thousand pounds per annum, required from the animal, vegetable and mineral kingdoms, to supply the waste which is so constantly going on in the body of an adult man.

The absolute requirements that our natural bodies may live, are, a due supply of air, water in some form, combustible materials, and substances which are capable of entering into and becoming a part of the various tissues of the body. These are required to sustain the loss which results from the unceasing activity which is everywhere present throughout the body, even in our sleeping moments, wearing away our very substance. Wherever there is activity in living animal structures, there is death, and particles which are dead are useless, and even injurious to the system; and, whether new matter is prepared to take the place of the old or not, they must be removed; for which purpose we have organs which remove or separate such substances from the blood and body. The liver, kidneys, bowels, skin and bronchia, are outlets for worn out and useless matter; and, that these various organs should be in a situation or condition to be able to perform their offices or functions faithfully, is quite as important for health and life, as it is that the organs of nutrition should be able to repair the waste. If the kidneys for a few days cease to secrete urine, death follows from the retention of the constituents of urine in the blood; and the cessation of the liver to secrete bile is attended by a similar, but less speedily fatal, result; and we are all aware of the commotion caused by a suppression of perspiration, and the result would perhaps be as fatal as a suppression of urine, were it not that either the kidneys or bowels usually take on a vicarious action. In fact, it is common among these secreting organs, when one of them becomes disabled from disease, for one or more of the rest to attempt to save the system from the pernicious effects which would result from the retained secretion, by taking on a vicarious action. Thus, when the liver becomes so diseased or deranged that it cannot remove the constituents of bile, bilious matter appears in the urine, and the skin becomes yellow, and it even sometimes escapes with the perspiration through the pores of the skin in sufficient quantities to stain the linen yellow. In cases of suppression of the urine, I have seen crystals of urea form upon the skin, which should have escaped with the urine, as one of its constituents. As the human body has no power to create a single atom of new matter, it follows that all the substances, discharged in the various secretions, have been taken into the system in the form of food or drink, or inhaled through the air passages, or absorbed from the surface of the body; but they have changed form, and passed off, presenting a very different appearance from the substances taken into the system. The human body cannot live upon mineral substances alone; it requires food which has been organized in the vegetable or animal kingdoms. In a chemical point of view vegetables are organizing, and animals are destroying machines; for animals and men receive organized food from the vegetable kingdom, but when such nourishment has fulfilled its use in animal structures, and is worn out and requires to be removed, it is not separated usually in the same form, that is as an organized substance, but is chemically changed or disorganized, and cast off a very different substance, even vile and offensive. Thus are the delicious vegetables and savory viands changed by the human organization.

The substances dismissed from the body, in the various secretions, are oxydized bodies; that is, they are the products of a slow combustion, which has supplied the body with animal heat; therefore the food necessary for man must contain a large amount of combustible materials. Combustion is caused by the uniting of the oxygen of the air, with the substance burnt, and in such a union heat is evolved. In the burning of a stick of wood, the oxygen of the air unites with the carbon of the wood, and a degree of heat which is perceptible to the senses and visible to the eye results, and the wood which is chiefly formed of carbon disappears in the form of carbonic acid gas, and various volatile substances, leaving but a small earthy residuum. Vegetable charcoal may be burnt without a blaze, and all disappear but a small quantity of ashes, in the form of carbonic acid gas. As we may have burning without flame, so we may have burning without visible fire. If a farmer's hay is too green when he stacks it up, it becomes hot—hot to the feel and imperfectly burnt.

The food we eat is to perform a double use. First, to nourish and build up the organism; Second, to be in due time oxydized or burnt up, to supply heat to keep up the temperature of the body. A portion of the food we eat is burnt up immediately, or unites with oxygen, and mostly escapes during expiration in the form of carbonic acid gas, without ever having become a part of the solid structures of the body; but the portion which enters into the formation of the various structures, is only oxydized or burnt when it is worn out; or ready to be removed; then this change takes place, and it is constantly going on in every part of the body, supplying warmth to the part. The carbonic acid generated by this process escapes through the pores of the skin, or is carried to the lungs and is thrown off, while the various other products of combustion, are carried in the blood to the kidneys, liver and bowels, and escape in the secretions from these organs. A small portion of the carbonic acid gas also escapes from these organs, especially from the kidneys.

In order for the oxydation, or combustion, of the worn out particles of substance throughout the tissues, or different structures of the body, also of the portion of the food taken into the stomach or bowels and absorbed and received into the blood, but not needed to build up or nourish the various structures, it is necessary for oxygen to come in contact with the particles to be oxydized; and this object is accomplished by the absorption of oxygen from the air during respiration. From four to six per cent. of the oxygen introduced into the lungs in the air we breathe disappears, or is absorbed by the blood. The air which is thrown off from the lungs during expiration is found to contain from three to five per cent. of carbonic acid gas, which has escaped from the blood in the lungs. The escape of this carbonic acid gas and the absorption of oxygen, together with other less important changes which occur in the lungs, change the whole appearance of the blood. From being dark venous blood it becomes of a bright crimson color, as it flows on in the pulmonary veins to the left auricle of the heart. By the contraction of the auricle it is forced into the left ventricle, and by the contraction of the latter it is sent through the aorta and its various arterial ramifications until it arrives into the minute capillary or hair-like vessels in every part of the body, bearing with it its precious load of oxygen, to burn up or oxydize the worn out particles of matter in the various structures; and also to consume the more combustible or heat-making portion of the nutriment received from the digestive organs, and flowing in the current of the blood itself, thereby imparting heat and warmth in the very substance of the entire organism. Thus are men and animals able to retain a uniform temperature, or nearly so, even when the surrounding atmosphere is much colder than the body; the latter remaining at the temperature of about ninety-eight when the mercury sinks below zero, in the surrounding air.

I have now called the attention of the reader to the necessity for, and the effects of food in heating the body, that the latter may retain a uniform temperature irrespective of a limited degree of external cold; but it is almost equally important that some provision should exist to relieve excessive heat, whether it arise from external or internal causes; for the body may be placed in an atmosphere much hotter than its natural temperature, or, by active exercise of body or even mind, thus causing active respiration and oxydation, a degree of temperature would often be generated far above the ordinary standard, if no provision existed for relieving the organism of the unnatural heat. In a cold atmosphere, the constant reception of cold air into the lungs, into the very center of the body, during respiration, tends to reduce the heat. This air, under such circumstances, absorbing a large quantity of heat in the lungs, leaves the air passages much warmer than the surrounding atmosphere. But if the air inhaled is above the natural temperature, respiration will tend to increase the heat of the body rather than to relieve it. There is a slight variation of the temperature of the body at different seasons of the year, and periods of the day, corresponding in a great measure with the changes of the surrounding atmosphere; but such variations are not as great as would be expected. Then the loss of heat by radiation from the surface of the body, and also by contact with the external air, is considerable when the atmosphere is cold; and in all cold climates men are obliged to protect the body by clothing, and thus guard against the loss of animal heat. The animals of cold climates are protected by dense coats of hair or fur, and the fowls by feathers. But by far the most important of all the cooling agencies to prevent excess of heat will be found evaporation. From the skin and air passages large quantities of the vapor of water are exhaled. There is poured out through thousands of little tubes, all over the surface of the body, a watery fluid; and as the internal or external heat rises, these little tubes, if in health, act with increasing energy, and pour out their excretion faster than it can be removed by evaporation, and it accumulates as drops of sweat upon the surface. To change water into vapor a large amount of heat is required, and the continual vaporization from the surface, when the skin is moist, and from the air passages, or change of water to vapor, is one of the most powerful sources of refrigeration or cooling of the body. The daily loss of water in this manner is estimated at about three and a half pounds, of which the pulmonary exhalation, or that from the air passages, constitutes about one-third, and that from the skin about two-thirds. The skin acts in a variable manner, losing more or less water as the external air is dryer or more damp. Three different organs are concerned in the removal of water from the circulation, the skin, the lungs and the kidneys. Of these the skin, as has just been remarked, acts variably according to the state of the atmosphere; but the lungs and respiratory passages, for the most part, act uniformly. It is true that the exhalation from the passages of the nose, and larger passages extending to the lungs, or trachea and bronchia, depends in a great measure, like that from the skin, upon the state of the atmosphere, and is therefore variable; but it is not so with that from the air cells, the temperature of which, and of the air they contain, is always nearly uniform; therefore water must vaporize into them at a uniform rate, and remove a uniform amount of heat as caloric of elasticity. As it is necessary that the daily average of water should be removed from the system, the variable action of the skin causes a variable action of the kidneys, for the excess which the skin cannot discharge must be strained off by these organs, as the lungs, as just stated, remove nearly a uniform quantity. The kidneys, therefore, in this respect, act vicariously for the skin. In hot weather, when the loss by perspiration is great, but little urine is discharged, but during cold weather, when the perspiration is diminished, the quantity is increased.

Thus it will be seen that the establishment of equilibrium of temperature in man, is effected by the mutual operations of the heating and cooling arrangements. By increasing or retarding the oxydation of combustible materials in the system, more or less heat, as the body requires, may be furnished, and by the cooling processes, to which allusion has been made, excess of heat is held in check.

Although man is born into the world more nearly naked than almost any animal, still by the aid of his superior intelligence he is able, by varying his diet, clothing and habitation, to withstand with comparative impunity, the change from the heat of summer to the cold of winter, which drives even the bear and a large number of hibernating animals, notwithstanding their hairy coverings, to their dens and to torpor. While man is able to live and flourish, and extend his dominion from the vertical sun of the torrid zone, where the elephant roams over ever green fields, and the lion and tiger, whose powerful limbs would be paralyzed by even the cold of our winter, lie in wait for their prey in forests and jungles which are ever alive with the warmth of a summer's sun, to the cold frigid zone which surrounds the poles, and there upon fields of never failing ice contends for the mastery with the polar bear, and contends not in vain. The white bear can no more withstand a tropical sun than the elephant can a polar winter. But man, by varying his diet, clothing, exercise and shelter, can withstand the never ending heat of the tropic, the sudden changes of the temperate zones, and the eternal frosts of the polar regions. To him is given dominion over the beasts of the field, the fowls of the air, and the fishes of the sea.

Although we have found that the body is warmed and cooled in accordance with certain chemical and physical laws, still, upon careful inquiry, we shall find that the indwelling spirit has much to do in holding in check or increasing the action of those chemical or physical changes, which tend on the one hand, to burn up, or oxydize, the very substance of the organism, or on the other, to cool down the body by allowing its fluids to escape, as sometimes happens, as in the cholera, when the minute capillary vessels of the skin and mucus membrane of the bowels, cease to retain the watery portion of the blood.

The natural body is but the clothing of the spirit, and it is the latter which moulds it into form, and sustains it in being. Although the chyle, and nourishment which is derived from our food, is poured into the mass of the circulating blood, and passes directly to the lungs, and thenceforth flows in contact with oxygen, yet the latter is restrained from burning up such particles as are needed to build up the various structures of the body, and they are directed to their proper place in the system and woven into living structures; at the same that unneeded particles of the chyle, and of the nourishment absorbed by the veins of the stomach, or such of these particles as are combustible, but not needed or adapted to enter the various structures, are permitted to be oxydized to warm the body. Nor is this all, particles which have entered into the different structures, are protected from the action of oxygen until they have fulfilled their use, or are worn out, then they are given over to this merciless destroyer to be used up as fuel, and new particles take their place.

The controlling power seems to be exercised, to a great extent, through the nervous system, but in a great measure independent of the will. Still love is the very life of man, and when his affections become active, excited, or warm, the body becomes also hot, so that animal heat is caused by spiritual influx into the material body, and, during a healthy state, it varies with the influx. But it is spiritual influx into appropriate material substances, and we can no more have animal heat without the physical conditions requisite for developing natural heat, as for instance, the presence of oxygen and combustible materials, than we can have a material body developed by such influx without the aid of appropriate material substances. When man's affections are moved the heart and lungs act with increased energy, and when man voluntarily brings into activity all the various parts of the body which are under the control of the will, this increased activity of the circulation and of the rest of the organism, will wear out the particles of which it is composed, and promote their oxydation, and that of the combustible materials in the blood, thereby increasing the temperature of the system. All this increased wasting of the various structures will increase the demand for food to supply the waste; so that man can use his various organs, wear out the materials of which they are composed, and increase the demand for a new supply, and thus sustain the activity and vigor of his organism in health, or he can do as the hibernating animals do during the winter, grow torpid or inactive and listless, and permit all the functions of life to sink to their lowest ebb, the respiration and circulation to become feeble, the extremities cold from the lack of vital heat, and the mind listless and inactive, until little more than simple organic life remains; incapable of resisting the various causes of disease, when ill health, suffering, and premature death, are sure to result sooner or later.

I have not as yet, except indirectly, called the attention of the reader to the important use which water performs in the animal economy. We have seen that by its evaporation from the surface of the body and air passages, the system is cooled when it would otherwise become too hot, still this is by no means the only, if it is even the most important office it performs. It acts as a solvent or vehicle to convey the more dense and less fluid substances from the stomach to their destination in the body; it gives fluidity to the blood, and conveys the dead and worn out particles, which cannot escape in the form of gases, out from the body through the kidneys, liver, bowels and skin. It is therefore essential to life, and it should be used as the system requires, and be unpolluted by poisonous drugs—pure water.

I trust the reader is now able to see, in some measure the important use the digestive organs have to perform. After calling attention, for a short time, to a hasty description of the functions which are performed by the different organs which make up the digestive apparatus, we will consider in the light of the uses which we have seen are to be performed by food and drink, what substances are proper and what improper for such purposes. This inquiry is one of vast moment to us, for health or disease, and even life or death of the body, depend more intimately upon the character of the substances used as articles of food or drink, than is generally supposed by the unthinking multitude, or even by the great mass of medical men.

I propose to call the attention of the reader in a separate chapter to the effects of alcoholic and fermented stimulants, and of narcotics, but there remains a large class of poisonous substances in almost constant use among us, which act, many of them at least, more directly upon the stomach, deranging its action, and causing disease.

THE DIGESTIVE ORGANS.

BEFORE the articles which are suitable for food are prepared to be absorbed and enter the circulation, certain preparatory processes are necessary, which it is important to understand before we can fully comprehend the extent of the abuses to which this department of our being is subject.

The teeth give form, fullness and beauty to the face, and aid materially the vocal organs in speech, so that their preservation is of great moment aside from their use in preparing food for the stomach. But at present we have to consider them in their relation to the process of digestion. Their first and most important use is to masticate or break down and divide our food, and prepare it for the stomach, and their preservation depends in a great measure upon their being required to habitually perform this use. When they are not used the gums become soft and spongy, earthy concretions from the saliva are deposited between them and the teeth, until the latter become loose and often drop out ; or unhealthy secretions and portions of food accumulate around and between the teeth, and cause them to decay ; so that the present habit of cutting up many articles of food very fine, and of rendering others very soft, so as to be able to swallow them without much chewing, is very injurious to the teeth. There are other reasons, aside from the preservation of the teeth, why we should never swallow our food without carefully chewing it. We have beneath the ears the parotid glands which secrete saliva, or spittle, which is poured into the mouth through a small duct above the back upper teeth of each side. Beneath the under jaw, at the sides, we have the submaxillary glands, and beneath the chin the sublingual gland, which all secrete saliva, which flows into the mouth through minute openings beneath the tongue. The first use of the saliva is to mix with, moisten and lubricate our food, that it may be readily swallowed; and, in order that it may do this, it is all important that we carefully masticate our food. Some may suppose that any other liquid will do as well to moisten our food with as saliva; this is a great mistake, and a serious one for the stomach and bowels. The saliva, when properly mixed with our food, materially aids digestion. This is especially true of all articles which contain starch, as bread and potatoes; the starch is changed into sugar by its contact with the saliva, and the latter, during the process of digestion, is changed into lactic acid, which is often important to aid digestion in the stomach, and is also an important heat producing substance. Instead of soaking crackers and bread in liquids we should eat them dry, and neither of them nor potatoes, nor any food which contains starch, should be swallowed until thoroughly masticated and mixed in the mouth with the saliva.

The saliva is not intended to be wasted, or thrown out of the system, and cannot be without danger to the digestive organs, therefore the habit of spitting is not only a very filthy and disgusting one, but it is also very injurious, and should never be practiced, except the secretion is the result of disease as in catarrh. We here can see one reason why the chewing of tobacco, gum, and other substances, is so injurious to health, it causing such a waste of this important fluid, which is needed to aid in the digestion of our food.

The Stomach. This organ, of which we hear so much, and to which we pay so little respect in our eating and drinking, performs a very important part in the process of digestion. From its internal surface the gastric juice is secreted by thousands of little follicles, from which this fluid exudes when food or irritating substances are taken into the stomach. The gastric juice is acid, containing either hydrochloric or lactic acid, and its use is to dissolve our food, and thus prepare it for absorption by the minute veins of the stomach, and the absorbents of the intestines. By the motion of the stomach, when food is received into it, the food is brought in contact and mixed with this fluid, and the portions which are capable of being dissolved by the gastric juice are prepared to be absorbed by the minute veins of the stomach, or to pass out of the stomach into the upper portion of the intestines. When it reaches the latter it presents the appearance of a semi-fluid called chyme, which varies in color according to the character of the food from which it has been made. About four hours, sometimes a little more or a little less according to the nature of our food, are usually required to complete the process of digesting solid food, and of preparing it to pass out of the stomach. Now the stomach is one of those organs which needs rest after labor, for at least two or three hours. When individuals abuse this organ by eating every three or four hours, thereby giving it no chance to rest, is it strange that sooner or later they become troubled with indigestion? Not at all, for it is only what they have a right to expect.

Fat and starch are not digested in the stomach, but pass into the upper portion of the intestines, where they are mixed with the secretions from the pancreas and liver, and from the glands of the intestines. The pancreatic juice resembles saliva, and like the latter is alkaline in its character. It acts upon fats, forming them into an emulsion, similar to that formed by lime-water and sweet oil, so that they can be readily absorbed; and it acts upon starch even more energetically than the saliva, changing it into sugar and lactic acid. The bile is alkaline in its character, and facilitates the absorption of fat by the lacteals or absorbent vessels of the intestines. This fluid is poured into the intestine a few inches below the stomach, and, after having performed its use in the process of digestion, a portion of it is re-absorbed, and the balance passes off with the excrement, giving a yellow color to the latter. The fæces or excrement, aside from a small quantity of indigestible substances which pass the bowels without being absorbed, are composed of a secretion, from the mucous membrane of the bowels, of worn out particles brought from the various parts of the body to be cast off.

As the object of this work is not to teach physiology, but to point out the chief avoidable causes of disease, suffering, deformity and premature death, the aim of the writer is to give the reader sufficient insight into the secret workings of his own organization to enable him to see, in the light of this science, when he violates physiological laws. If the reader desires, as I trust he may, to obtain farther knowledge of this interesting science, he will obtain in a small compass much useful knowledge from the small works written for schools; or, if he has leisure, from the more extended works of Draper or Carpenter.

Two great ends, or objects, are to be obtained by the use of food; one is to obtain substance, and the other to obtain heat for the body. "Viewed as regards this physiological distinction food is generally considered by physiologists, of two kinds. Histogenetic, or tissue-making, and Calorifacient or heat-making. Histogenetic food furnishes the chemical substances—carbon, hydrogen, oxygen, nitrogen, sulphur, chlorine, phosphorus, iron, potash, soda, lime, &c. Calorifacient food furnishes carbon and hydrogen mainly. In consequence of this chemical constitution, tissue-making food is sometimes called nitrogenized, and heat-making, non-nitrogenized food." (Draper.) The former is also sometimes called nutritive, and the latter respiratory food.

But, although there results a practical advantage in bearing in mind this division of food, still it is in a great measure arbitrary, as there is no such absolute natural division; for most articles suitable for food, partake more or less of the character of both tissue and heat-making in their chemical composition, although one may predominate in different articles; and, for this reason, we may select one in preference to others, as an article of diet. Yet non-nitrogenized, or heat-making food, is equally essential to nutrition as tissue-making material; for organization can only go on by the aid of heat, and in the presence of calorifacient, or heat-making substances.

Then again, food which has entered into the tissues of the body, when it has fulfilled its use, and is to be removed, is oxydized, which change produces heat; so that in the end, even tissue-making food, becomes also heat-making, before it leaves the organism. But the predominance of the one or the other quality, in various articles suitable for food, enables man, by varying his diet, to do much towards adapting himself to the various latitudes of the earth. If he is to live far north, in an excessively cold climate, he needs, and must have, food which will give him, not only substance or tissue-making material, with an ordinary amount of heat-making substances, but he must have that which will give him an excess of the latter, that it may be burned up, or oxydized, to supply heat to sustain the body at a living temperature. Such food the Esquimaux finds in the fat and oil of the seal, walrus, whale and white bear; and he obtains the tissue-making material he needs, aside from the small quantity which is contained around the fat and oil, from the muscle or flesh and viscera of these animals. Next to oil and fat, sugar is one of the most important heat producing articles of diet; it requires to be taken in connection with articles which contain more tissue forming material. Then in cold climates, and cold weather in temperate climates, fat and sugar become useful articles of food; whereas in hot climates, and hot weather in temperate climates they should be used sparingly.

BREAD.

Bread made from wheaten or rye flour, or from corn or oatmeal, has justly been called the staff of life. Few simple substances contain more perfectly all the qualities necessary to nourish the body of man. The gluten, or vegetable fibrine, is the nutritive or tissue-making portion of the grain; and the starch, by being changed into sugar, and from thence into lactic acid by the saliva and pancreatic juice, furnishes heat-making material. But bread, especially wheat, rye, or oat meal bread, is somewhat deficient in the heat-making element, especially for cold climates, or winter in temperate climates; therefore the proverb says: "It is good to have bread, but it is better to have bread and butter." It will be seen that this is true, and that there is a reason for this proverb, and that is, because butter contains in excess the very elements which are deficient in bread; namely, carbon and hydrogen—combustible materials. Now, if in cold climates, and cold weather, we add to bread and butter sugar, together with fruits and vegetables, we shall, perhaps, have the very best diet man has ever used; and by lessening or increasing the amount of butter and sugar, a diet adapted to almost every climate, except, perhaps, the very arctic regions of the earth, where, if men must live, we will leave them to prey upon the walrus, seal, and white bear; for sugar, butter and grain they have not, and it would be easier to ship the Esquimaux to a temperate climate than to send them the productions of our zone.

The importance of bread as an article of diet, renders an inquiry into the various processes by which it is prepared from the grain both interesting and useful.

Wheat is composed of water, gluten, starch, sugar, gum, oil and bran, with salts which are left as ashes when it is burned. The relative quantity of each varies slightly in different samples of wheat, but the following is about the average; water 11 per cent. gluten 13, starch 60, sugar 8, gum 4, oil 2, bran 2. The bran is simply the external hull or husk. The other elements of the seed are not equally distributed throughout its mass. This is a very important fact which we shall need to bear in mind. Immediately beneath the external hull is a layer of darkish colored matter, which is not easily reduced to a fine powder, or to superfine flour, and in the ordinary process of grinding and bolting, a large portion of it is cast off with the middlings and bran; and yet this very portion is rich in gluten, and most of the oil in the wheat exists in minute drops inclosed in its cells. Beneath this dark portion is the heart of the seed, which is whiter and more readily pulverized. It is composed chiefly of starch, and from it is formed the finest and whitest flour. There is more or less gluten in this portion of the kernel, and of starch in the dark portion, but they are each found in excess in the parts indicated. The mineral ingredients in wheat exist also unequally in different portions of the seed. About 2 per cent. of ashes remain when wheat is burned. These are composed of phosphoric acid about 46 per cent., potash 30, soda 3, magnesia 3, oxide of iron about three fourths of one per cent., sulphuric acid less than half of one per cent., and a small quantity of common salt, and of silica. These mineral ingredients are found distributed about as follows in the different products of our mills: fine flour a little over one per cent.; the next grade between 3 and 4 per cent.; still coarser, about 5, and bran 7. So it will be seen that fine flour contains but about one half, or a little over, of the quantity of these mineral ingredients, which is found in the wheat before grinding, the rest is cast off with the bran and coarse flour.

Now the mineral ingredients existing in the vegetables we use for food, are as indispensable to life as any other portion, and it has been found by experiments upon the lower animals, that when they are withdrawn as far as possible from the vegetable food upon which they are fed, that animals actually perish from starvation. These minerals are the very nourishment which important parts of the body require, and when the organized compounds in which they are contained are oxydized, or burned up, the mineral ingredients, or ashes, are not removed immediately from the system, but remain dissolved in the blood, and are withdrawn at points where they are needed to nourish local parts. The bones require phosphate of lime, the muscles the phosphates of magnesia and potash, the cartilages soda, the brain phosphorus, the hair and nails silica, while the red globules of the blood and the black coloring matter within the eye require iron. Notwithstanding the importance of these mineral substances, by our system of bolting and separating, our fine flour contains as we have seen, but a little over one half the quantity which has been provided for the wants of our systems, in this important grain. The almost universal use of the fine flour of wheat or rye, instead of unbolted flour, is doubtless a fruitful cause of imperfect development, if not of disease; in fact it is quite certain that here is to be found one of the most fruitful causes of consumption, and I would suggest to physicians, if it would not be more sensible to feed their patients with unbolted flour, and thereby supply phosphorus as it exists in organized food, than it is to give them the various phosphates, with the expectation of preventing or curing consumption; which treatment bids fair to be the next hobby for this disease. It is doubtful whether these minerals, directly from the mineral kingdom, can be appropriated so as to supply the wants of the organism in the slightest degree.

The attention of the reader has already been called to the fact that the external or dark portion of the kernel, is composed, in a great measure, of gluten, and the central or white portion, of starch.

Now in the process of bolting, the dark portion is separated almost entirely, and yet the gluten is the nutrious portion of the grain; it is that which in a great measure nourishes the muscles, and gives strength to the system; whereas starch is of but little use, except as a heat producing agent; and in this respect it is far inferior to oil, or fat; and most of the oil in wheat is contained in the dark or external portion of the kernel. The reader will bear in mind that the white central portion of the kernel, although chiefly starch, contains some gluten.

Dr. Bennett in an article published in the January Number of the *Ohio Cultivator* says:

"Now if there is a well established fact emanating from experimental analysis, it is this. That superfine or very finely bolted wheat flour will not alone sustain animal life. This fact has been repeatedly demonstrated by Magendi the greatest physiologist that ever lived. Having ascertained that the muscular and nervous tissues, including the whole brain or cerebral mass, was composed of nitrogenous matter, he readily concluded that starch or the fecula of wheat would not alone sustain animal life, for the reason that it contains not a particle of nitrogenous matter. Consequently, he found by experiment that animals fed exclusively on very finely dressed flour, died in a few weeks, whereas those fed on the unbolted thrived.

"Then, again, by the repeated analysis of both American and European Chemists, it is abundantly demonstrated that the portion immediately beneath the external covering, contains a very large per cent. of nitrogenous matter which should be mixed with the internal, or non-nitrogenous, in order that the muscular and nervous systems be properly nourished. Add to this well known fact, that the inhabitants of Scotland, Germany, Russia, as well as families and individuals in all parts of the world, who use almost exclusively unbolted flour, are seldom troubled with dyspepsia or indigestion, enjoy better health generally, and are possessed of much greater powers of endurance, and we have an array of facts, which, if universally heeded, would consign the use of superfine flour unmixed with this most nutritious or nitrogenous part, to oblivion."

The worst case of scurvy I have ever had to treat, occurred in a little girl five or six years old who lived entirely on toast, made of bread from superfine flour. She would eat no fruits or vegetables nor any animal food, nor could she be persuaded to change her diet in the least, and it was only by using potatoes freely with the flour in making her bread, that she obtained relief; but at the end of about a year this expedient failed, and symptoms of scurvy returned, when by starving and urging she was induced to eat fresh meat, potatoes, and other vegetables, when she rapidly recovered again.

It will be seen that we actually feed to our swine, horses, and cattle, the most nutritious and important part of the grain, and also the oil, and retain for our own use an inferior heat producing material, with a smaller amount of nutritious matter than was intended for our benefit. We also lose the sweetest portion of the grain; and all this is sacrificed to simple whiteness and fineness, notwithstanding our teeth are perishing for the want of use. Surely there is more show than substance in this, and if the useful ever comes to take the place of the superficial, we may expect a change for the better.

Mr. O. P. Stevens, of Cleveland, Ohio, has invented a machine with which, after moistening the wheat, he removes mechanically the external hull, and then grinds the grain without sifting it afterwards, so that his process furnishes unbolted flour without, or with very little of the harshness of the ordinary Graham flour. This I conceive to be as near perfection as we can ask in the way of grinding grain. There is no advantage in retaining the hull, for it is indigestible, and passes the bowels with little or no change, and can only be useful in extreme cases of constipation; whereas in not a few cases it is too irritating to the delicate mucous membrane of the stomach and bowels.

In regard to Mr. Stevens' process of hulling wheat before grinding, Prof. J. Brainerd, of Cleveland, says:

"The fatty matter and starch afford the carbonaceous portions of our food, the gluten furnishes the real nourishment for the muscle and nerve. The value of food, therefore, for human consumption, depends not upon the quantity of starch which affords material for the accumulation of fat, but chiefly upon the quantity of gluten contained in the grain. Any course of preparation, therefore, which tends to waste this important element, (gluten) must be objectionable. It is a singular fact, that in all the seeds of wheat and other grains, the principal part of the gluten lies near the skin, bran, or berry, it should therefore be a desideratum in the preparation of wheat for food, to preserve as much of this nutritious quality as possible.

The present mode of preparing flour, by refining it to its utmost possible extent, diminishes somewhat its value for food.

In addition to the gluten, the phosphates, (important ingredients in human food,) lie near the surface. The epidermis, or outer covering of the berry of wheat, is composed principally of silex, (flint,) which is indigestible in the stomach of a person, and will even withstand the action of concentrated nitric acid. The *setæ*, or hairs seen in the lower end of the wheat berry are also of a silicious structure, and therefore indigestible.

It therefore becomes a matter of no small moment, how wheat may be best prepared for the purposes of food.

Flour manufactured from wheat from which the silicious coating has been removed, is much more valuable than that prepared by the common method. This improved process, saves all of the nutriment which is wasted in the bran by the common method."

In regard to the relative value of unbolted and superfine flour, the writer of an article on the "Frauds in Food," in the *Eclectic Review*, says:

"Many of the most important aliments of our blood, brain and bone, are found in the greatest abundance in the colored, outward part of the wheat, which we deem fittest for pigs; so we fatten them, and suffer ourselves. The difference in nourishing properties between whole meal flour, and very finely dressed flour, amounts, in many cases to fully one-third."

I give this notice of Mr. Stevens' machine with great pleasure, for, I am sorry to say that he has thus far found its introduction to public favor an up hill business, although it is certainly one of the most meritorious inventions of the age. I have ate bread for the past few months made from flour manufactured by Mr. Stevens, and it has answered my expectations in every respect.

RAISING DOUGH.

VARIOUS methods are employed for this purpose, and as some of them are very objectionable, this subject requires at least a hasty notice in this connection. Dough is raised by the formation of gas throughout the mass, distending it and forming small cells, thereby rendering it spongy and light. In the process of raising by the aid of leaven, yeast, salt or milk risings, carbonic acid gas is generated by the commencement of fermentation, which process is checked by baking.

The use of leaven, or a portion of sour dough kept from a former baking, is objectionable, as it almost always communicates to the bread a sour taste, caused by the presence of lactic acid. Beyond all question the best methods at present in use for raising bread, are by the aid of yeast and salt or milk risings; as by these methods we obtain the end in view without contaminating the bread by leaving in it any injurious substance; and experience has abundantly demonstrated the wholesomeness of bread thus prepared. But the same cannot be said in regard to the various chemical substances used for raising bread, for they are all objectionable, and should never be used, either for raising bread or biscuit. The use of saleratus or bicarbonate of potash, and sour milk is objectionable, as it is difficult to get the exact quantity required to neutralize the acidity of the milk, and if enough is used to prevent a sour taste an excess is very sure to remain in the biscuit, often sufficient to change the color and affect the taste. It is the opinion of some medical writers that the habitual or frequent use of this salt is a fruitful cause of consumption. The use of bicarbonate of soda and muriatic acid would, perhaps, be the least objectionable of that of any of the mineral substances used, if we could always obtain them pure, and use the exact proportions; as we get from their action upon each other carbonic acid gas, water, and common salt, so that the bread is both raised and salted. But if the acid be in excess there will be sourness, and that caused by one of the most powerful acids we have, whereas, if the alkali be in excess the bread will be stained yellow, and have a disagreeable, hot, bitter, alkaline taste. Bicarbonate of soda and tartaric acid are frequently used to raise bread, but if either is in excess we have it left in the bread, and even if the exact proportions are used, we have from their mutual decomposition tartrate of soda, a pernicious salt, remaining in the bread.

E. L. Youmans, in his "Hand Book of Household Science," which contains more useful knowledge than almost any other book of its size in the English language, says:

"The class of substances thus introduced in the bread are not *nutritive*, but *medicinal*, and exert a disturbing action upon the healthy organism. And although their occasional and cautious employment may perhaps be tolerated, on the ground of convenience, yet we consider their habitual use as highly injudicious and unwise. This is the best that can be said of the chemical substances used to raise bread, *even when pure*, but as commonly obtained they are apt to be contaminated with impurities more objectionable still. For example, the commercial muriatic acid which is commonly employed along with bicarbonate of soda, is always most impure—often containing chloride of iron, sulphurous acid, and even arsenic, so that the chemist never uses it without a tedious process of purification for his purposes, which are of far less importance than its employment in diet. While common commercial muriatic acid sells for three cents per pound wholesale, the purified article is sold for thirty-five. Tartaric acid is apt to contain lime, and is frequently adulterated with cream of tartar, which is sold at half the price, and greatly reduces its efficacy; while cream of tartar is variously mixed with alum, chalk, bisulphate of potash, tartrate of lime, and even sand."

I am satisfied that the use of these mineral substances is doing much toward preventing and impairing the physical development of the young, and that it is a fruitful cause of disease. These poisons have no business in the kitchen, and should be speedily banished.

Milk is a valuable article, and, with the addition of bread and fruits, it may well form no inconsiderable share of the diet of man, and especially of the young. No better diet can be found during the days of childhood and youth than good coarse bread and milk.

We have in peas and beans the most concentrated form of vegetable nourishment, and when they are used in connection with less nutritious food, such as bread, potatoes, and other vegetables, they constitute cheap and wholesome articles of nourishment.

As it is my aim more especially to point out what is improper in our present manner of living, I shall not notice in detail, if at all, the great variety of fruits and vegetables in use, which are harmless, grateful to the taste, and more or less nutritious, and especially valuable as containing certain mineral ingredients which are somewhat deficient in grain and bread. A large portion of our food should be composed of fruits and vegetables when practicable, and we need to make special provision for a supply the latter part of winter, and fore part of spring, or we are liable to suffer from disease, for the want of such nourishment.

ANIMAL FOOD.

The reader will reasonably expect a few words in regard to the use of meat, or animal food. It is well known that we have a class of writers who condemn the use of meat, as entirely unnecessary and injurious. Without spending much time or space in the consideration of this subject, I will frankly state my own convictions. I believe that the time has been, in the far distant past, in the golden age of the world, when the men of our earth did not use meat. We are thus taught by revelation; and reason, I think, teaches that the time will again come, in perhaps, the not very far distant future, when the glorious promise shall be fulfilled of the establishment of the prophetical

New Jerusalem, even in the earthly and sensual planes of man's mind, when the wilderness shall blossom as the rose, and peace, good will, temperance and obedience to spiritual and natural laws, will fill the earth with a population so dense, that the entire soil will be needed for the nobler purpose of raising grain, fruits, and vegetables for the sustenance of man. It requires as much vegetable food to rear an ox to the age of five years as it does to feed several men, and yet the men will eat the ox in a few weeks; so that it is a great waste of food to live on meat or animal food.

One of the strongest arguments, to my mind, against the use of animal food is to be found in the fact that our Creator has established in the mind of every child born into the world, an antipathy to taking the lives of animals to make food of their flesh. Doubtless every one can bear witness to the strength of this feeling in his or her younger days; and I am free to confess, that more than forty summers have not so far eradicated this feeling, but that if I had to do all the slaying of animals, and had the ability to do it, a majority of those who now use meat so freely, would have a chance to try a lighter diet; from which change I do not imagine that they would suffer any serious injury in the end, for I know that man can live without the use of meat. In my native town, lived a young man who never used meat, or any kind of animal food from his childhood, not even butter or milk, and yet his system was well developed, and he was one of the most muscular men I have ever seen.

In Hayward's History of Massachusetts, is to be found an account of a man, living in Worcester County, who was able to go into the hay-field and mow, at the age of one hundred and sixteen years, and yet he had ate no meat from early childhood. The Hindoos live to a great extent on rice, and are capable of enduring strong muscular exertions, and are healthy; while the flesh-eating foreigner suffers severely from the heat of day, and the air of night; and is very liable to disease of the liver, and digestive organs. The natives of Sierra Leone who subsist on boiled rice and fruits, are strong, healthy and long lived, notwithstanding they live in one of the worst climates; and many of the vegetable eating African laborers, on the coasts of that country, are said to possess great muscular power, and good health.

"In Humboldt's description of the Indians of Peru, Mexico, Quito, and New Grenada, they are represented as peaceful cultivators of the soil, remarkably exempt from disease, and free from physical deformities. They live almost entirely on vegetable nourishment. In his narrative of himself, he gives the same decided testimony as to the character and habits of various other South American tribes. Our American Indians, who, in their savage state, live entirely on flesh, are short-lived, and greatly subject to epidemic and contagious diseases. Whole tribes are sometimes swept off by measles, small-pox, and other maladies. In Nantucket and Martha's Vineyard, in 1764, a fever appeared among the Indians dwelling there, which swept off 202 out of 340. in the course of six months. Its fatality was confined to those of entire Indian blood, and Indian dietetic habits. The inhabitants of the Pacific Islands, in their heathen state, were well built, fine featured, mild and pleasant; and their physical strength and activity was such that captain Cook's men stood no chance with them in boxing and wrestling. Their diet was almost entirely of vegetables. The Hottentots and New Hollanders, on the other hand are ill-formed, stinted, sickly and short-lived. Their living consists almost entirely of animal food. They live on lizards, serpents, frogs and other reptiles, and are without intellect, or a sense of right and wrong."—PHILOSOPHY OF HEALTH, (by L. B. Coles, M.D.)

"FLESH EATING AND VEGETABLE EATING.—To consider man anatomically, he is decidedly a vegetable-eating animal. He is constructed like no flesh-eating animal, but like all vegetable-eating animals. He has not claws like the lion, the tiger, or the cat; but his teeth are short and smooth, like those of the horse, the cow, and the fruit-eating animals; and his hand is evidently intended to pluck the fruit, not seize his fellow animals. What animal does man most resemble in every respect? The ape tribes, frugiverous animals. Doves and sheep, by being fed on animal food (and they may be, as has been fully proved,) will come to refuse their natural food: thus has it been with man. On the contrary, even cats may be brought up to live on vegetable food, so they will not touch any sort of flesh, and be quite vigorous and sleek. Such cats will kill their natural prey, just as other cats, but will refuse them as food. Man is naturally a vegetable-eating animal: how, then, could he possibly be injured by abstinence from flesh? A man, by way of experiment, was made to live entirely on animal food; after having persevered ten days, symptoms of incipient putrefaction began to manifest themselves. Dr. Lamb, of London, has lived for the last thirty years on a diet of vegetable food. He commenced when he was about fifty years of age; so he is now about eighty,—rather more I believe—and is still healthy and vigorous. The writer of the Oriental Annual mentions that the Hindoos, among whom he travelled, were so free from any tendency to inflammation, that he has seen compound fractures of the skull among them, yet the patient be at his work, as if nothing ailed him, at the end of three days. How different is it with our flesh-eating, porter-swilling London brewers! A scratch is almost death to them!"—FLOWERS AND FRUITS, (by J. E. Dawson).

The increased liability to acute diseases among meat-eaters, and tendency to decomposition of the fluids and solids of the body, may depend, in a great measure, upon the fact that man receives his nourishment second-handed when he eats meat; and, when he eats carnivorous animals, third-handed. The nourishment for the structures of both men and animals, is derived from the organized substances of the vegetable kingdom. The same process of nutrition, sustenance and waste, are unceasingly going on in animals as in man; and while some of the particles of which the flesh of an animal is composed are fresh from the vegetable kingdom, others have fulfilled their use or are worn out, and are being decomposed and are nearly ready to pass out of the system through the kidneys or bowels.

But most members of the adult population of our country have eaten meat, and their fathers, for many generations before them, have done the same, so that their digestive systems are accustomed and accommodated to the use of meat, which is generally more stimulating and more easily digested than vegetable food; therefore, it is not every one who can leave off eating meat with impunity, and enjoy good health, or even live. I have not unfrequently been compelled to recommend the use of meat to my patients. But there is no doubt but that many will find themselves better in body, and clearer in mind if they will use less meat than they do. And if we eat meat at all, we shall do well to take the Word of the Lord as our guide, and abstain from the use of the flesh of those animals which the Jews were prohibited from eating. We may rest assured that an infinitely wise Creator never declared swine's flesh unclean without a good reason; and, if it is unclean for the Jews, it is certainly unclean for us. We have no warrant in the Bible for its use, and many physicians and writers claim that its use is a fruitful source of scrofulous diseases. Although I cannot regard the use of pork as being as pernicious as that of alcoholic drinks, tobacco, coffee, tea, or many of the condiments in use, for multitudes who use it are robust and healthy, still the hog is a low, groveling, filthy animal, and it seems difficult to avoid the conclusion that the use of such an animal must tend to debase man morally and physically. I do not care to have my body built up of such materials, still I would eat pork, as I would many other articles, sooner than starve, or go hungry, but not when other kinds of meat are accessible.

The attention of the reader has already been called to the use which sugar performs in the organism. This substance is grateful to the taste, and its moderate use, in our food, when pure, is unobjectionable; but to the use of sugar candy there are serious objections. "Candy is commonly adulterated with flour, and frequently with chalk."—(YEOMANS.) But far more pernicious ingredients are found in the poisonous subtances used for coloring and painting the various kinds of candy. Among these Dr. Hassall found various preparations of lead, copper, and arsenic, also bisulphuret of mercury, cobalt, and gamboge. The Doctor remarks: "It may be alleged by some that these substances are employed in quantities too inconsiderable to prove injurious; but this is certainly not so, for the quantity used, as is amply indicated by the eye alone, is often sufficient, as is proved by numberless recorded and continually recurring instances, to occasion disease and death. It should be remembered, too, that these preparations of lead, murcury, copper, and arsenic, are what are termed *cumulative*, that is, they are liable to accumulate in the system, little by little, until at length the full effect of the poison becomes manifested.

"Injurious consequences have been known to result from merely moistening wafers with the tongue; now the ingredients used for coloring these include many that are employed in sugar confectionary. How much more injurious, then, must the consumption of sugar thus painted prove when these pigments are actually received into the stomach."

COMMON SALT.

THIS substance is in almost constant use as a condiment. When taken freely it impairs digestion by its action on the gastric juice; but used with moderation it is useful; as, by its decomposition, it furnishes hydrochloric acid, which is an important constituent of the gastric juice, and it furnishes soda to the bile. Man instinctively craves more or less salt, nor is it altogether a cultivated habit, for even those noble animals, the horse, ox and sheep, animals who are above using tobacco or whisky, also crave salt. Deer and other wild animals visit salt springs. When man is deprived of salt, lactic acid, which is furnished by the decomposition of milk, starch or sugar, takes the place of hydrochloric acid, in the gastric juice; so that man can live without the addition of salt to his food, but there is no objection to its moderate use.

Food and drink may be tolerated by a healthy stomach at almost any temperature, unless it is scalding hot, but ice-cold water, or food, is objectionable, and if used at all it should be used cautiously, as injury is liable to result. Very hot liquids should be avoided. If food or drink is too hot for the mouth, we may rest assured that it is too hot for those organs which are comparatively destitute of sensibility, or feeling, therefore we should never think of swallowing it, for it will scald the æsophagous or passage to the stomach, and the stomach, as badly as it will the mouth, although the former may not tell us of it, only by after disease; for the æsophagous and stomach are not furnished, to any considerable extent, with nerves of sensation; and therefore, they may be burnt or cut without our scarcely feeling it; still, when these organs become diseased we often suffer severely; even very acute pain.

COFFEE AND TEA.

THAT these substances are yet to be banished from use is perhaps certain, for if the inhabitants of our earth ever come into true order, they will certainly cease to use, as articles of food or drink, disease-creating substances. But coffee and tea are not as poisonous as alcohol and tobacco, and perhaps many other articles in use, and I shall be content with simply pointing out a few of the symptoms caused by their habitual use. The reader will please bear in mind that healthy articles of food do not cause specific diseases, but I shall call attention more fully to this point hereafter, when considering the use of tobacco and alchohol.

Coffee, causes a great variety of symptoms. It causes a peculiar form of headache which commences in the morning, gradually increases until the middle of the day, or later, and then declines. Both coffee and tea palliate the symptoms they cause, and patients always suffer from such symptoms, for several days, when they discontinue their use. Coffee excites the bowels to unnatural activity, and consequently weakens the digestive organs. It often entirely destroys the appetite for breakfast, especially with children. It excites more powerfully than almost any other substance in use the sexual propensity, and is a fruitful cause of licentiousness; and this over excitement is followed by premature impotency.

Tea causes headache, violent palpitation of the heart, and a peculiar gone feeling at the pit of the stomach. These symptoms are worse when the patient has been some time without tea, and are ameliorated when he again partakes.

It is said that the tea drinkers of China, who indulge freely, are thin and weak, of a leaden complexion, with black teeth, and are very subject to diabetes. Who can say that the use of tea, during successive generations, has not been one of the chief causes of the physical and moral degradation of the inhabitants of that land?

Coffee and tea excite the nervous system and brain, and hasten on a premature, but consequently imperfect, development of both body and mind. If parents will persist in using these injurious substances themselves, I do not think they have a moral right to give them to their children, thereby polluting their natural appetites, giving rise to an unnatural craving for these substances, the use of which will do incomparably more injury to the growing organizations of the young than to those of adult men or women.

These drinks not only hasten on a premature development, and consequently premature decay of the body and mental faculties, but their use also engrafts upon the organism the particular diseases which, as we have seen, they are capable of causing. Multitudes suffer from nervous and sick headaches, palpitation of the heart, goneness at the pit of the stomach, loss of appetite, derangement of the stomach and bowels, &c., from the use of coffee and tea, without ever suspecting that these beverages injure them; in fact, feeling all the time that they do them good, because they suffer when they attempt to leave them off, for they palliate the symptoms they have caused, as do all poisons.

If parents have no regard for their own health and lives, may it not be a duty which they owe to their children to set them a better example than to use these substances before them? Every one can but see, upon reflection, that it is very wrong to allow children to use these poisons.

But we are told by some that tea and coffee contain more or less nourishment. Well, supposing they do, and so do the body and head of a rattlesnake; but if we were to steep up his snakeship, head, poison and all, and drink the tea, we might perhaps pay dearly for our folly. The deadly nightshade, hemlock, henbane, and all poisonous plants, when analyzed may be found to contain more or less of materials which are useful for food, but they also contain substances which are poisonous, and therefore they are unsuitable for food or drink. The nutritious portion of tea, is in a great measure, if not entirely, insoluble, so that if we do not eat the leaves, we fail to get the nourishment they contain.

An article on Coffee and Tea, in the *Atlantic Monthly* for January, 1859, advocates the use of these beverages, not because they are nutritious, for it is admitted that the supply of nourishment can be better obtained in solid food, but because they stimulate the mental faculties, and prevent, or retard the wasting of the tissues, and thereby lessen the demand for food. That they produce such effects, is beyond question; and, if an individual had a limited supply of food, with no occasion for activity, he might live longer, perhaps, with than without them. But is it desirable to lessen the waste and the demand for a fresh supply of nutritious materials in the human body, and that by the use of articles, the cost of which would supply substantial food to take the place of worn out particles? If it is desirable to arrest this change, there are various methods for accomplishing this end without taking pernicious substances. A life of indolent inactivity will very effectually accomplish this; also living in a warm climate, and warm air, and the use of warm drinks. But all these tend to debilitate and weaken the body, even when no obnoxious substance is taken to accomplish the object. Health, strength and vigor, depend on using the organism, and increasing rather than retarding this change; for this reason active exercise, wearing out the particles of which the body is composed, increasing the appetite for food, or a new supply of nutriment, does not debilitate, but invigorates the body. What a violation then of nature's laws, or the laws of health, to use, instead of the substantial food, for which our structures call, articles which retard the change on which health and vigor depend; and especially when such substances cause unnatural excitement, which must, necessarily be followed by corresponding depression. Is it strange that our coffee and tea-drinkers are thin-faced, delicate and nervous, and lack the plumpness, and firmness of structure of those who increase, rather than retard the metamorphosis of the structures of the body, and use, to supply the waste, substantial food, instead of these exciting drinks? But this is, perhaps, not the worst effect which results from these drinks, for they cause specific diseases. Even the writer in the *Atlantic Monthly* admits that tea in excess is well known to "produce an exaltation of the actions of the heart, amounting in some persons to a painful and irregular palpitation." He also admits that the active principles of coffee in excess cause "increased action of the heart, rigors, headache, a peculiar inebriation, and delirium, also perspirations, augmented activity of the understanding, which may end in irregular trains of thought, restlessness, and incapacity for sleep." Now healthy, nourishing, life-giving food, causes no such results; yet multitudes are suffering from these, and many other symptoms every day, not from what this writer would call an excess, but from the steady persevering use of about a given quantity, month after month, and year after year, and can never be cured until they give up these drugs entirely, for the smallest quantity will often keep up the symptoms. Cold drinks are more invigorating than warm, and are generally preferable except at meals. There are persons who are in the habit of drinking freely at their meals (a bad habit by the way,) who cannot use cold drinks with impunity, and, perhaps, they are best for no one; but surely there is no excuse for taking tea and coffee so long as hot water, milk and sugar are more plenty, and cheaper than either. And as for the sociability, and excitement, caused by such stimulants, we want a different kind of sociability and excitement than that which results from unnatural sensual indulgences. We want the cheerful, playful innocence of childhood, coupled with the wisdom of manhood, to flow forth from warm hearts — warm not from the fires of earth, but from the Divine Love, which is ever seeking a habitation in the human heart or soul; seeking to flow forth in smiling words, kind acts and innocent social recreations and amusements. Who would think of adding to the joyous happiness of early childhood, by administering whisky, tobacco, coffee or tea to the young child? Surely no one. If we would be happy like children, we must diligently cultivate, by permitting them to flow forth into act, those innocent, kindly and cheerful affections which make the child happy, and which we are smothering by unnatural sensual indulgence, and selfishness, until we become cold-hearted and almost dead, so far as their existence is concerned. One hour spent in the performance of kind acts, or enjoying active social amusements, if the old adage be true—" Laugh and grow fat"—will do more towards clothing the muscles with fat, than a pound of coffee or tea.

The physician who is aware of the symptoms and diseases which tea and coffee so frequently cause, and has seen such symptoms and diseases gradually abate when the use of these beverages has been discontinued, as I have, can have no doubt about their being improper articles, especially for children, to use.

CONDIMENTS.

We come now to the consideration of a large class of substances, which are almost constantly in use, under the name of condiments, which man during health should never use, and their use certainly is rarely required during disease, as every physician will testify. Among the most prominent of these pernicious substances, will be found black and red pepper, allspice, cloves, mustard, horse-radish, ginger, nutmeg, cinnamon, together with many other irritating substances, which are in some form or other mixed up with the food of which we are daily almost compelled to partake, especially if we eat at a public table, for we will scarcely find a dish that does not contain more or less of one or more of these miserable irritants. Our cooks cannot be satisfied to leave to every boarder to season his own food with such trash or not, as he may prefer, but must take upon themselves the liberty of seasoning our food with these vile drugs, until it has become an unbearable nuisance to every one who desires to live as we all should live, with his stomach uncontaminated by these poisons. It is the duty of every one of us to set our faces resolutely against this abuse, and by the time the cooks in our public boarding houses and hotels, find they are under the necessity of cooking a second dish, when they have put their pepper and the like into the first, a few times, they may be led to see that it does not pay.

Does any one question that to put such irritating substances into the delicate organization of the stomach is wrong? Let him put them into his eyes, or nose, or even retain them in contact with the mucous membrane of the mouth. Yes, more, let him moisten them with water and apply them to the external gross organization of the skin, and even there he will find that they will all create an unnatural irritation of the surface, and several of them will even blister the skin, and cause deep and troublesome ulcerations. Is it reasonable to suppose that man can put such substances into his stomach with impunity? He may not feel a similar irritation, smarting and pain in his stomach, to that which he experiences in his mouth, or on the skin, simply because, as I have already said, the stomach is not supplied with nerves of sensation; but the effect upon the stomach will not be the less on that account; for many of the troublesome cases of dyspepsia, and of chronic inflammation of this organ, which are so common, are caused by these irritants. When taken even in moderate quantities, they act directly as local stimulants, causing an unnatural flow of blood to the mucous membrane of the stomach, increasing the secretion of gastric juice, producing a morbid or craving appetite, which results in the individual over-eating, or taking more food than is required by the system; and often more than the stomach and bowels can digest. The undigested food, when an excess is taken, acts as a foreign body, causing diarrhœa and various other derangements of the bowels and stomach, and the poor victim wonders what should have made him sick. But this unnatural excitement caused by the use of these stimulants, even if they are not used in sufficient strength to blister the stomach, or cause inflammation, is necessarily followed by depression, or debility; and by a constant repetition of the stimulant at almost every meal, the vital energies of this organ are exhausted, and it is prematurely worn out; of course the whole organism, failing to receive due nourishment, fails; the skin becomes wrinkled, the flesh soft, and premature old age, and death follow. Even if the subject escapes disease and death from some attack supervening as a consequence of the debility caused by these stimulants, he is liable to be cut off by the diseases which these poisons cause, for their effects are not spent entirely upon the stomach, but they are absorbed and enter the circulation, and flow throughout the entire body, exciting and irritating the various tissues and organs, exciting the passions, and making man more earthly, sensual and evil. Is it strange that man cannot restrain the outbursts of his already perverted passions, while he is constantly stimulating the organism through which such passions are manifested, by the very substances which are the natural types of these perverted passions? Have parents a right to expect that their children will grow up virtuous, temperate, and good, to say nothing of their physical health, when they allow them to use such unnatural stimulants?

If space would permit, the various symptoms and diseases which are caused by the different poisons now under consideration, might be pointed out, so far as they are known, as they are described by medical writers. But there are some symptoms which are common to several of these substances, to which I will call the attention of the reader; and one of the most marked, is the effects which they produce upon the red globules of the blood. Few poisons so certainly and rapidly destroy the red blood, as several of those under consideration. Whether this is done by the direct action of the poison upon the blood, or upon the nerves of organic life, or by causing debility and weakness of the digestive organs, thereby preventing the development of red blood globules, it is difficult to say.

They destroy the natural acuteness of the taste, and render plain, wholesome food insipid; they therefore lessen the enjoyment which it was intended man should realize during the act of eating. He alone who lives on plain wholesome food, can realize the loss in this respect. For many years, while sitting at our own table, I used none of these substances, and now avoid them when I can, and not go hungry. I never add them to food, and am never satisfied when I find them mixed up in dishes which are set before me. A mince or apple pie without these spices, is as far superior, to one with them, to the unperverted taste, as can possibly be imagined. In the former we taste the apple and meat, and they are much more natural to the healthy palate than spices. Pies filled with these substances taste like chips in comparison with plain pies. Place the two kinds for the first time upon the tongue of a young child, and you will soon see which he would prefer; no healthy palate would ever be satisfied with most of these substances, and it is only by sprinkling them upon, or mixing them up with other articles of wholesome food, that the palate becomes reconciled to their use; and it only craves them when its natural sensibility becomes so far impaired, as to lose the delicate natural taste. So that nothing is gained by their use, save loss of taste, and of a natural appetite, and of health.

All alkalies, except such as are naturally contained in our food, should be avoided during health; for they neutralize the natural acidity of the gastric juice, and impair the power of the stomach to digest food. Soda water should be avoided, for if the soda is in excess, it injures the stomach by interfering with the process of digestion.

Acids, if used at all, should be used sparingly. They are perhaps less objectionable than alkalies, and the appetite sometimes craves them, even when they are not habitually used, and in certain states of the system, as in scurvy, the use of vegetable acids is very beneficial. Tart and acid fruits are also useful, and grateful to the taste. Vinegar, to say the least, is a very doubtful article of diet. It is, like alcohol, a product of decomposition, and not of life; and in its concentrated form it is a powerful corrosive poison. Ordinary strong vinegar contains about four or five per cent. of the pure acid. If vinegar is used at all, it should be used very moderately. It is undoubtedly better, as far as possible, to substitute for it the living vegetable acids, or those derived from fruits and vegetables, and which are not the product of decomposition, but of life.

Americans generally eat too fast, and certainly should eat slower, that they may have time to more perfectly masticate their food, and more intimately mix it with the saliva, and also to give the gastric juice a chance to mix with the food as it is swallowed, and thus that the sensation of hunger may be appeased without the individual taking more than is necessary to duly nourish the body.

FREQUENCY OF MEALS.

How often should we eat, is a very important question, and one which we shall do well hastily to examine; for health and even life are often sacrificed through ignorance, or willfully disobeying physiological laws, by eating more frequently than is compatible with the healthy process of digestion. We eat to nourish and sustain the body, and we should never have as an end, simply to gratify the appetite, for if the latter is our object, we become gluttons and sensualists. To the truly wise man,—who witnesses around him the consequences of abusing the digestive organs in the way of eating and drinking, in the wrinkled faces, and bowed forms of dyspeptics, in the swollen and stiff joints, and almost infernal tortures of the gouty, or in the bloated faces of high-livers—no question pertaining to eating and drinking can be unimportant, for he sees positive evidence that he cannot violate the laws of his being with impunity.

The reader has already learned that the food which is taken into the stomach, has to pass through certain processes preparatory to entering the circulation to nourish the body. It should be well masticated in the mouth, and it must be mixed with and dissolved by the gastric juice in the stomach, and portions of it with the bile and pancreatic juice in the upper portion of the intestines, before it can be absorbed by the veins of the stomach, or the lacteals of the bowels. For food to pass through these preparatory processes, and to be absorbed, time is required; and the period of time required for digesting different articles of food, varies; but upon an average, about four hours elapses before the stomach has disposed of the entire meal, and carried it into the duodenum, or upper portion of the intestines. The stomach is one of those organs which requires seasons of rest, and at least an hour should be allowed for this purpose, before the next meal;

so that no two meals should be nearer together than five hours. When food enters the stomach, it stimulates thousands of little secreting organs to pour out the gastric juice, which comes in contact with the food, and by the incessant motion of the stomach itself, this fluid is gradually mixed with the entire mass, dissolving it, and preparing it gradually to be passed on by the action of the stomach to the duodenum; the central portion of the contents of the stomach of course, will be acted on last. Every one can but see what confusion must be caused by taking additional food before the stomach has got rid of the preceding meal. It must, of course, to a greater or less extent mix with the latter, or portions which are already digested, and is liable to be hurried along into the intestines undigested, there to ferment and give rise to flatulence, colic, and diarrhœa. Children which are nursed, or fed, every hour or two are very sure to be thus troubled. These are not the only troubles which result from frequent eating, for upon the reception of more food, the secreting organs and vessels are stimulated to secrete more gastric juice, and an increased flow of blood is excited to the stomach, and at an improper time, when the muscular coats of this organ are hard at work; congestion and unnatural excitement result, which, often repeated, may give rise to chronic or even acute inflammation, or to debility in other cases. The process of digestion being partially arrested, by the gastric juice being absorbed and acting upon the food last taken, the first may ferment and give rise to nausea, sour stomach, belching or even vomiting. Such are a few of the evils resulting from eating too often, or eating between meals. Three times a day is as often as any individual can safely take food, especially food in substance, like bread and meat, potatoes and the like; and this is true whether the individual be well or sick. The practice of eating little and often, during sickness, has destroyed many lives. The sick may sometimes take fluids which are slightly nutritious, but do not tax the digestive organs much, more frequently than three times a day, but never substantial food, like rice, cracker, bread and meat, without great risk. It is surely unreasonable to suppose that the stomach of a sick man can stand an amount of abuse which will make a well man sick.

CHEWING GUM.

THE habit of chewing spruce, or other kinds of gum, is becoming very prevalent, especially with children and young persons. This is a very bad habit, not only filthy and unpleasant, but also destructive to health; and parents cannot be to careful to guard their children against it. Few substances, in the mouth, excite a more profuse secretion of saliva than gum. If the chewer spits the saliva from his mouth, its loss weakens and exhausts his whole system, and seriously impairs his digestion; for the saliva contains important alkaline properties, and is not a fluid which can be wasted with impunity, for it is all needed in the stomach to aid in the process of digestion. If the saliva, impregnated with the stimulating properties of the gum, is swallowed into the stomach, it may cause inflammation of this organ; and I have seen troublesome and even serious disease of this character thus caused. I have also known pain, soreness and lameness of the chest, caused by this practice, as well as general debility. There is also danger of its leading the young to the use of tobacco.

COSTIVENESS.

A CONSTIPATED state of the bowels is represented by patent pill manufacturers as the cause of innumerable ills, and is regarded by some medical writers, and many physicians, as a very dangerous condition; and one justifying and often requiring the use of cathartic and laxative drugs. But careful observation for many years has satisfied me that costiveness, when not aggravated by the frequent use of cathartic remedies, is rarely the cause of disease; and that the danger from this source is very much overestimated. I have sometimes known piles connected with costiveness, not often caused by this state of the bowels, but arising from the same cause which has given rise to the latter; most frequently from sitting, sedentary habits, and improper diet; or undue mental application, interfering with the process of digestion. I do not fear disease being caused by the absorption of effete substances which have once been cast into the bowels from the circulation, for I have no satisfactory evidence that any such absorption occurs; I know very well that the water is absorbed, and the fæces become drier, the longer they remain in the lower bowel.

In a state of health the bowels should move once a day, and if proper attention be paid, such as attending to them at a regular hour, and never varying the hour, which is all important, with suitable exercise, and care in regard to diet, they will rarely fail to move once in twenty-four hours. But no very serious consequences will result if they do not move daily. One of our most intelligent medical writers says, that "costive people generally live to grow old if they do not commit suicide by taking physic;" and certain it is, that many tailors and indolent and sedentary individuals do not have a passage more than once in one or two weeks, and yet enjoy good health otherways. I have known a man to go forty days without a passage from the bowels, and perform duty as a sailor, without disease resulting. Such a state of the bowels surely is not desirable, and can and should be avoided, and that without taking cathartic remedies. Nor is the frequent action of the bowels so essential in fevers and other acute diseases as many suppose. I have known a patient go without a passage from the beginning to the end of a run of typhoid fever of three weeks duration, and get along well; and I have frequently known them to go, in this disease, after a previous diarrhœa, one, two, three, and in one instance even four weeks, without a motion, and get along well, and no inconvenience result, nor injurious consequences. In peritonitis, or inflammation of the external membrane which covers the bowels, and lines the walls of the abdomen, the safety and even the life of the patient, often depends upon the bowels remaining costive until the inflammation is subdued; for the least motion towards a discharge rubs the inflamed surfaces together, and thus adds to the suffering and danger, and no truly intelligent physician would think of giving a cathartic, or urging a passage from the inflamed portion of the intestines, any more than he would think of rubbing the two surfaces of menbrane together, in a case of acute inflammation of the knee-joint. Not a few patients have lost their lives by an ineffectual attempt to force a passage in acute inflammation of the bowels, who would have recovered if the bowels had been let alone, and measures taken for subduing the inflammation. The bowels are generally costive in such cases, and it is often impossible to force a passage until the inflammation has been subdued; and yet the ignorant often suppose that the chief difficulty lies in the want of a passage, and, without a moment's thought, dose themselves or friends, when thus attacked, with all sorts of cathartic remedies. During acute inflammatory and febrile diseases the appetite is generally in a great measure destroyed, very little solid food is taken, consequently there is very little to be discharged, without exciting an unnatural secretion from the mucous membrane, which secretion will rapidly debilitate the patient: therefore we have not a right to expect that during the continuance of such diseases, the bowels will be as regular as during health. My aim is to discourage the use of cathartics in domestic practice, and not to prevent their being taken when recommended by physicians, who are better qualified to judge as to their safety and utility than the uneducated in medical lore.

Costiveness is not desirable, as has already been stated, for the escape of the hard passages which result is often difficult and attended with suffering. To prevent and cure costiveness, eat coarse bread, or that made from unbolted flour or corn meal; use fruits and vegetables freely at your meals, drink little while eating, but a glass of cold water half an hour before eating, and at bed time; exercise freely; walking is good exercise in such cases; knead the bowels several times a day with the hands or fists, and above all, make an attempt to have a passage at a regular hour every day, and never fail to do this, unless your bowels have been long costive; in that case if they will move once in two or three days, it will be all you can expect; so attend to them regularly every second or third day. If the bowels are very costive, and especially if cathartics have often been used, for a few days take an injection of warm water one hour before the attempt to have a passage; but discontinue this practice as soon as possible, as it will not cure the disease, for it is only palliative like cathartics; a cure depends upon the measures above indicated.

DOMESTIC DRUGGING AND QUACK MEDICINES.

I CANNOT close my remarks on the abuses to which the digestive organs are subject, without calling the attention of the reader to the class of poisons which are so extensively used as medicines for the cure of the various ills to which we are subject. That poisons are useful as remedies for the cure of the sick in the hands of a skillful physician, I cheerfully acknowledge, but for them to be of any service they must be given when indicated; and for any safety to attend their use, or any reasonable prospect of obtaining relief from them, their administration must be guided by the hand of science, and large and poisonous doses must not be given empirically and recklessly; especially is this true of emetic and cathartic remedies. I have known within my own observation several patients lose their lives from a single dose of cathartic remedies. In our autumnal and typhoid fevers, there is generally a predisposition to irritation of the mucous membrane of the stomach and bowels, and a single cathartic given at the commencement of these fevers, will not unfrequently develop this predisposition into a formidable disease, from which state, all the skill of the ablest physician will not always be sufficient to rescue the patient from death. The patient may linger, in such cases, for a few days, or even for three or four weeks, and yet die as surely from the effects of the cathartic, as he would drown with his head under water.

Then my advice, which is the result of observation, is, never take cathartics, unless it may be under the direction of a physician in whose skill the reader may have confidence, who can watch, and, if needs be, restrain their action. I have rarely given cathartics to my patients for many years, and yet I have never failed to give them when I have honestly thought I could do better with than without them.

He is unworthy the name of a physician who will let theory, or a favorite idea, stand between himself and his duty to his patients, and so is the man who will blindly confine himself within the narrow precincts of his own experience, in this age of progress and conflicting views, and thus obstinately refuse to heed the discoveries made by others, and the results of their experience.

The hundreds of patent medicines, especially cathartic pills, which are scattered over the country, from which their manufacturers make splendid fortunes, are doing an immense amount of injury, not only in many instances destroying life directly by the irritation and inflammation of the mucous membrane which they cause, but in a far greater number of cases, they weaken the digestive organs, causing costiveness and piles, together with dyspepsia, and a steady and gradual decline of the general health and strength, until at last the patient falls a prey to some acute attack, dysentery, cholera-morbus, and other acute diseases, or he dies from some chronic disease of the lungs, liver, or stomach and bowels.

I have no hesitation in expressing the opinion that if the skulls of all those who have been hurried to an untimely grave, by the use of some of the most popular patent pills now in vogue, could be accumulated in one pile, they would be sufficient to form the walls of a palace of far greater dimensions, than the splendid mansions of marble and stone which may have been erected by some of these pill venders, from the profits derived from the sale of their miserable compounds. Shun these poisonous masses then, for the stomach and bowels are vital organs; if they fail our time has come, and we must go. They are not like an old brass kettle; and we cannot irritate, scratch, and rake them out with drastic cathartics with impunity, as we would the kettle with soap, sand and rushes. Patients may often take cathartics with comparative impunity, and sometimes feel some temporary relief to feelings of fullness, as they would, in such cases, from the loss of a pint or a quart of blood, when, perhaps, no intelligent physician would think of bleeding. The physician when he seeks for palliative relief, duly considers which the patient will suffer from most—the present symptoms or the secondary effects of the remedies which he may use as palliatives. I have no doubt but that if all cathartic remedies were banished from domestic use, we should have far less sickness, and fewer deaths than at present. A patient stands many times the chance to do harm by their use, that he does to do good; better, far better, do nothing. Why use these substances? What do patients expect to gain by their use? Why, say some, the stomach and bowels are foul, they need cleansing; but did such individuals ever suspect that if they were half as foul as the miserable cathartics they put into them to cleanse them, that their contents would be likely to create as much of a muss as do their cathartics, and they would be very sure to have a diarrhœa? Cathartics cause a diarrhœa by the irritation which they produce, but the contents of the bowels are not, at the time when patients generally propose to take cathartics, sufficiently irritating to produce such an effect; which, then, is the most foul? But, say some, we take cathartics to cleanse our blood. Did such ever think that an organ would be quite as likely to faithfully perform its functions during a state of health, as during a state of disease? if they did not, let them put a small quantity of the physic, which they are so anxious to put into their stomach and bowels, into their eyes, and watch its effects, and see it cleanse the blood. This experiment can be made here, where we can very readily watch the effects, without any danger to life; the eyes may be destroyed, to be sure, but they are not vital organs. The presence of physic in the eyes will stimulate the lachrymal glands to secrete tears profusely, to wash away the irritating substance, and the conjunctiva, or mucous membrane of the eyes, to secrete an increased quantity of mucous; and if the irritation is continued, even matter or pus will be formed, and there will be a profuse quantity of tears, mucous, and pus flowing from the eyes. Now does any one suppose that all this would cleanse the blood? and yet we have, perhaps, even more reason to suppose that it will, than we have that cathartics do, for, with the exception of the pus, we shall have only increased the natural secretions from the parts; whereas from the bowels, by the use of cathartics, we get watery passages, when it is not the office, or function, of the bowels to secrete water to be thrown off. But the idea of cleansing the blood by the use of emetics and cathartics, is the remains of an exploded system of medical practice, and should have been uprooted centuries ago, when that system ceased to command the respect of the medical profession. But say some, we take cathartics for the headache, or for some disease away from the stomach and bowels; but did such ever stop to inquire whether there is any sense in making their stomach and bowels sick to cure their head?

Health and life are of too much consequence to every one, to justify trifling with them; and the unskilled run too great a risk of impairing the one and destroying the other to justify their ever using emetics or cathartics, unless it may be upon the recommendation of an educated physician: and I am happy to say that our most intelligent physicians are rapidly discontinuing the use of these drastic remedies; and are substituting, to a great extent, milder measures; and it is high time that the people, who usually are not behind their leaders in matters of medical reform, should follow in their wake. Costiveness can never be cured by cathartics, for the reaction of the organism is in the wrong direction, and diarrhœas are often dangerously aggravated by their use. Cathartics are like double-edged swords; handle them not.

Nor are the other patent nostrums in use much more safe than those we have been considering. Any remedy which is capable of curing the sick when properly used, is also capable of doing great injury when indiscriminately used in large doses, as is recommended by the venders of such compounds. The safe and true way is to let them alone unless prescribed by an intelligent physician.

CHAPTER IV.

VIOLATION OF THE CONDITIONS REQUISITE FOR PHYSICAL DEVELOPMENT AND PRESERVATION.

THE infant's physical organization possesses the capacity to receive nourishment from the natural world to build up the material body; first from the maternal breast, and afterwards from the various organized substances of the vegetable and animal kingdoms which are suitable for food; together with water from the mineral kingdom, oxygen from the air, and light and heat from the sun. All these are indispensable for the development of the natural body.

Water gives fluidity to the blood, holding in suspension, or solution, the red globules, fibrine, albumen, and all the various substances which enter into the different structures, for the entire body is formed from the blood. Not only the soft parts of the body, but also even the very bones, or the materials of which they are composed, have at one time flowed in the current of the blood, suspended, or held in solution, in water; and water enters extensively into all the various structures of the body; it is therefore indispensable for life and health. How important then, that the water which we use should be pure—free from all poisonous substances, that it be not a vehicle of death rather than life to the organism.

AIR.

AIR is quite as important as water. It is composed principally of oxygen and nitrogen gases, in about the proportion of twenty parts of oxygen to eighty of nitrogen; it also contains a small quantity of carbonic acid gas. It has always floating in it more or less of the vapor of water, and emanations, arising from vegetables, animals, and the earth. The effects of air on the human body vary according to its greater or less density, temperature, moisture, proportion of carbonic acid gas it contains, etc. It performs an important office in supplying the system with oxygen through the lungs during respiration, and in the removal of carbonic acid gas. Let a person be deprived of air for the short space of five minutes, by being confined under water, and recovery rarely results from the most skillful treatment; the minute capillary vessels of the lungs, refuse to circulate the blood because it neither parts with its carbonic acid, nor receives its due supply of oxygen. It is not arterialized, and the lungs and entire venous system become congested and the patient dies. If the atmosphere contains an excess of carbonic acid gas, if the quantity is very great, life is speedily destroyed. Instances are quite common of the destruction of life by the placing of burning charcoal, or simple coals from a fire, in a tight room; the oxygen of the air uniting with the carbon of the coal forming carbonic acid gas; and so insidiously may the effects of this poisonous gas steal over a person, as to destroy life without awaking him from sleep. Many an individual, ignorant of the danger, has gone into a slumber from which he has never awakened in this world, from simply placing in his bed room, on a cold night, a pan, or kettle of burning coals from the fireplace or stove. Let the young remember this. Both the mind and body become gradually benumbed, even when the quantity of carbonic acid gas is not sufficient to destroy life.

During respiration the oxygen of the surrounding air is gradually disappearing, and carbonic acid gas is taking its place, and it is this change, together with exhalations which arise from individuals, which makes the air of a crowded room, when not properly ventilated, unwholesome and suffocative. Every one has felt fullness and oppression of the head on entering a small tight room, even when it was occupied by only one or two individuals, especially when the room has been warmed by a stove,—in such cases the delicate organization of the brain and nervous system takes cognizance of the presence of an excess of this gas, when it is not sufficient to seriously interfere with respiration.

Carbonic acid gas is not only being constantly given off by men and animals into the atmosphere, and oxygen being absorbed from the air, but the same occurs in the combustion and decomposition, or decay, of all vegetable and animal substances; so that the air, from the absence of oxygen and the presence of carbonic acid gas, would soon become too impure for men and animals to breathe, and they would all, as at present constituted, be destroyed, were there no provision for counteracting this tendency to deterioration of the atmosphere. But this deleterious gas which will destroy men and animals, carries, as it floats along in the currents of the atmosphere, substance and life to the vegetable kingdom. The leaves of trees and plants are their lungs; they decompose the carbonic acid gas and set free the oxygen for the use of men and animals. The carbon is carried in the sap, which is as it were the blood of vegetables, to the various parts of the tree or plant, where it is needed to build up the solid structures of the vegetable organism.

Some may be surprised to learn that a large portion of the solid structures, of even the mighty trees of the forest, has been derived from the atmosphere, that the carbon which has been a constituent of our very bodies, which is every moment uniting with oxygen, and is being expelled during every act of respiration in the form of carbonic acid gas, will, sooner or later, floating in the currents of the atmosphere, be absorbed by the leaves of trees, or by water, (a point perhaps not fully settled yet) and entering through the roots, be decomposed in the leaves, and the carbon converted into woody fibre in the part where needed, and may in due time be used to warm ourselves and children; or it may enter into the fruits, vegetables, and grain which we shall eat. Organization takes place in the vegetable kingdom to sustain men and animals, but in passing through the systems of the latter organized substances are disorganized.

The reader will now be able to see the importance of fresh and pure air, both for the development of the human body, and also for sustaining the organism in health. And yet how little attention is paid to this subject; but as much of this neglect results from ignorance, I will endeavor to point out some of the existing abuses. It is estimated that on an average we inhale about a pint of air during every act of respiration, and we breathe about twenty-five thousand times in twenty-four hours. The air which has been once used during respiration is not fit to be used again for this purpose, until it mixes with other air and comes in contact with vegetation; for in the lungs it has parted with about one fourth, or one fifth of its oxygen, which goes to oxydize the worn out and combustible materials in the system and to warm the organism, and has received as a product of such combustion, in the place of the oxygen which it has lost, from three to five per cent. of carbonic acid gas, which, in excess in the atmosphere, is destructive to life. Dr. Franklin found that when an adult confined himself more than one minute to the same gallon of air, he suffered very severely. In this case he breathes the same air over about twice or a little more. The second time the air is very impure and if long breathed will endanger health, the third time even life is endangered, and beyond a certain point death ensues from the absence of oxygen and the presence of carbonic acid gas. The reader has heard of the Black Hole, at Calcutta, where out of one hundred and forty-seven persons confined in a dungeon, eighteen feet square, with little or no ventilation, one hundred and twenty-four perished in less than twenty-four hours, and the rest came very near dying before they could be removed.

Carbonic acid gas is heavier than air, and when there is no current, or the air is not agitated, and there are no vegetables to use it up, it sometimes accumulates in low situations in a quantity sufficient to destroy life. The reader has heard of the famous Grotto del Cane, in Europe, in which a human being may walk uninjured, while the faithful dog at his side perishes from a layer of carbonic acid gas, which is deep enough to poison or suffocate the dog, but not deep enough to affect the master. It is this gas which accumulates frequently in wells, especially in those from which the water is not constantly drawn in buckets, and also in those in the immediate vicinity of recent fires, where this gas, which is generated by combustion, frequently settles. Our newspapers occasionally remind us of the fact that it is no uncommon occurrence for one man to descend into a well, containing more or less of this gas, and, as he becomes insensible and silent from its influence, for his ignorant or thoughtless friend above ground, fearing that some accident has befallen him, to descend but to share the same fate. Before descending into a well it is always best to pass down a lighted candle or lamp, by the means of a string or cord, to the bottom or to the water, and if that grows dim or goes out, let no human being descend, for the lamp of life will surely go out under such circumstances, if the sufferer is not immediately rescued, which is not always easily accomplished.

IMPURE AIR.

A PROPER supply of pure, fresh air, as we have seen, is all-important for the preservation of life and health. Although life may not be suddenly destroyed by breathing an impure atmosphere, still the vital energies are slowly but surely impaired under such circumstances; and this is especially the case with the young.

Dr. Alcott, in his excellent work on the laws of health, which every reader will do well to consult, says: "There is much more suffering in our schools, from the want of a due regard to ventilation, than is generally supposed. The very young pupils first begin to yawn, and give signs of distress, both because they have less employment than those who are older, and because they sooner breathe the denser carbonic acid gas. And they not only yawn on the one hand, or become restless and troublesome to the teacher on the other, but they are all excited to do positive mischief. Or, if they are too well educated in the school of obedience and good manners to do anything worse, they soon fall into the habit of picking their nails, or other vulgar movements, for the mere sake of relief. With the blood half renewed they cannot be quiet; and to do something to relieve themselves is almost inevitable. Many a ferule is plied, and not a few rods are broken in a fruitless endeavor to reduce to order, and bring into subjection, where nature most loudly remonstrates. The teacher may feel very comfortable, and so may not a few of the older pupils; while the little children are half immersed in the ærial poison. Every school-room, and indeed every other room, where there is no natural or intentional provision for ventilation, is a Grotto del Cane to its occupants. It is so, to some extent, in our very best school-houses. Too often they are something worse than this, and would almost rank with the Black Hole of Calcutta."

This is a serious objection to the present cruel method of confining young children five or six hours a day to the school-room, to which I shall again allude in the chapter on education, for most of our school-houses are very imperfectly ventilated, and none of them, when occupied by so many respiratory organs, are at all suitable for such confinement, if there were no other objections to it. But, as we shall hereafter see, there are insuperable objections to such lengthy confinement, even aside from bad air.

Our churches, public halls and parlors, are generally imperfectly ventilated, during the time they are occupied; and often scarcely exposed to fresh air or light any considerable part of the time when not occupied. Air tight stoves, which afford a chance for very little circulation of air in a room, are frequently used in sitting rooms and parlors, and women and children by thousands, breathe an atmosphere containing an excess of carbonic acid gas; which, although not sufficiently poisonous to destroy life immediately, is sure to cause debility and disease with the adult, and with the child, to prevent a healthy development of the body. Let husbands and fathers, who care for the health and lives of their families, watch the increasing paleness, delicacy, and nervousness of their wives and children; the disposition to peevishness, neuralgia, and headache, which is sure, sooner or later, to manifest itself, and they will not be long in casting air-tight stoves out of their doors.

If stoves must be used in parlors, sitting rooms or school-rooms, some provision should always be made for ventilation. A very cheap and quite an effectual method for ventilating stove rooms, can very readily be adopted by all who have any regard for health. Cut a hole, at least one foot square. through the zinc and floor beneath the stove ; let this communicate with the out door air, as high above the earth as practicable, by the means of a tube, of boards or any other material, one foot square running between the joice, or beneath the floor. Then surround the stove with a box as high or higher than the bottom of the stove, and a few inches larger than the stove; and cut a hole, much smaller than the one in the floor, in the opposite side or end of the room, for the escape of the warm air into a flue of the chimney or out doors; and the room will be ventilated by a current of fresh air which will be warmed by coming in contact with the stove, and all risk to health from a current of cold air, will be avoided.

Our bed-rooms are often too small, and not properly ventilated at that. Physiologists estimate, that, to preserve health, an adult requires at least seven cubic feet of pure air a minute; this is at the rate of four hundred and twenty feet an hour. Now if a sleeping room is but seven feet by ten, at this rate it would take but one hour to spoil the air, or render it unfit for respiration, to the depth of six feet, if the room were perfectly air-tight; but, as our rooms, when no special efforts are made to ventilate them, are not perfectly air-tight, more or less fresh air is received, but not enough to prevent the health of the occupants being slowly impaired by a poisonous atmosphere. If children are permitted to occupy a lower bed than adults they suffer first and more. If individuals are compelled to sleep in small rooms, a door should be left open, or a window let down or raised. The cold night air should not blow directly upon the sleepers, something should be placed before the open window, to interrupt the current of air.

It not unfrequently happens that dogs and cats are permitted to occupy, even small rooms, in company with human beings, especially with children, and to rob them of the needed pure air; this is an unnecessary abuse, and should be avoided.

Carbonic acid gas is nearly or quite inodorous; and, therefore, the fact that a room does not smell bad, is no evidence that the air in it is wholesome. We all know that a person who has occupied a room several hours, whose system has been gradually accustomed to bad air, suffers at the time very little, even when the atmosphere is very oppressive to a new comer. There may be no very offensive odor which disturbs the latter, but he suffers from oppression of the brain and lungs from the effects of this poisonous gas, and the absence of oxygen in the air.

There are several other injurious gases. Carburetted hydrogen gas is offensive to the smell, as well as poisonous. It results from the spontaneous decomposition of vegetable substances, and is found about sinks, wells, pumps, and cellars, when proper attention is not paid to cleanliness. It arises in bubbles from mud-puddles when they are agitated in hot weather. It is inflammable and very similar to the coal gas, with which our cities are illuminated; and also to the fire-damp of coal mines, which was so destructive to the lives of miners by its explosions, before the invention of the safety lamp by Sir Humphrey Davy. This gas, when breathed for a short time, often causes nausea, giddiness, and great general and nervous prostration. Severe forms of fever, and other diseases, have not unfrequently been traced to decomposing vegetables in the cellar, or to an offensive sink.

Sulphuretted hydrogen gas.—This is more offensive and poisonous than either of those named above. It is this gas which gives the offensive smell to a decaying egg. It arises from the vaults of privies, sewers, &c., when suitable care is not used to prevent it. It also frequently escapes from the stomachs of gluttons, and individuals of weak digestion. Dr. Carpenter, in his Principles of Physiology, informs us that air containing one-fifteen-hundreth part of this gas, if inhaled, will kill a bird in a very short time; and that it will kill a dog if it contains but little over double that amount. When inhaled in a diluted form, by human beings, sulphureted hydrogen gas, lessens the force of the circulation, causes great prostration of strength, and mental torpor.

BREATHING AND LIVING IN HOT AIR.

Heat rarifies the air, or renders it less dense; and, of course, a given volume of heated air contains less oxygen than the same quantity of cool air; and yet the activity and vigor of the organism, as well as its ability to generate animal heat, depends to a great extent, on the amount of oxygen received during respiration. Every one who has spent any considerable length of time in the Torrid zone, is aware of the debilitating effects of a hot climate upon the natives of cooler latitudes; and, as a general rule, the inhabitants of such sections of the earth are less robust and energetic than those of colder regions; although they do not suffer as much as strangers, from the fact that their organizations are adapted to the climate.

Few in our climate realize the importance of breathing a cool and dense atmosphere; not too cold, but much colder than is generally to be found in our parlors and sitting rooms, during the winter season. During cold weather, to be able to withstand with impunity the cold to which we are all more or less exposed, and the sudden changes of our climate, as well as the change from in-door to out-door air, we need a vigorous circulation, and a rapid oxydation of combustible materials within us, such as we can only obtain by constantly breathing a cool atmosphere.

Every one is familiar with the fact, that if we occupy a room at 60 degrees, which is comfortable to us and our friends, and we alone remain in the room and gradually raise the temperature until it reaches 80 or even 90 degrees, we may not feel the change, nor be any warmer than we were when it was at 60 degrees, but let our friends enter the room, and the first exclamation is: "Why, how hot the air is in your room!" While the external heat has been steadily increasing, the animal heat has been as surely decreasing, and the extremities will be found much cooler than those of the new comer, perhaps even cold and clammy. It will be seen, at once, that such an individual, with the heat-generating function thus debilitated, and his vitality exhausted, is in no condition to withstand the sudden change caused by a current of cold air, or by stepping into a cold hall, or passing into the open air. Is it strange, then, that those who confine themselves most of the time to hot rooms, are so subject to colds and inflammatory diseases? that so many of our Northern people, especially children, who live in rooms kept excessively hot by stoves and furnaces, die of bronchitis, croup, and inflammation of the lungs; or suffer from rheumatism and other inflammatory diseases? When we learn to substitute proper clothing and exercise for our hot rooms, such diseases will become comparatively rare. When hot rooms do not directly destroy life, by rendering the individual susceptible to acute diseases, they gradually exhaust the vital energies, and cause a predisposition to innumerable chronic diseases; and they are certainly among the most prominent of the various causes which are destroying the women and children of our land. Feeble and delicate persons, if not otherwise instructed, are very sure to injure themselves by external heat, it is so grateful; but no course can be more destructive and injurious to such, than to crowd to the fire or increase the heat of the room; proper clothing, exercise and cool air, are all important for such. If we desire cold feet habitually, let us use a foot stove or hold them to the fire continually, or whenever we have an opportunity, and we shall surely have cold feet. In very cold weather we certainly need more or less artificial heat, but the less we can do with, and be any way comfortable, the better; the more animal heat and vigor shall we have. I would by no means encourage fool-hardy exposure to cold air, or weather, ice cold water, or snow, or even very cold water, especially for feeble persons, or for any one; for there are two sources of danger from such exposure; one from not being able to get up a reaction, and thereby causing disease or death, and the other by causing similar results by inducing excessive reaction. We should avoid the extremes into which enthusiasts are liable to run.

MOIST AIR.

I HAVE already alluded to the fact that the air contains more or less of the vapor of water, diffused through it, which renders it moist and unirritating to either the surface of the body or the delicate lining membrane of the lungs. If a room is kept very hot, a larger quantity of water is required to preserve the necessary degree of moisture, in the atmosphere it contains, than would be necessary at a lower temperature. Stoves and furnaces not only increase the liability to keep rooms too warm, but they also tend to deprive the air of the requisite degree of moisture, and to render it irritating to the air passages and skin, often causing the latter to chap and to become dry, harsh and scaly. In all instances, when a room is warmed either by a furnace or a stove, proper provision should be made to supply moisture to the air. This would be almost as important if not equally so, when a room is warmed by a fire-place, if the air could be kept as hot and ventilation could be as carefully prevented; but we know that with a fire-place or grate, we rarely get such a uniformly hot air throughout the room as from a stove or furnace. It is important to remember that, when we depend for moisture upon the evaporation of water from a vessel, everything depends on the extent of the surface of water exposed, and little or nothing on its depth.

BREATHING.

Having considered the uses which air performs in the animal economy, and the importance of having it pure, at a proper temperature, and moist, it will be well to consider how we should use it to develop the lungs and walls of the chest, and to ward off a tendency to deformity or disease.

It is no uncommon occurrence to see in children a prominence of the breast-bone or sternum, which resembles almost as much the keel of a ship as a portion of a well-formed human chest; there is often depression of the ribs a few inches from this bone, and the breadth of the chest is less than natural. This deformity, if the child lives to grow up, often grows less when he comes to use the muscles about the chest freely, but it rarely disappears entirely, and should receive attention during childhood while the bones are pliable. The increasing tendency to disease of the lungs in our country, renders a consideration of the present subject important to every one. Consumption is much more frequent among females than males, which is not strange, when we take into consideration the prevailing practice of tight dressing, or doing violence to the organs within the chest, which is nearly universal, and the other habits of the female portion of our population; such as secluding themselves from the light of the sun, and air, and their avoidance of active exercise. Not only do more females die from this disease, but it also generally commences earlier in life with them, and is more rapid in its progress. But the subject of our present inquiry is, what can be done, in the way of breathing, to prevent this and inflammatory diseases of the lungs and air passages, and deformity of the chest, and overcome the tendency to the same?

The lungs require educating, and this is especially true with Americans at present, for the many causes to which I have already alluded, interfering with their natural action, prevent their full development; and where actual deformity or debility of these organs and the walls of the chest already exists, or a predisposition is inherited, it is only by systematic training that disease can be prevented, and a healthy development and symmetry of form secured. In order for a full development of the walls of the chest, it is all important that there be not the least restraint from the clothing at any point between the shoulders or arms, and the hips; for the muscles extending between these points must have the utmost freedom for acting, and this is also essential for the full expansion of the lungs. Dr. Alcott after alluding to the fact that the man who has the largest lungs, and keeps them best supplied with pure air, all other things being equal, is the most healthy, says: "It has been shown that the lungs will hold in some instances a gallon of air. Farmers, laborers, soldiers and sailors, who have a large amount of out-of-door exercise, have, in general, the largest lungs. There may, of course, be here and there an individual, of this description, the capacity of whose lungs is somewhat greater; but in a country where there is so much compression by dress, and so many consumptive people, the chests of thousands of people will scarcely hold as many as three quarts. From the beginning of the present century—perhaps earlier—the capacity of the human lungs has been diminishing. If it has diminished most rapidly in the female sex, still our own cannot be far behind. If mothers have small or feeble lungs, the inheritance of the next generation must be immediately affected. There is no possible escape. The late William Sullivan, a distinguished lawyer of Boston, and author of the Moral and Political Class-Books, in view of the prevailing customs of female dress, was accustomed, many years before his death, to say, that if the existing state of things should continue three hundred years longer, the present race of mankind must become extinct. Now, it is difficult for me to admit, for one moment, the bare possibility of such a result; and yet, I confess I am not wholly without forebodings. The prospect is certainly discouraging, clouds and darkness are round about us; yet, let us remember, that, in some instances, it is 'the darkest time just before daybreak!"

In treating of the importance of exercise, I shall call the attention of the reader to those exercises of the muscles of the arms, neck and body, which are of use in developing the chest, and for curing or preventing deformity; at present I propose simply to notice respiration. This act is performed by the aid of various muscles which expand the walls of the chest and increase the space which the lungs occupy, which distends them, enlarging the air cells and causing the air to rush in through the mouth, nose, windpipe and bronchia to prevent a vacuum being formed. The principal muscles concerned in the act of respiration, are the muscles between the ribs, those which form the abdominal walls, and the diaphragm, or midriff. The latter is attached to the lower edges of the ribs and is concave beneath, somewhat like an umbrella. During inspiration when the capacity of the chest is to be enlarged, the midriff contracts; which causes it to assume more nearly a plane figure and press down upon the contents of the abdomen; the muscles between the ribs contract, and thus raise and expand the external walls of the chest. During expiration, the muscles composing the abdominal walls, which were relaxed when the chest was being filled, contract and press up the midriff and draw down the ribs, thus expelling the air from the lungs.

Although breathing is in a great measure an involuntary action, still it is to a certain extent under the control of the will; for we can stop breathing for a limited time, or we can breathe more, rapidly and with greater energy than usual. We can simply breathe in a torpid lifeless manner, because we cannot help it, as we do during sleep, or we can breathe with a *will*, which will purify the blood and send it throughout the system, giving life and activity to both body and mind. Full and vigorous breathing brings into activity and strengthens all the muscles whose healthy action gives form, beauty and capacity to the chest and body, and it constitutes one of the most efficacious measures we have for the relief and prevention of deformity of the chest. It is safe to say that it constitutes by far the most important part of the treatment required for eradicating any hereditary or acquired predisposition to disease of the lungs, or consumption; and without persevering voluntary effort in this direction by the patient, the most skillful treatment by the physician, will generally fail to prevent, where a predisposition already exists, or to cure consumption even in its incipient stages.

The child then should be taught to breathe freely, and to make it a part of his duty to expand the chest by full breathing, and frequent deep inspirations. He should be taught that health and life depend upon the amount of air he uses, especially if he has any hereditary tendency to disease or deformity. He should not be allowed to speak or read with his lungs empty, for it tends to exhaust and weaken the lungs and even the whole chest, and frequently causes stammering. To cure stuttering, require the child always to draw in a full breath before he commences to speak, and often while speaking, and not allow him to continue speaking without breathing until the chest is empty, or comparatively so.

There is perhaps not one teacher in ten in our public schools who ever thinks, or even is aware, of the importance for the preservation of health, or in order to be able to read well, of keeping on hand in the lungs a full supply of air; and of course such teachers neglect to give the necessary instruction to their pupils, in regard to the importance of full breathing, or of keeping the "lungs at the top of their condition." How often is it that pupils in our schools read too fast, and without taking the least pains to keep the lungs expanded, or the body erect with the shoulders thrown back, so as to be able to breathe freely while reading. The pupil may commence in a loud voice, perhaps with the lungs half filled, he neglects to replenish them at suitable intervals with air, or not more than half does it, but rushes on to the end of the paragraph, which he reaches with his lungs exhausted of air and a voice scarcely above a whisper. The same fault frequently occurs with singers; the lungs are not kept adequately filled with air, and when they are not, both reading and singing exhaust and weaken them, and increase the liability to disease; whereas energetic reading and singing, when practiced with the lungs fully expanded, are among the most useful means for both preventing and curing incipient disease by giving strength and vigor to the lungs.

LIGHT.

Few are aware of, or begin to realize the importance of sunlight for physical development and preservation. I will therefore call the attention of the reader to a few facts to impress upon him the importance of light—the light of the sun with its conjoined heat. We may, as is well known, keep the seeds of plants and trees in a dry place for years, and they will not germinate, or sprout; their vitality is dormant. But if the seed be kept damp, and the temperature be raised to that of a summer's day, they do not fail to germinate if sound and healthy. Under the influence of air, heat and moisture alone, the new germ or plant consumes the nourishment stored up for it in the seed; its parts are gradually unfolded, a root is put forth, a stem rises from the ground, and leaves make their appearance. So heat, air and water, have enabled the seed to become a plant, but they can only enable the plant to feed upon the store of nourishment laid up in the seed. The plant is feeding on the seed, and without the aid of light, or while kept in darkness, it cannot add anything to its substance from any other source; therefore, it can only grow to a certain extent, and its stem and leaves are of a sickly yellowish hue so long as light is not admitted; and if the resulting plant be carefully dried and weighed, it will be found to weigh even less than the dry seed from which it came. Its development ceases entirely when it has exhausted the store laid up for it in the seed, and its leaves, unaided by light, have no power to decompose carbonic acid and appropriate its carbon to form its woody structures. But expose the newly organized plant to the solar rays, and its leaves and stem soon become of a green color, and the weight of the plant increases. We see then that the living force, or if you please, the spirit within the seed or germ, possesses the power, when aided by heat, moisture, and air, to organize a new plant, in the form of the old, from the stock of nutritive material which the parent had stored up for this purpose in the seed, but it possesses no power, unaided by light, to gather nourishment beyond. If the seed of a plant is covered so deep with soil, that the stock of nourishment in the seed is exhausted before the leaves reach the surface, the plant, after sustaining a sickly existence for a season in its earthly habitation, dies; but if planted at a proper depth, when the leaves reach the surface of the ground and are exposed to light, "all the day long and with the more activity as the day is brighter, the leaves which are the collecting organs, are absorbing material from the air;" (DRAPER) they cease to do it at night, and even to a slight extent reverse the action which has been going on during the day, by absorbing oxygen from the air, and yielding carbonic acid gas. The sunbeam enables a plant or tree, through its leaves, to take from the air, carbon, hydrogen, and nitrogen, which the vital force of the vegetable moulds into its organic and living structures. Although, as we have seen, vegetable organization may take place, the development of such organization cannot continue to maturity, or to the state of bearing seed so as to perpetuate the species, without the aid of light. We have even seen that vegetables feed by day, and fast by night, during their ordinary lives.

Light is scarcely less important for the development of the animal kingdom than for that of vegetables, athough a feeble, delicate and sickly development of animals and men, may take place in the dark, without the aid of light, for the reason that the latter feed upon substances which have already been organized in the vegetable kingdom. But a very few facts, among the many which might be adduced, will show us the importance of light for animal development.

In decaying organic solutions animalcules do not appear if light is excluded, but are readily organized when light is admitted. The tadpole, kept in the dark, does not pass on to development as a frog, but lives and dies a tadpole, and is incapable of propagating his species. In the deep and narrow valleys among the Alps, where the direct rays of the sun are but little felt, cretinism, or a state of idiocy, more or less complete, commonly accompanied by an enormous goitre, prevails as an epidemic and is often hereditary. Rachetis or rickets, or deformities, crookedness and swelling of the bones, are very common among children who are kept in dark alleys, cellars, factories and mines.

Also, crookedness and deformity of the spine, and other bones, are very common not only among the poor who are kept in the damp and dark places to which I have alluded, but also among the rich, who live in fine dry and airy houses, provided the children are confined in-doors any considerable part of the time, secluded from the sun's light; and this more certainly results if they are also deprived of an opportunity for active exercise. Even the teeth of such children will be found more delicate and subject to decay. Thus we see that the development of the most solid structures of the body is affected by the absence of the light of the sun, and the soft structures are still more manifestly affected by this cause. The skin loses its healthy, ruddy and fresh appearance, loses its color, and becomes of a sickly pale hue; the muscles become soft and delicate, the nervous system becomes deranged and diseased, the digestive organs enfeebled, and even the very blood becomes watery and loses its red globules—a change very similar to what takes place with vegetables when they are deprived of light, for they lose their healthy colour.

It has been found that, during the prevalence of certain epidemic diseases, the inhabitants who occupy the side of the street, and houses, upon which the sun shines directly, are less subject to the prevailing disease, whereas those who live on the shaded side are more liable to contract it.

The following has been clipped from a newspaper without knowing who is responsible for the statement:—

"Sir James Wylie, late physician to the Emperor of Russia, attentively studied the effects of light as a curative agent in the hospitals of St. Petersburg; and he discovered that the number of patients who were cured in rooms properly lighted was four times greater than that of those confined in dark rooms. This led to a complete reform in lighting the hospitals of Russia, and with the most beneficial results. In all cities visited by the cholera, it was universally found that the greatest number of deaths took place in narrow streets, and on the sides of those having a northern exposure, where the salutary beams of the sun were excluded." How important then the direct light and heat of the sun, not only for physical development, but also for health. I have noticed within my own observation that families who live in houses much shaded by trees, are more subject to asthma, dropsy and scrofulous diseases, than those whose dwellings are freely exposed to the sun. Shade trees should be at a little distance from the house that they may afford a grateful retreat for hot days, but they should never be so near a house as to shade the windows, or even the building. No one organ suffers more from the absence of light, the light of the sun, than the eye. I shall hereafter call the attention of the reader to the fact, that in the fish that swim in the dark waters of the Mammoth Cave, not only is vision impaired, but the eyes themselves are in all cases deteriorated in their very structure until, in some instances, there is scarcely a vestige of these organs remaining. How clearly does this fact teach us that the human body is but an organism of use, and that the sluggard's life tends to death. Light is the natural stimulus for the eye, and it is not necessary that the latter be deprived of it entirely, in order to impair both its function and structures.

Amaurosis, or at least partial paralysis of the optic nerve, is very common among young ladies who spend much of their time in our dark parlors, and rooms from which the direct rays of the sun are excluded by the means of blinds, and curtains, and in most of such young persons the eyes are more or less weak, and often troubled with chronic inflammation. Children who are kept in such shaded rooms, are liable to be afflicted with scrofulous inflammation of the eyes and lids. It must, on reflection, be manifest to every one, that the development and preservation of the eyes must depend much on a due amount of light. Of course, no one, for the sake of strengthening the eyes, should attempt to look directly at the sun, for to do so will cause blindness. Our eyes want reflected light, but they want the strong light of day, and not the dim light of twilight. Light which is reflected directly from bright or dazzling objects should be avoided, as it is liable to injure the eyes. When the eye is inflamed it will not always bear strong or even a dim light, any more than an inflamed joint will bear motion, although in health adapted to motion. When the eyes are weak the transition from a dim to a strong light should be made gradually. If the day ever arrives—with some I am happy to say it has already arrived, and for the benefit of such I write—when the wives and mothers of our land shall care as much for their own health, and the lives of their children, as they do now for their carpets, furniture, cool rooms, and the absence of flies, and will admit as freely as possible the cheerful, life-giving light of the sun into every room of their houses, during the entire day, to give and sustain the vitality of their occupants, and dissipate the causes of disease—dampness, mould, and the effluvia from human bodies—we shall have fewer gloomy family circles; fewer mothers made slaves by the care of sickly children; fewer husbands compelled to make nursing an important business of life, for some of the most important causes of disease will have been removed. If a husband and father cares not for his wife and children, and would as soon be rid of them as not, and a little sooner, let him do what thousands are doing, ignorantly and thoughtlessly; let him build a large house, so as to confine his wife indoors to take care of it most of the time; let him furnish blinds and curtains to afford her a chance to gratify her love for excluding the light of the sun, and then place carpets upon the floors, a little nicer than the neighbors possess; let him permit the monthly visits of the fashionable periodicals of the day, or the yellow covered literature, which are continually harping about the beauty of a delicate skin and form, with plates to illustrate; having done all this, let him encourage his wife, and permit his children to remain indoors most of the time. I have forgotten an important item—let him be sure and furnish his house with stoves, if possible, air tight stoves, or with a furnace. All this will give him the name of a kind and indulgent husband—which may be of future use to him—let him thus, in a sheep's clothing, act the wolf towards his family, and if he does not have an opportunity to marry as many wives, without the violation of the laws of the land, or the religious sentiments of the community, as most of the Mormon elders do, in violation of both, it will not be his fault; and this result will be the more sure, if he will only be careful and select his wives from among those who have been reared in the manner described above—and the children, if any are born, will be far more certain to be short-lived; a majority of them will soon cease to trouble the unfeeling parent. There is no habit against which I feel compelled to speak more earnestly than that, so prevalent in our cities, of excluding light from the dwellings where women and children spend too much time.

The reader is now prepared to understand one of the chief causes why the women and children in the huts, and even log-cabins of the west, which contain one or two rooms, and those small, remain healthy and strong, but the moment the settler builds a nice house, and is able to furnish blinds, and curtains, the women and children become pale faced, bloodless, nervous and sickly; and the daughters begin to die from consumption, and the wives from the same and female diseases, while the adult men remain comparatively healthy. Women and children, as well as men, in order to be healthy and well developed, must spend nearly all, or certainly a majority of their time during day light where the solar rays can reach them directly. During very hot weather for a few hours during the excessive heat of the day, the shade of a tree, grove or even an airy house, without blinds, or curtains, may be sought without serious injury; but never our dark parlors and rooms, for the cold "damp of death" is within them. Houses are only fit for occupancy during the night by being purified and dried by the solar rays during the day.

Dr. W. W. Hall, in his Journal of Health, says:

"A New York merchant noticed in the course of years that every book-keeper that came to him got sick, however healthy he appeared on his arrival. One day it occurred to him all at once, that the room occupied was on the first floor, and was so situated that the sun never shone in it. He at once changed it for an upper story apartment, which freely admitted the sun light, with the result of healthy book-keepers ever after."

EXERCISE.

It is a law of both mental and physical development, that, to be able to receive new substance, and thereby gain new strength, we must diligently use that which we already possess. This is true of both the affections and intellect, as well as of the body. To man is given the capacity to choose, use, abuse, or neglect, and upon his action will depend, not only his development and strength, but also the quality of his life, whether it be good or bad, healthy or diseased.

The affections grow strong by being cultivated and used, as manifestly as the body. The man who voluntarily makes the love of money his ruling affection, and the acquisition of wealth the great aim of life, strengthens this love, or affection, by every new effort and acquisition, even during a long life; nor does this passion grow weaker as old age approaches, or the final hour draws near, when it is evident that he must soon leave his wealth behind. The miser clutches his gold with his dying breath, and only permits it to pass into the hands of others, or to be applied to use, after he is dead, when it is impossible for him to retain it longer. The love of approbation or of glory grows stronger the more it is cultivated, or exercised and gratified. The young man may be as nearly satisfied if he can excel his near neighbor as the middle aged is if he can excel all in his city or state; let him attain to the position of the latter and is he satisfied? No;

but like Alexander the Great, who, when told that there were other worlds, wept to think that he had not yet conquered one, he will never be contented, even though he could excel the whole world. Such affections are selfish and infernal, and can only end in disappointment. They can only be reformed by a voluntary effort, for disappointment scarcely blunts their edge, as was manifested in the last acts of Napoleon, when he desired once more to behold his glittering uniform. Nor does inability to gratify destroy the passion, so long as the desire is harbored in the soul, as is manifest in the filthy thoughts and obscene words of the licentious old man.

If good and true affections are harbored; and if they are fed or strengthened, by being exercised by the performance of good and true acts, such affections grow stronger every day, until as the last hour of a long life approaches, the good man comes fully to realize that his treasures are not on earth, and that his heart is not in the selfish pleasures and gratifications of this world, and he looks with joy beyond the grave, but contented to wait until the hour of his deliverance draws nigh, when he is ready to exchange earth for heaven, his final abode. As our affections grow stronger by our exercising them, so for the want of exercise they grow feeble.

The same is true of the intellect. If the young man or woman continues diligently to acquire knowledge, and apply it to use, and if during adult and advanced age, a man continues to read, think and exercise his memory, he will retain his intellectual faculties to old age; and will often be able to stand with intellect unimpaired, when his poor old trembling physical organism is tottering on the brink of the grave, as the late venerable John Quincy Adams was able to stand in the halls of Congress—the old man eloquent—an intellectual giant, even to the very hour when he was stricken down. When the physical organism of the old man, especially the brain, is not impaired by disease, I do not think a second childhood so far as the intellect is concerned, should occur. The perception of surrounding objects will fail, if the perceptive organs fail; sight, touch, hearing, taste and smell, also the ability to speak may fail from the gradual wearing out, or loss of substance of the various organs through which these faculties are manifested; but the brain, which is the organ through which the affections and intellect are manifested, is inclosed within a bony cavity of a certain capacity, which cavity, from atmospheric pressure, must ever remain full; therefore, the brain, if undiseased, must retain not only its fullness of form, but also even of substance, to the last hour of the life of the old man—a merciful provision for the chief habitation of the noblest faculties of man.

Not only is the brain itself invigorated by mental exercise, but also the entire organism is sustained in a healthy condition by mental activity. A writer, in the *Independent* says:

"It is demonstrable, both by philosophy and observation, that intellectual pursuits are not only compatible with, but actually tend to promote physical health and long life. Cato was eighty when he learned Greek, and Plutarch about as old when he acquired Latin. Benjamin Franklin's philosophical studies were begun when he was nearly fifty; and Isaac Walton wrote some of his most interesting biographies in his eighty-fifth year. Michael Angelo evinced his creative genius in extreme old age; and Sir Christopher Wren retired from public life at eighty-six, and after that spent five years in literary engagements. The widely prevalent notion that intellectual labors necessarily tend to break down health and abbreviate the term of natural life is erroneous. People do not die of hard study as a primary cause, a thousand and one obituary notices to the contrary notwithstanding. The great Humboldt, if he had lived a few months longer, would have reached the age of ninety; and yet where shall we look for an example of manifold intellectual toil more illustrious than we see in him?"

But students and sedentary men do die from neglect of the physical man, even when not accustomed to an amount of "hard study" which would do them the least harm, if it was accompanied by proper bodily exercise, and mental recreation and amusements.

Then the man who uses his faculties to acquire knowledge,

continues to possess the capacity to acquire, even to the very hour when the organs of sensation fail to convey impressions to the brain; but let the young man cease to use these faculties for acquiring knowledge, or his memory for retaining it, and he will gradually but surely lose his ability both to acquire and retain knowledge, until at the age of forty or fifty, even, it will be very difficult to learn at all. Nor is this all, if a man neglects to use the knowledge which he already possesses, it will gradually fade away. A young man may acquire a knowledge of Latin, Greek, or French, and if he fails to use that knowledge, or to read, write, or speak the language, he will steadily lose his knowledge of it.

It is equally important for the development of our physical organizations, and for sustaining that development, that we use our various organs; and the body as a whole can only be sustained in vigor by active exercise. Even all the senses are quickened by their legitimate use. Let a man lose his sight, so that he is obliged to depend upon the senses of touch, hearing, taste and smell, and these faculties become more acute than natural. Whereas let an eye be drawn out of the axis of vision, or crossed, so that a person cannot use it without seeing double; as he ceases to use it, the eye will gradually lose its power of vision; whereas let both eyes be crossed, so that the individual uses one when he looks in one direction, and the other when he looks in the other, as is usually the case when they are both crossed, and both eyes will alike retain the power of vision, although each is out of its true axis. Let an individual have paralysis of an arm or leg, or disease of the shoulder or hip, so that he cannot use his arm or leg, and it will grow small, delicate and flabby, compared with the extremity on the opposite side of the body which is used.

But we have much more manifest examples upon a larger scale; showing the absolute necessity for active exercise to develop and sustain well organized structures and substantial bodies. Behold our men of sedentary habits, or the indolent, or those whose occupations do not require them to take much exercise, and who neglect exercise; feel of their soft flesh, of their delicate, imperfectly organized structures; witness their want of capacity for endurance, their poor health, and compare them with our active farmers, or mechanics, or even the day laborers in our streets. Enter the parlors of the rich and fashionable, more especially of such as bring up their daughters, without requiring of them to engage in active employments, but allow them to live in fashionable idleness; behold their delicate hands, soft flesh, pale, semi-transparent skin, sickly countenances; then pass through the parlor into the kitchen, or into the basement, and compare the young ladies who spend their time in the dry, wholesome air of the best part of the house, with the servant girls, who do the hard work in the damp, often unwholesome basement, with their strong, firm flesh, and useful hands; and we will find no comparison, in the capacity for physical endurance, health and happiness, between the daughter and maid-servant.

"In the sweat of thy face shalt thou eat bread." Active useful labor, or active exercise of some kind, is indispensable for physical development, health, enjoyment and happiness. There is not a single muscle in the body that does not require exercise for its development and preservation in a healthy state; and not one but becomes deteriorated in structure, and feeble from indolence.

The muscular system is not the only portion of the organism which is developed and strengthened in structure, and invigorated in function, by exercise; and which deteriorates in every respect by inactivity. The same is true, as we have seen, of the eye, and brain, and in fact of every portion of the body, even to the very bones. Dr. George H. Taylor, a New York physician, in a letter from Stockholm, Sweden, to the New York *Independent*, dated May 30th, 1858, says:

"The anatomical cabinet of Prof. Regius, of Stockholm, who is extensively known among scientific men for his ethnological researches, affords some excellent confirmations of this statement, from which I select two or three instances. A person, who, from a trifling and transient lameness in one limb, took up the occupation of begging, sat at the end of a bridge receiving alms the rest of his life. The favored limb was used as little as possible in the mean time. The thigh-bone of this limb is nearly *three quarters of an inch less* in circumference than the other, and more than one inch shorter. A criminal who was confined by a chain attached to one ankle for five years, died by frost, in making his escape. Although the bone of the unused limb had not materially changed its size, it *feels* to be not more than half as heavy as the other. It seems in handling as light as pine wood. * * * The vertebræ of a carpenter, or of any one who has followed any similar occupation, are shown here by numerous examples, to be not only larger, but much heavier in proportion to size, than those of a shoemaker or tailor.

"Facts exactly similar to these really exist in every living community, but are only dimly seen or entirely neglected by the common mind, and often ignored in the practice of physicians. They ought to lead the mind to suggestions of the utmost importance. With them constantly before our eyes, we should place less reliance upon the power of drugs to correct the result of our physiological faults. Let me ask my countrymen, since so much is begun in Sweden, where the natural temperament of the people, as well as the institutions of the country, are so averse to change, what ought to be done in the United States toward retrieving men from the ills they are at present so prone to encounter?"

Exercise, then, is, as has already been intimated, indispensable for physical development, preservation, and health. "Most truly did Theodore Sedgewick say, that it is the man of robust and enduring constitution, of elastic nerve, of comprehensive digestion, who does the work of life. It is Scott with his manly form. It is Brougham with his superhuman powers of physical endurance. It is Franklin at the age of seventy, camping out on his way to arouse the Canadas, as our hardiest boys of twenty now camp out on the Adirondacks or on the Miramichi. It is Napoleon, sleeping four hours, and on horseback twenty. It is Washington, with his splendid frame and physical strength."

General exercise increases respiration, and the activity and force of the circulation. The effect of exercise on individual organs and parts, as well as upon the entire body, is to increase, the rapidity of the oxydation and decomposition of the particles of which the various parts and structures are composed, and their removal from the body, and to give an increased demand for nourishment to repair the waste, which causes an increased appetite and demand for food. If a due supply of the latter is furnished, a steady increase of exercise adds to the development and strength of the whole body, and of individual organs, and powerfully counteracts any tendency to disease.

If the exercise of individual muscles or organs is steadily increased, they increase in substance and ability to perform their functions. When the valves, situated at the commencement of the pulmonary artery, which conveys the blood from the right side of the heart to the lungs, or of the aorta which conveys it to the rest of the body, become gradually indurated, so as to afford a partial obstruction to the flow of blood through them, the walls of the ventricle, which forces the blood through these valves, become thickened and heavier than natural.

METHODS OF OBTAINING EXERCISE.

If exercise is so essential for development, preservation and health, an inquiry into the proper methods of taking it, becomes important.

Man is compelled to take a certain amount of exercise from necessity, to supply his bodily wants. He is born naked, and must have clothing and shelter; and is compelled to seek, or cultivate, materials suitable for food and drink. He is also endowed with social and moral faculties, through which he is brought into certain relations with others of his species; and if he faithfully performs his duties as a husband, father, neighbor, or citizen, so far as the physical man is concerned, he is obliged to take more or less exercise. The various kinds of exercise which are necessary to provide for the physical wants and comforts of himself, his family, neighbors, countrymen, or species, are called labor, or work, and are certainly among the most, if not the most important kinds of exercise; for the different forms of labor not only exercise the body, but they also enable man, if he so wills, to exercise and strengthen the nobler faculties of the soul, by performing acts of kindness and benevolence to others. Useful labor may well constitute no inconsiderable share of the exercise which is necessary for physical development and health. If there were no idlers, and all were to labor, a very few hours daily devoted to active work, would supply the physical wants of all, and not give the amount of muscular activity which is required for health. There would be time and strength remaining to engage in other avocations, aside from providing for physical wants; time to devote to teaching the laws of health and life, as well as natural sciences, to the young; and especially time to teach, both by precept and example, the duty of man to his fellow man, and of man to his Creator.

But neither ordinary labor, nor teaching, brings into activity all the muscles of the body, nor all the faculties of the mind; and, while parts are duly, or perhaps over exercised, other parts are torpid and inactive. A symmetrical form of either body or mind depends upon the development of every part in harmony with the rest; and such development is most conducive to health, both physically and spiritually. We see in the mirthful playfulness of childhood what provision, aside from the necessity for labor, our benevolent Creator has made for the development and health of the human body, and even for that of the soul; for the faculty which prompts recreation and amusement is pre-eminently a social faculty. The child may play alone, but it does not satisfy his nature—he wants companions to share his sports. The days of childhood constitute man's innocent, happy hours, and during this period of his existence, his angels which do ever behold the face of our Father in heaven, yearn to give of that happiness to others which he enjoys; and who that has witnessed the unceasing efforts which children often make to amuse and please their little companions, has not felt that angelic influences were descending to earth? The heart that is so cold and lifeless as not to long for a return of the innocent joyous days of childhood, accompanied with the wisdom of manhood, is about fitted for the regions of darkness, for it is dead to heavenly light and life. This faculty of the soul is one of the chief corner-stones upon which the hope, both for the physical and moral regeneration and development of the child, rests; and as he arrives at manhood, it should not be stifled by selfishness, or labor to make money, gratify vanity, or to acquire dominion; but should at suitable seasons be permitted to flow forth in active social recreations, and amusements, which exercise both body and mind, and give pleasure and profit to others, as well as benefit to the individual.

Our needed exercise should be obtained, and in a true order of society would be, by engaging in active labor and amusements, to satisfy the demands of our own being and to do service to others. But in the present artificial state of society, fashion deters multitudes, especially females, from engaging energetically in the performance of active physical labor, and unjust religious prejudices put down, to a great extent, those active amusements which are so much needed both by the body and soul, and thus vanity has joined hands with nominal Christianity, and thus united they wage a successful war against the physical and moral welfare of our race, until delicacy and consequent ill health have become fashionable, and are sought after by the simple; vice of course following in the train of idleness. And, in our cities, the importance of play grounds, even for children, to say nothing of adult men and women, has been entirely overlooked or neglected in the miserly grasp for wealth, by the original owners and layers out of our town plats, who have been made rich, not by any labor or merits of their own, but by the hard labor and earnings of others, and to a great extent, of poor men. The principles of eternal justice, and the claims of humanity have been disregarded in the scramble for wealth, until the hovels of the poor reflect the light of that sun, which sheds its life-giving rays on the poor as well as the rich, on the glittering palaces of wealth —until human beings clad in rags walk the same streets with those dressed in purple and fine linen, and even enter the house of God together—of Him who has commanded man to love his neighbor as himself.

As no provision, in the way of proper play grounds for our men, women and children, has been made in our cities and large villages, it has become necessary to seek other methods for obtaining exercise—artificial methods. Being deprived of an opportunity for athletic sports, and games, few in our cities are aware of the different motions which the human body and its numerous organs are capable of making, and which the health of the various muscles and parts, and the symmetry of the whole body, require should be made, to prevent diseases and deformity. For this reason a competent teacher of physical exercises, has become almost a necessity, even more necessary than is a teacher for many of the branches taught in our schools; nor is the occasion and necessity for such teachers, confined to our cities and villages, for the female portion of the population of our rural districts, have so long neglected active out-door amusements, that disease and deformity are to be seen on every hand, as consequences of such neglect. It is not fashionable for young girls, and ladies to engage in active out-door sports, such as running, jumping, wrestling, playing ball, rambling over the fields, sliding down hill, skating, &c.; and if young girls engage in such necessary sports, they are cruelly called tom-boys, and romps,—which are regarded as terms of reproach—as though girls have not as good a right to air, light, exercise, amusements, and consequent health, symmetry of form, and beauty, as boys. Nor is it fashionable for the young ladies to engage in any of the out-door employments which give vigor and health to young men. I would not wish to see them engaged in the performance of the hardest kinds of labor, side by side with men, but I would like to see, in the vicinity of every farm-house, a large garden and orchard, with all kinds of fruit trees, grape vines, and bushes for the growing of fruits and berries, and to see the ladies, young and old, spending less time in useless, and even pernicious, cooking and sewing, and spending most of their time in the cultivation of fruits, berries, useful vegetables and flowers, in the open air; and thus making the homestead a paradise, where shall abound health, beauty, and happiness, instead of the present discontent, deformity and disease, which we so commonly witness among the occupants of our gloomy, prison-like, farm-houses. Such a change would cause the young men of our land, to seek happiness in the quiet and peace of the domestic circle of a home, in the arms of a loving wife, surrounded by happy children, the pledges of love; instead of their being repelled, by the fear by being yoked to lazy, extravagant, and sickly wives; and by imaginary ghosts of starving, sickly, and dying children, rising up in the foreground, and thus being sent off to seek their fortunes amid the pollution of our cities, or the gulches and river beds of the Rocky Mountains; as though their neighbors had no daughters, and a domestic circle were not more desirable than a golden chain; which is very liable to drag both soul and body to destruction, even if they do not reach perdition by a shorter cut than by the acquisition of wealth.

The ladies, even in our farm-houses, at present, perform very little productive labor, however industrious they may be in cooking pies, cakes, and high seasoned dishes—which so far as health is concerned, were all better uncooked—or at fancy sewing, or knitting. It is thought, I am sorry to say, by many of our farmers, more genteel, and cheaper to buy cloth already manufactured, than it is to have the wife and daughters make it from the wool and flax, even when the ladies are dying for the want of the exercise which they would thus derive. It would, undoubtedly, be cheaper, and perhaps better, if the ladies were engaged, in the mean time, at any other productive labor, which would pay the manufacturer, especially if it were out-door labor, such as has been suggested; but when, as at present, idleness, useless cookery and sewing, take the place of the spinning and weaving, thus destroying health and happiness, and producing nothing in exchange, it only throws a double burden on the gentlemen; and a young man, who has not a fortune, may well hesitate before he takes upon himself the obligations of a husband and father, with a knowledge that he is expected to provide all the food and materials for raiment, and manufacture most of the latter, and with the almost certainty, that he must spend no inconsiderable portion of his time, either directly or indirectly, in nursing a wife and children, made sick by needlessly violating natural laws.

It is time we have a change. Our ladies are very ready to

follow the foolish, destructive, and absurd fashions set them by a few vain, silly women in Paris; why can they not follow the worthy and dignified example of their noble sisters of France?

Says Dr. Shelton McKenzie, in the Philadelphia *Press:*

"French women, from the middle class down, are generally happy, because employment prevents their being afflicted with *ennui.* They are busy, they are useful, they help, they regulate, they rule—in a word, they have a far wider sphere of labor than an American or English woman, and they voluntarily not only take, but are delighted to make this field of employment. In France, from the middle class inclusive, female education has an utilitarian complexion. The women among these classes—which are seven-eighths of the whole—can read, write and cipher. They are independent, and will exercise their freedom. Instead of remaining at home, lazily lounging on rocking-chairs, over sensation novels, or sensation weeklies, or airing their clothes in the street, marvels of crinoline expansion, they assert their right to be useful, and will have that claim allowed. For a French girl has as much pride in earning a becoming cheap dress as an American 'young lady' has in wearing a costly one.

"French women are earnest, active beings. They may earn little, but they are usually good economists, and, content with simplest wholesome food, do not covet culinary luxuries. Neither do they indulge in expensive attire. Dress, with them is rather a means than an end. Plain materials, neatly made and well put on, sufficiently satisfy them. A young Parisian whose class wear cottons and muslins, merinos and de laines, would be regarded very suspiciously by her associates if she were to flaunt about in silk dresses, illimitable hoops, and fly-away bonnets, such as even *our* shop women and milliners' girls so greatly affect.

"There may be difficulty in this country as well as in England, in providing women with suitable employment. It is to be done —but it will take time. Women must be brought up to it. We suspect that the French system of employing women, and thereby keeping them out of want and immorality, will be in full vogue in England, long before American females will *condescend* to it.

But, in truth, the political principle of equality which here prevails, has got so personally extended that our young American 'ladies,' no matter how reduced their parents' circumstances, too often think it derogatory to work. That word 'lady,' by the way, has a great deal to answer for. It puts false ideas of gentility into young women's heads, and puts them far above being useful. It is dreadfully misapplied, too. Only the other day we saw it stated, in a leading New York paper, of the two females (of her own class) who were in company with Virginia Stewart, when she was shot by McDonald, a week ago, that the coroner had committed her 'two lady friends' to prison, to appear as evidence when required. '*Ladies*,' indeed."

THE GYMNASIUM.

For reasons, which have already been given, it is all-important for the preservation of our race, that calisthenic and gymnastic exercises, should be taught in every school district of our land, and that every city and village should be furnished with its gymnasiums, and that all, both male and female, old and young, who have not other forms of active exercise, should resort to them regularly. When practicable it is important that such exercises should be in the open air, and a well arranged gymnasium should have both in-door and out-door accommodations, for both bad and good weather.

I have made the following quotation from a report of an excellent address, delivered by George E. Hand Esq., at a gymnastic exhibition, at Merrit's Gymnasium, in Detroit, reported in the Detroit *Free Press*.

"He said, that the attendance of so many ladies and gentlemen was accepted as a manifestation of their interest in, and as a recognition of their appreciation of the value and importance of gymnastic exercise. There were, however, unfortunately, too many who did not duly appreciate the importance of such exercise, and its bearings on the developments of actual life. The mere abstract idea of gymnastics would convey no definite impression to the mind. It is necessary, therefore, to witness some of the manifestations and results of such exercises—the muscular development produced, the vigor imparted, and the elasticity communicated—to judge of their favorable effects in all the paths of life. Many imagined that there was no necessity for gymnastics, because they were a novelty introduced of late years, and had never been heard of in former generations. Why should they depart from the good old customs of their forefathers? Was it not enough to follow in the footsteps of their predecessors, in such matters? But, the fact was, times had changed, and people had changed with them, and it was precisely in consequence of this change, which had come over the whole of the civilized world, but, more especially, over the American community, that they needed something of this kind to build up, strengthen, and develop the muscular energy of the present generation. All could see at a glance, the great, the wide difference between the times of their forefathers—the days of the revolution, for instance—and those of the present time in regard to the habits, manners, customs employments and pastimes of the people.

It was that change which rendered it so imperatively necessary to have something to counteract the evil effects of sedentary life in the present generation. No such need had been felt in the times of their forefathers, who were a simple race, mostly agricultural and living in villages. They had no large cities. There were then few workshops, no factories, and few places where people were gathered into masses. The whole country was open. All or nearly all were engaged in agricultural pursuits, and were thus accustomed to daily toil and to constant employment in the open air.

Their habits were frugal, they dieted simply, appropriated a portion of their days to labor, and a good portion of their nights to sleep. Under such circumstances there was no great difficulty in maintaining a healthy condition both of mind and body. The same observation applied in the case of ladies. Their mode of life was simple—there was none of the luxury of the present day. They were constantly employed, for at that time cotton was unknown, power looms were unknown, spinning jennies were unknown, and the factories which now turn out such quantities of textile fabrics were unknown. They were then obliged, in every household, and in every community, to produce themselves, principally from wool and flax, every article of apparel required for their own use. It was no simple matter for the females of the family to spin and weave all the fabrics of wool and linen which were required for the use of the family. These, their ordinary avocations, kept them in constant employment, and tended to develop in them a vigor corresponding to that acquired by the males in the labor of the field. Then there were no stoves, and very few carpets. Houses were built in such a manner that there was generally a current of fresh air from one end of them to the other. The dietetic errors of the present generation, such as bird suppers, were unknown. But now all this had passed away—a new time had come upon them, and the affairs of practical life, consequent on the introduction of spinning and weaving by power, had been so entirely modified, that, the other day, when some friends of his who desired to illustrate, by a tableau vivant, a scene from the Courtship of Miles Standish, endeavored to procure one of the little spinning wheels of former times, they sought in vain through the whole town, and at last only succeeded in obtaining it by the kindness of a German friend, who had very thoughtfully brought one from Germany. In place of the invigorating employments of former times, ladies now occupied themselves with embroidery, knitting, sewing, or crochet, and sat the whole day with their feet on a footstool two feet high. This, combined with late hours, luxurious living, and vitiated atmosphere, was steadily undermining female health. Gentlemen, on the other hand, did things which were equally imprudent and bad for the system. The use of tobacco, which was now becoming universal, was the greatest curse ever introduced into a civilized community. It was deteriorating the whole race, and doing more to destroy the tone and vigor of the rising generation than almost all other vices put together. Now that large cities had grown up, town boys were deprived of suitable places for the exercise and recreation necessary for their proper development. A necessary consequence of that want was the introduction of gymnasiums. Although the gymnasiums came to them from Germany, where they had them in the highest perfection, they were no new things in the world. Long before Germany was known to the civilized world—long before Alexander the Great marched into Persia—before the Romans conquered Hannibal, or overran Spain and Gaul—before Great Britain was known, gymnastic establishments were well known, highly appreciated, and in the highest state of perfection in the most civilized nation of the ancient world—in Greece.

"Among the Greeks, the various gymnastic games were publicly celebrated at regular intervals in different cities, and made the occasion for great public festivities, and the meeting together of all the principal citizens from the different provinces, or rather colonies, which had been planted in Asia Minor, Italy and Africa. Here the competitors came and struggled for the mastery in these gymnastic exercises; and the simple wreaths and crowns which were appropriated to the victors on these occasions were considered of as much importance, received as much applause, commanded as much distinction, and were as highly prized, as the highest offices and public trusts. As a consequence, the whole nation engaged in these exercises, and every city, village and hamlet had its gymnasiums, where the practice of wrestling, boxing, running, leaping and throwing the discus and javelin was taught to every youth of proper age. Those exercises required a strict diet and regimen, and produced a nation of hardy and vigorous men, who carried the fame of the Grecian arms throughout Asia, and to the borders of Italy. They were the men whose hardy nerve and daring courage, developed by such training, had met the invader at Thermopylæ, Marathon and Platea, and driven back their countless hordes from the soil of Greece—who under Alexander carried their arms through Asia to the Indus. The same men, in the time of Cyrus the Younger—a small band of 13,000 strong—went to the centre of Asia, fought a great battle against 900,000 of the enemy, on the plains of Babylon, where they lost their leader. They were then 500 leagues from home, and had no way of retreat but by cutting their way back through the hosts of Persians who opposed them. Such was the valor, vigor and discipline exhibited by these men during months of constant hostilities that 10,000 of them reached their homes in Greece.

"Xenophon, who was one of the officers, has given an account of the return, which is known in history as 'The Retreat of the Ten Thousand,' and is justly considered the most remarkable military expedition on record. That expedition would never have been successful but for the Grecian training and discipline. So in Rome; though the gymnastic exercises were not so distinctly marked, yet every Roman soldier underwent a discipline which enured him to every toil and every hardship, and every Roman citizen was by birth a Roman soldier. Thus, when Hannibal and Amilcar led their Carthagenians to the gates of Rome, they were repulsed, the war carried into Africa, and the Carthagenian government and kingdom entirely destroyed. These Romans overrun the whole of Europe, and finally discovered and conquered a little island which had never before been heard of, and to which they gave the name of Britain. All these things had happened much earlier than the time of our forefathers, and the discipline, development and exploits of those nations were sufficient to show the importance of gymnastic exercise. It was a matter of fact that every nation which had enjoyed liberty and personal indepéndence had been distinguished by constant and vigorous exercise, either in their daily avocations or in their accustomed sports. As soon as luxury and sloth usurped the place of such exercise, the overthrow of their liberty and institutions had speedily followed."

No Christian, or philanthropic man would desire the cultivation and development of the body, by gymnastic exercises, by the inhabitants of our land, to enable us to carry on successfully an offensive warfare against neighboring nations, or for the sake of encouraging degrading personal combats, in which are manifested the lowest passions of our nature. But surely no higher motives for action, can be found than already exist, and which should drive the inactive residents of our cities and villages, to the gymnasium, as a duty, not to be neglected under any circumstances. To gain strength with which to be useful to others, ability to keep the Divine Commands, capacity to be happy, and enjoy rationally the good things of earth; to obtain freedom from disease and consequent suffering, to give activity and harmonious action to all the organs of the body, and faculties of the mind, so as to be able to restrain the passions, as well as counteract the present tendency to fanatical excitement on beholding the imaginary or actual evils of others, are not these motives worthy of a man—of a Christian? When a man is so circumstanced that he can neither obtain the needed exercise from either ordinary labor, or proper amusements, to preserve the balance between the different organs of the body and faculties of the soul, these motives exalt the exercises of the gymnasium to the dignity of true labor, not less important, or less a Christian duty, than the most important employments denominated labor. It is as important to develop the brain and muscle with which to guide and move the pen or needle, as it is to write or sew; and so of all other employments.

EXERCISE AS A CURATIVE AGENCY.

Very many of the diseases, especially those of a chronic and nervous character, to which we are at this day subject, are caused by the want of exercise, either of the whole body, or of individual muscles and parts. Without proper general exercise the circulation of blood becomes languid, and if particular organs or parts are not duly exercised, the blood is excited to flow more freely to the parts which are exercised, of course less to such as are not. While, in the parts exercised, the circulation may be comparatively active, and the blood vessels strong and healthy, in other parts, from the languid circulation, the vessels may become unduly contracted, leaving the parts cold and lifeless for the want of a due supply of blood; or for the want of healthy tone and vigor, which results from activity, the blood vessels may become dilated and over disturbed with blood, causing congestion in the part, attended by pain and soreness, which may very readily pass on to a state of inflammation, with increased suffering and danger. Thus we may have health and life endangered by following occupations which only exercise a part of the muscles and organs of the body, provided we neglect to duly exercise the remaining parts. In this way sedentary men, tailors, dressmakers, shoe-makers, and those who follow many other mechanical pursuits, destroy their health and shorten their lives. If high living is added to the want of exercise, this but increases the suffering and danger, either by causing derangement and disease of the digestive organs, or by adding to the circulation more nutriment than is needed to supply the languid organism, and thus overtaxing the organs of secretion in its removal, and causing disease of such organs; or, again, giving rise to the gout and other diseases which result from such a course of life.

Exercise prevents disease by giving vigor and energy to the body and its various organs and members, and thus enabling them to ward off or overcome the influence of the various causes which tend to impair their integrity. It cures disease by equalizing the circulation, and nervous energy, thus invigorating and strengthening weak organs, and removing local torpor and congestion. It is not often compatible with acute inflammation ; and even in chronic inflammation, it requires to be used, if at all, with caution, but in very many diseases, which are unattended by inflammation, proper exercise is far more important than medicine, and without it medicine can only afford palliative relief.

Exercise has long been known to be a valuable remedial agency. Galen, who was born in the year 131, and was one of the most celebrated physicians of antiquity, whose opinions bore almost undivided sway among medical men until the beginning of the seventeenth century, says, that he is the best physician who is the best teacher of calisthenics or gymnastics. He was himself in feeble health until he was thirty years old, after which by devoting several hours every day to gymnastic exercises, he became strong and healthy. Lord Bacon expressed the opinion that "there was no disease among pupils that gymnastics and calisthenics could not cure." Dryden sung long ago: "The wise for cure on exercise depend."

Dr. Taylor, in a letter from Sweden, to which I have already referred, speaking of the gymnastic institution established under the patronage of the government of that country and other similar institutions, says:

"Many chronic invalids only require a proper training of their defective powers in order to secure a recovery of health. hence there is a medical department of this institution, and as the members in the community who have not learned the art of self-preservation are exceedingly large, this has become by far the largest school. Its medical purpose is soonest appreciated, since it responds to the immediate necessities of the people. The success of the treatment corresponds with the rational simplicity of the theory, and there follows a great and constantly increasing demand for it. This method has spread widely in other countries, so that there are now twenty-five or thirty institutions in Europe devoted to the treatment of diseases by medical gymnastics. In Sweden, the physicians, who are frequently the representatives of traditional science, bow gracefully to the decree of public opinion, for this opinion is generally in favor of new physiological methods of treatment. So that Stockholm, which has a population of about one-seventh of New York, with a thinly peopled country about it, and is of no commercial importance, has three institutions for the practice of medical gymnastics. At Professor Bronting's there are yearly about one thousand in all departments, three hundred of whom are invalids. Of the others, the one under Dr. Satherberg is much renowned, and is devoted exclusively to invalids, of whom nearly three hundred and fifty were treated during the year. Dr. Satherberg is orthopedic professor in the Carolinian Medical Institution, of which Prof. Regius is the well-known head, which indicates his standing in the profession. He also enjoys a large government stipend, in consideration of maintaining a medico gymnastic clinique for the poor. With the third institution here I am not well acquainted, but it is not unreasonable to suppose that more than fifteen hundred people belonging to this city alone, yearly avail themselves of the advantages of this method of training and treatment."

The following graphic picture of the effects of regular gymnastic exercises, by Horace Mann, is scarcely over drawn:

"It requires, indeed, no very strong imagination to see the horrid forms of the diseases themselves, as they are exorcised and driven from the bodies which were once their victims, and are compelled to seek some new tenement. Those prodigious leaps over the vaulting horse, how they kick hereditary gout out of the toes! Those swift somersets, with their quick and deep breathings, are ejecting bronchitis, asthma, and phthisic from the throat and lungs. On yonder pendant rope consumption is hung up like a malefactor, as it is. Legions of devils are impaled on those parallel bars.

"Dyspepsia lost hold of her victim when he mounted the flying horse, and has never since been able to regain her throne, and live by gnawing the vitals. There goes a flock of nervous distempers, headaches, tic-douloureux and St. Anthony's fire; there they fly out of the window, seeking some stall-fed alderman, or fat millionaire, or aristocratic old lady. Rheumatism, and cramps, and spasms sit coiled up, and chattering in the corner of the room, like satanic imps, as they are; the strong muscles of the athletic having shaken them off, as the lion shakes the dew drops from his mane. Jaundice flies away to yellow the cheeks and blear the eyes of my fair young lady reclining on ottomans in her parlor. The balancing pole shakes lumbago out of the back, and kinks out of the femoral muscles, and stitches out of the side. Pleurisy and apoplexy and death hover round; they look into the windows of this hall, but finding brain and lungs and heart defiant of their power, they go away in quest of some lazy cit, some guzzling drone, or some bloated epicure at his late supper to fasten their fatal fangs upon him. In the meantime the rose blooms again on the pale cheek of the gymnast; his shrivelled skin is filled out, and his non-elastic muscles and bones rejoice anew in the vigor and buoyancy of youth. A place like this ought to be named the Palace of Health."

The reader who may desire to obtain a practical knowledge of applying gymnastic and calisthenic exercises, for the development of the body, and preservation of health, can obtain such information in Dr. Trall's Family Gymnasium, published by Fowler & Wells, 308 Broadway, N. Y. Every gymnasium should have a competent teacher, not only to teach the proper exercises, but also to restrain and prevent excessive exercise, which is equally as injurious as lack of exercise.

In concluding this subject, I will introduce the testimony of an intelligent and venerable physician as to the value of a single form of exercise, as a preventive and curative agent, which is accessible to all. I do this with more pleasure, as from an acquaintance of many years, I am able to vouch for the writer's qualifications for judging correctly in regard to the effects of the practice, and his entire reliability as a witness. I will simply hint, "for the benefit of all whom it may concern," that this is a form of exercise admirably calculated to benefit the deformed waists, shoulders and spines of our fashionable young ladies.

THE SWING AS A CURE OF CONSUMPTION.

"I WISH to say a few words 'to whom it may concern,' on the use of the swing—one of the gymnastic exercises—as a preventive and cure of pulmonary disease. I mean the suspending of the body by the hands by means of a strong rope or chain fastened to a beam at one end, and at the other a stick three feet long convenient to grasp with the hands. The rope should be fastened to the center of the stick, which should hang six or eight inches above the head. Let a person grasp this stick, with the hands two or three feet apart, and swing very moderately at first—perhaps only bear the weight, if very weak—and gradually, increase, as the muscles gain strength from the exercise, until it may be freely used from three to five times daily. The connection of the arms with the body (with the exception of the clavicle with the sternum or breast bone) being a muscular attachment to the ribs, the effect of this exercise is to elevate the ribs and enlarge the chest; and, as nature allows no vacuum, the lungs expand to fill the cavity, increasing the volume of air—the natural purifier of the blood—and preventing congestion or the deposit of tuberculous matter. I have prescribed the above for all cases of hemorrhage of the lungs and threatened consumption, for thirty-five years, and have been able to increase the measure of the chest from two to four inches within a few months, and, always with good results. But especially as a preventive I would recommend this exercise. Let those who love life cultivate a well-formed capacious chest. The student, the merchant, the sedentary, the young of both sexes—aye, *all* should have a swing upon which to stretch themselves daily; and I am morally certain that if this were to be practiced by the rising generation, in a dress allowing a free and full development of the body, thousands, yes, tens of thousands, would be saved from the ravages of that *opprobrium medicorum*, consumption."

LAWSON LONG, M. D.

Holyoke, June 8, 1859.

CHAPTER V.

CHILDREN AND THE CAUSES OF THE MORTALITY AMONG THEM; THEIR DISEASES AND DEFORMITIES.

INFORMATION upon no subject is more important to our race, than a knowledge of the causes of infantile diseases, and the mortality among children. A distinguished writer, more than a century ago, said:

"When we reflect upon the many painful and dangerous maladies to the attacks of which children, from the earliest period of their existence, are liable, and by which so large a proportion of them are annually destroyed; and when we consider, also, that in many, perhaps in the majority of cases, these attacks might easily be avoided by a proper attention to those external agents, to the influence of which the infant is subjected from the moment of its birth, and which, while they are essential to its existence, become, when counteracted or mismanaged, the cause of nearly all its infirmities and diseases; the physician can scarcely be considered as fulfilling all his duties, when he neglects to point out and urge the administration of the means by which the occurrence of disease may be prevented, as well as those, which, when disease is already present, are adapted to remove it." (FAUST.)

If, as this writer intimates, it is easy when in the possession of the requisite knowledge, by proper attention, to avoid in a majority of cases the attacks of diseases, which cause so much suffering and so many deaths among children, is it not clearly the duty of every parent, and all who expect to have the care over children, to spare no efforts to obtain the knowledge which is so requisite for the welfare of the helpless and innocent little ones committed to their charge. Yet how many parents are so thoughtless, and reckless, as to the welfare, suffering, and even lives of their children, as to spend their time in reading the last novel, or making comparatively, useless embroidery, or grasping for riches or show, and spend their money freely for the yellow covered literature of the day, for fine clothes, worse than worthless luxuries, such as tobacco, coffee, tea, etc., but neglect to spend the few hours in reading which are required, to obtain the knowledge indispensably requisite for the safety of their children; or, who perhaps, think they cannot spare the money to obtain suitable books from which the required information may be derived. They can pay doctors, and spend nights in nursing, and see their children suffer, and die, but not a dollar, nor an hour are they willing to spare, for such information as will enable them to preserve the health, and lives of their little ones.

One of the chief causes, of the fearful mortality among children, is to be found in their inheriting delicate organizations from their parents, which are, at birth, predisposed to disease, and sometimes already diseased. Parents who possess delicate constitutions, or, who are in poor health, cannot transmit substantial, vigorous organizations to their children, with all the care possible; but they may, by proper care and attention, do much toward giving their children even better organizations than they possess; or by unlawful indulgences, negligence, and abuse, they may, by exhausting their own vitality, and deforming their persons, transmit delicacy, deformity, and disease, to their offspring. It is all important for young persons who intend to become parents, if they wish to transmit healthy organizations to their children, so to live as to preserve their own organizations in a vigorous and healthy condition; for if they fail, or neglect to do this, their children must inevitably suffer from their folly. The conditions requisite for the preservation of health and life, have been pointed out in the chapters on the use and abuse of the digestive organs, on air, light, exercise, amusements, fashions, narcotics, stimulants, etc., and they need not be repeated here. But it is important that a few special suggestions should be made in this connection. And, first; it is important for the young to bear in mind that nothing before marriage, so certainly impairs their own vitality, and destroys their ability to ever transmit healthy, and substantial organizations, to their children, as self-abuse. Let them read carefully, and ponder well, the section on this subject in the author's work on "Marriage and its Violations," and shun it as they value their own lives, and the welfare of their race. Scarcely less destructive to parents, and their offspring, are excesses after marriage. None but physicians can form the least conception, as to the amount of suffering from this cause alone. If husbands and wives will not regard their own welfare, they certainly should feel some compunctions of conscience, in impairing, in this manner, the vitality of their children, and causing them to suffer and die. Let those who desire to do right, read carefully the work above named, and they will find many useful suggestions, which, if heeded, will save them, hereafter, from years spent in useless regrets, for past acts. During pregnancy, especially during the latter months of this period, the entire vitality of the mother is needed to give a healthy substantial development to the child; and, for some months after confinement, it is needed to supply nourishment of a proper quality, and of sufficient quantity, and should not be squandered in sensual indulgences; and all this is especially true of our delicate women of fashionable life. The habit, which many ladies have, of compressing, during pregnancy, the waist, and even abdomen, by corsets, and dresses, is a frequent cause of miscarriage, or abortion; and when it fails to produce this result, it may cause club-feet, and other deformities of the child; not that I suppose every case of such deformity is caused in this way, but the danger of such a result, is so great, that mothers who desire well-formed children, may well beware how they voluntarily produce the least compression of the waist, or abdomen during pregnancy, for a single hour. A loose dress, fresh air, light, nourishing food, regular exercise, and cheerful amusements, are all important during pregnancy. These are the conditions which are necessary to give health and vigor to the mother, without which it is impossible for her child to receive a substantial and healthy organization, which will with any certainty survive the days of childhood.

WANTS OF VERY YOUNG CHILDREN.

THE child, after birth, requires great care to preserve it from suffering, and even from great injury. Its eyes are unaccustomed to the light, and not able to tolerate a strong light with impunity; if light is admitted too freely, inflammation and blindness may ensue. The room should be quite dark at first, but daily the light should be increased, until the full light of day can be borne. The surface of the body and the air passages are unaccustomed to the air, and if great pains is not taken to keep the room warm, especially during the first few washings, cold in the head, or even inflammation of the bronchia, and of the lungs, are liable to result. Even when the room is warm, it is well not to expose the whole body of the child while washing, but keep it carefully covered, except the part where the washing is in progress. The child's stomach is unaccustomed to food. Up to the time of birth it has derived its nourishment directly from the mother, without taxing its digestive organs to any considerable extent, if at all. Now it is to be nourished by the means of food taken into the stomach. The first nourishment which the child should receive, when there is no insurmountable obstacle to it, should be drawn from the mother's breasts, for that which is therein contained is prepared expressly to answer to the demands of the infant's digestive organs; and no nourishment supplied by art, can answer equally well. It is slightly laxative, and this quality is useful to move off the secretion which has accumulated in the bowels during fœtal life. If the baby is allowed to nurse as soon as it seems hungry, and the mother has obtained rest, there will be no need of giving it any other laxative, or cathartic, such as molasses, castor oil, &c., for nature has made all the provision, in this direction, which is necessary. For the last twelve years I have not given, in a single instance, any form of laxative medicine to new born infants, aside from that nourishment provided in the mother's breasts; and I am satisfied that children do much better without, than with, such articles as are frequently given to them to move the bowels. The nearer we can follow nature the better. Mothers, at present, often object to nursing the child soon; and ignorant nurses still more frequently object to the mother's nursing, until about the third day, when the breasts begin to "fill with milk;" and very serious consequences to both mother and child frequently result from such neglect. They suppose that during this period there is nothing in the breasts, or secreted, for the child. This is a mistake, for there is always some secretion, and the little that is secreted is always precisely what the new born child needs. Then, if the infant is fed a few times before nursing, it often loses the faculty of nursing; and it is, in such cases, exceedingly difficult to induce it to nurse. The child is often fed with improper substances, and is frequently made sick before it is a day old. If allowed to nurse, it will often obtain all the nourishment it needs from the commencement; if not, a very little milk and water, sweetened with loaf sugar, is all that is needed in addition to what nature has provided. Nor does the child alone suffer from its not being allowed to nurse during the first two or three days, the mother's breasts become distended, and the nipples are rendered less prominent, and it becomes more difficult for it to lay hold of them, even when it retains the faculty; as a result inflammation and abscess of the breast frequently occur from this cause; or if the child nurses readily sore nipples frequently result from such delay; whereas if it is allowed to nurse from the commencement, it will retain its faculty for nursing, the breasts will be kept empty, the milk fever will be prevented, or lessened, and the nipples will gradually become accustomed to being used, and far less liable to become sore. For the first two days the child should not be nursed more frequently than once in six hours, on the same breast; which by changing will allow it to nurse once in three hours. Nor should nursing be continued more than a minute or two, or only until the mother feels that the breast is empty. If the nursing is continued when the mother begins to feel uneasiness in the breast, there will be great danger of causing the very evils we are seeking to avert by early nursing, viz.: sore nipples and inflammation of the breast.

The practice of giving a cathartic to the mother during confinement, within a day or two after labor, is very injurious to both the mother and child. If let alone the mother will not usually have a passage from her bowels until from five to eight, or ten days. This gives time for the enlarged uterus to approximate its natural size; and the soreness of the parts involved in labor, to abate; whereas if a cathartic is taken soon after labor while the parts are distended and sore, from the exercise which is necessary, and the passage of the contents of the bowels through the rectum and anus, or lower portion and outlet of the intestines, we are very liable to have produced inflammation of the womb, puerperal fever, piles, or prolapsus uteri, which may cause much present and future suffering. I have known a single dose of castor oil, given to a woman soon after the commencement of confinement, who was doing well without it, cause the most intense suffering, which was not even mitigated, by treatment, at the end of six months. The infant's bowels are often disturbed by colic, griping pains, and diarrhœa, from nursing the mother after she has taken cathartics. All these dangers to both mother and child can be, and should be, avoided by letting cathartics alone soon after confinement, as every physician can testify, who has tried this method; and yet, so strong is the prejudice among both mothers and nurses, in favor of giving a cathartic as soon as the second or third day, that one is often taken, without even consulting the attending physician, if he has not given special directions to the contrary; and if he has, he often finds it exceedingly difficult to satisfy mother and nurse and prevent their administration. If, at the end of eight days, the bowels do not move spontaneously, a copious injection of tepid water should be administered, and repeated at the end of twelve hours, if necessary; and, if a passage is not procured, the attending physician should be consulted on the ninth or tenth day, which will rarely be necessary. In all cases where the bowels have not moved for seven or eight days, it is well to take an injection of tepid water, a few hours before they are expected to move, so as to render the contents of the lower bowel less hard.

It is not uncommon for the skin of the infant to become yellow, or jaundiced, within a few days after birth, and for nurses to give saffron tea for this difficulty. I know of no reason for its administration except the correspondence in color, which does not seem to a medical man at this day, however it might have seemed to physicians at one period in the past, a very satisfactory reason. As this yellowness generally disappears spontaneously without treatment, in a few days, saffron tea as a remedy for it, has gained some reputation, like various pernicious applications for wounds, which do not permanently prevent their healing, however much they may retard the efforts of nature. But saffron tea is not a harmless remedy, as it sometimes causes violent nausea and vomiting, with diarrhœa; therefore it should never be given to young children in such cases, as it can do no good. If the yellowness of the skin does not disappear in a few days, it is better to apply to a physician, than to dose the little one with a remedy which has no true relation to the disease.

The infant requires proper nourishment, at regular intervals, but does not often require herb-drinks, and other strong medicines, and its organization is too delicate to justify parents, and nurses, in the administration of such drinks, cathartics, anodynes, ect.; and I am satisfied that many children lose their lives from this domestic drugging; and, not a few who are not destroyed are thus rendered delicate and feeble during life. If parents desire to have crying children, let them commence the use of anodynes, and cordials, especially such as contain opium, and they will soon have this kind of music to their heart's content; for these remedies palliate, for the time, but keep up a disposition to the same trouble for which they are given, and soon add innumerable aches and pains by their own poisonous action; and the babe soon comes to cry for its accustomed dose, and suffer as intensely when it is withheld, as the confirmed opium eater of adult life. By the use of such poisons, the various functions of the body are rendered torpid, and the organism partially paralyzed, so that a healthy development is prevented. These remedies act specifically upon the brain, impairing its functions, and giving rise to various nervous diseases; and even comparative mental imbecility is sometimes undoubtedly caused by their use.

If a young child cries excessively, or seems ill, we have good evidence that the laws of its organization are being violated in some direction or other: and instead of palliating the suffering by an anodyne, we should seek out and remove the cause of the evil. The point of a pin may be irritating the skin, or the band may be pinned too tight around the body. I have in more than one instance been called to see children suffering from this latter cause, and have seen all suffering cease, the moment the bandage was unpinned. It should never be pinned tight around the body, but loosely. The child may be too hot, or too cold, or it may be suffering from improper nourishment.

NURSING BY THE MOTHER.

If there is no serious objection which renders it improper, or impracticable, every mother should undoubtedly nurse her own children; and where mothers do not care more for their own gratification and pleasure than they do for the welfare of their children, they are generally very ready to do this: but there are many circumstances which may render nursing impossible, or not expedient. It sometimes happens, that, owing to tight dressing while young, or some other cause, the nipples are sunken in to such an extent as to render it impossible ever to draw them out, so as to enable the infant to nurse. The structure of the breasts may have been so far destroyed by abscesses or disease as to destroy their capacity to furnish nourishment. Owing to fever, or some acute or chronic disease, the milk may spontaneously "dry up," in spite of the utmost care. All these, and various other conditions may render it altogether impossible for the mother to nurse her own child. Then there are many cases where it is not expedient for the mother to nurse her babe, on her own account, even though the child may thrive. Some mothers, especially in cities, have a free flow of milk, but are excessively exhausted to the extent of endangering life by nursing; others while nursing become subject to what is called "nursing sore mouth," which is a disease of debility. This disease can generally be prevented, and cured when it exists, by exercise, air, light and a nourishing diet; but more especially by an out door life; aided, perhaps, after it is developed, by proper remedies; but it not unfrequently happens, that it is allowed to continue unchecked, until the irritation extends to the stomach and bowels, causing vomiting and diarrhœa, and thus preventing nutrition, destroying the red globules of the blood, and giving rise to a train of symptoms which it may be impossible to arrest in time to save the patient from death; and if from death, at least not from a serious impairment of health for years afterward. The infant generally thrives until the mother becomes very much exhausted; but it is much better for both that other nourishment should be sought, than that her vitality should be too much exhausted; for, beyond a certain point, which is easily reached, a cure is with great difficulty accomplished. It is better then, if the disease is not soon checked by the means I have suggested, and such remedies as the attending physician may recommend, to wean the child before the bowels become too much disturbed, or the countenance very bloodless. This disease generally soon abates after weaning the child, provided it is not delayed until too late an hour.

If there is a strong predisposition to consumption in the mother, especially if there are incipient symptoms, it is not well for the mother to nurse her child. Nor is it well for the child to nurse the mother in such cases, and the same is true where the mother is suffering from scrofula, cancer, severe chronic eruptive diseases, or serious acute diseases.

The return of the menses, or monthly turns, during the period of nursing, does not render it necessary to wean the child as a general rule; and never so long as the milk agrees with it. The same is true if pregnancy should occur, while the child is too young to wean, especially if the mother is strong and healthy; but it is not well, perhaps, to continue the nursing longer than three or four, or at most five months, in any case, after the commencement of pregnancy.

FREQUENCY OF NURSING.

Regularity in receiving its nourishment, is as important to the infant as to the adult; and the comfort and happiness as well as health of both mother and child, depend so much upon the cultivation of regular habits that this subject is worthy of attention. Some sacrifices may be required on the part of the mother, in order to establish such habits as are for the child's best good. The following just and useful remarks, I have taken from the pages of a work entitled, "Mothers and Infants," by Dr. Al. Donné, recently translated from the French, and published by Phillips, Sampson & Co., of Boston; which work I can cheerfully recommend to parents, as containing much useful information, important to them and their children. In speaking of the importance of regulating the care which a mother lavishes on her child, in order to promote its physical and moral welfare, the Dr. says:

"It is necessary to love him, first of all for himself, through regard for his future, more than his present well-being; and to avoid manifesting, to his detriment, excessive sensibility of heart, yielding to weaknesses pleasant to gratify, but dangerous for the child, or purchasing repose by an absence of all restraint, the fatal effects of which recoil upon the child himself. These considerations, to which I will here only advert, present themselves already in respect to nursing as to all questions relative to the education of infancy. But this is not the place to dwell upon them now. Suffice it to say, that the mother must have system and calmness enough to introduce a little of these two qualities into the performance of her functions, and not alarm and disturb herself for the slightest untoward circumstances. Nursing requires to be conducted with a certain method. It must take place at intervals as well regulated as possible; the caprices which manifest themselves thus early, must be wisely resisted, and bad habits must be avoided; and when the mother is certain that her child has all which he needs, that he has nursed sufficiently, and that he does not suffer, she must know how to divert his attention and even be able to bear his cries, without yielding to new importunities. This last point is so essential that I do not fear to make it a veritable axiom in saying, that every mother who cannot bear to hear her child cry, is incapable of bringing him up well.

"The cries of the child are in the first place one of his functions, as necessary to be exercised, from time to time, as every other; and what is more, every mother may be assured that, from the moment she cannot command herself enough to bear them, when it is necessary, without impatience, trouble or fright —without wishing to put a stop to them at any cost, and by all possible means, such as giving him the breast when he cries for it without needing it, and, still later, by yielding to every demand of his—that, from that instant, the control over him, that is so necessary to maintain, is lost. There is no further hope of regulating his physical any more than his moral education. It is no longer the mother who will govern the child; it is she who will be governed by him."

It is not necessary to lay down any fixed rule, as to how often a new born child should nurse; yet it should not be permitted to nurse too frequently, and the intervals should be somewhat regular. Perhaps at intervals of from two to three hours, during the day, and from three to five hours during the night, would be the average, as to frequency, best adapted to the wants of children, until the age of three or four months. The child should never be allowed, night or day, to remain at the breast continually, nor should it ever be given the breast simply to quiet its crying; for, as Dr. Dewees truly remarks:

"If this system be pursued, much inconvenience will result; for one or two things must happen.

"First: If the child do not cry from absolute pain, a bad habit will be generated; for the child will cry for the mere gratification of being nursed; this will not only create a great deal of trouble, but will be highly injurious to the stomach itself, by occasioning it to be overloaded, and thus producing vomiting, purging, or colic.

"Secondly: If the child cry from actual suffering, the food may not do any possible good, or it may much increase the evil, by its being given at an improper or unnecessary time."

Let an adult take even a small quantity of food often, say every two or three hours, and an unnatural craving soon results, and the digestive organs soon become deranged; pains in the stomach, flatulence, colic, and, not unfrequently, diarrhœa, ensue. With how much more certainty must the delicate organs of the child be deranged by too frequent nursing or feeding. The infant may take liquid food more frequently than an adult can solid food, without injury; but its stomach must have seasons of rest, or disease will result, as surely, as in the case of the adult. Some writers recommend nursing children, even young infants, but three times a day, and they tell us that they thrive well, when thus nursed. That this is much better than it is to nurse them every hour or two I do not question; still, experience has shown, that they may be nursed more frequently than this without harm, say once in three or four hours, during the day, after they are three months old.

Regular sleep is all important for the health of the mother, and it is very important that the child should be got into the habit of sleeping at night; and by a little care in not allowing it to sleep much during the afternoon, and evening, there is generally no difficulty in getting it into the habit of resting all night, without waking more than once or twice at most. It is neither necessary, nor desirable, that the youngest child should nurse more than once or twice during the eight or nine hours the mother requires for sleep; and, after a few weeks, if nursed at the hour for retiring, it is quite as well for it to sleep until morning; or, at most, not nurse more than once during the night. If the mother can have her regular rest, she will be much more certain to have a good supply of nourishment, and of a good quality, for her child, than she will if she is disturbed several times during the night.

DEFICIENCY OF MILK.

It not unfrequently happens that mothers, owing to some constitutional defect, or from debility, ill health, or from mental emotions, have not a sufficient secretion of milk to supply their children; in other cases they may have enough at first and it may gradually fail; or perhaps not increase with the increasing growth of the child. In such cases it is not uncommon for mothers to resort to the use of certain stimulating drinks, for the purpose of increasing the secretion of milk. In regard to the propriety of such a resort Dr. Condie, in his work on the "Diseases of Children," says:

"The only drink of a nurse should be water—simply water. All fermented and distilled liquors, as well as strong tea and coffee she should strictly abstain from. Never was there a more absurd or pernicious notion, than that wine, ale, or porter, is necessary to a female while giving suck, in order to keep up her strength, or to increase the quantity, and improve the nutritious properties of her milk. So far from producing these effects, such drinks, when taken in any quantity, invariably disturb, more or less, the health of the stomach, and tend to impair the quality and diminish the quantity of the nourishment furnished by her to the infant."

Another medical writer, speaking in regard to the use of such beverages, says:

"The constitutions of both are stimulated by them beyond what nature ever intended that they should be. The laws which govern the animal economy are positively infringed, and it is impossible that either mother or infant can escape the penalty of that infringement. Both will suffer to a certainty in some shape or other, if not immediately, at a future period. * * * * Thousands of infants are annually cut off by convulsions, etc., from the effects of these beverages acting upon them through the mother."

Dr. Wm. B. Carpenter, the most celebrated English physiologist, in his Prize Essay on the use and abuse of Alcoholic Liquors, says:

"The regular administration of alcohol, with the professed object of supporting the system under the demand occasioned by the flow of milk, is 'a mockery, a delusion, and a snare.' For alcohol affords no single element of the secretion; and is much more likely to impair than to improve the quality of the milk."

In regard to the use of fermented liquors, after detailing a case in which the use of a single glass of wine, or a tumbler of porter, per day, was followed by a speedy and marked improvement in the condition of both mother and child, he says:

"But it may be questioned whether the practice *is in the end* desirable; or whether it is not, like the same practice under other

other circumstances already adverted to, really detrimental, by causing lactation to be persevered in, without apparent injury at the time, by females whose bodily vigor is not adequate to sustain it. Such certainly appeared to be the case in the instance just referred to; for the system remained in a very depressed state for some time after the conclusion of the first lactation; and on subsequent occasions it has been found absolutely necessary to discontinue nursing at a very early period of the infant's life, owing to the inadequacy of the milk for its nutrition, and the obvious inability of the mother to bear the drain. Hence it may be affirmed with tolerable certainty, that the first lactation, although not prolonged beyond the usual period, and apparently well sustained by the mother, was really injurious to her; and the inability to furnish what was required, without the stimulus of alcoholic liquors, was nature's warning, which ought not to have been disregarded. Considering, then, that lactation (unlike pregnancy) may be put an end to at any period, should it prove injurious to the mother, the writer is disposed to give his full assent to the dictum of Dr. Macnish; that if a woman cannot afford the necessary supply without these indulgences, she should give over the infant to some one who can, and drop nursing altogether.'—'The only cases,' continues Dr. M., 'in which a moderate portion of malt liquor is justifiable, are when the milk is deficient, and the nurse averse or unable to put another in her place. Here of two evils, we choose the least, and rather give the infant milk of an inferior quality, than endanger its health, by weaning it prematurely, or stinting it of its accustomed nourishment.' Now upon this the writer would remark, that a judicious system of feeding gradually introduced from a very early period in the life of a child, will generally be preferable to an imperfect supply of poor milk from the mother; and that if the mother be so foolish as to persevere in nursing her infant, when Nature has warned her of her incapacity of doing so, it is the duty of the medical man to set before her, as strongly as possible, the risk—the almost absolute certainty—of future prejudice to herself. The evils which proceed from lactation, protracted beyond the ability of the system to sustain it, may be to a certain degree kept in check by the use of alcoholic stimulants; but the writer is convinced from observation of the above and similar cases, that its manifestation is only postponed. Under no circumstances, therefore, can he consider that the habitual or even occasional use of alcoholic liquors, during lactation, is necessary or beneficial."

Then, when the mother does not furnish a sufficient supply of milk for the wants of her child, instead of resorting to alcoholic or fermented drinks, it is better that a wet nurse should be obtained, if a suitable one can be found. The next best course is to commence making up the deficiency by feeding cautiously, and at proper intervals, with cow's milk, instead of striving to increase the secretion from the mother's breasts, beyond what will result from a good, nourishing, plain, unstimulating diet, and out-door exercise. If no effort is made to excite an unnatural flow of milk, it will not generally do the mother any harm to continue to nurse, even although she may not have over one-third or one-half enough for the child; and such an amount may be sufficient to sustain the child, and preserve its life, in case of serious derangement of the stomach and bowels. It is desirable that the aliment which the infant receives, in addition to the mother's milk, should approach as near the latter in quality as practicable; and, in this country, cow's milk, when proper precautions are used, is the best substitute for that from the human breast we have. Among the most pernicious kinds of nourishment for a young infant, may be named those miserable compounds of flour and milk, cracker, or bread and water, or oatmeal and water which are fed to children under the names of pap, panada, and water-gruel. The powers of the infant's stomach are inadequate to digest properly these substances. Dr. Eberle truly says:

"Let the infant's stomach be once or twice filled during the twenty-four hours with gruel, or any of the ordinary preparations prepared by nurses for this purpose, and the chances will probably be as ten to one, that acidity, vomiting, colic, griping, and jaundice will supervene."

A frequent cause of failure in the secretion of milk is to be found in the use of an unusually stimulating diet, under the plea of having to support two. This is especially true of hired wet nurses, when they are taken into the families of the wealthy. The change of diet from a coarse, plain, perhaps rather scanty diet, to rich, stimulating food, with the free use of meat, and unusual in-door confinement, is very sure to make the system feverish, and lessen the quantity of milk, as well as impair its quality. In all such cases instead of seeking to increase the milk by the use of porter, or ale, the nurse should be put upon a plain, coarse diet, as near like that she had formerly used as possible, and required to take active exercise especially out-doors.

"I have always observed," remarks Dr. Marley, "that if a woman who is nursing, eat heartily, but not immoderately of plain food, avoiding that which is stimulating, she will, generally speaking, preserve her health, the result of which will be a plentiful secretion of milk. I consider meat once a day as quite sufficient."

WEANING.

UNTIL the child is at least six or eight months old, he should receive no food except from the breast, provided the mother or nurse has a supply; and if she has not a full supply, nothing in addition but cow's milk should be received, unless a physician, for some particular derangement, should prescribe some substitute for milk. After this age, children may be allowed to partake once or twice a day of rice flour, arrow-root, potato-starch, or tapioca, prepared with milk and sweetened. Two or three months later, if the child has made some progress in getting its teeth, stale bread, or cracker may be crumbled into the milk of which he partakes; and still later, roasted potatoes, carefully mashed up with cream, may be added to the articles of which he partakes. As a general rule it is well not to give much if any meat, or animal broth too soon.

"Until after the first dentition is completed," remarks Dr. Condie, "solid animal food, in our opinion, should form no portion of an infant's diet; it is apt to increase the febrile excitement to which the system is already predisposed, and to augment the irritability of the digestive organs, which is an almost invariable attendant, to a greater or less extent upon the process of teething."

The proper period for weaning the child entirely from the breast, is, generally, at the age of from twelve to fifteen months. Strong and healthy children may sometimes be weaned with safety earlier, and delicate children who have not made much progress in teething, may require nursing longer. In doubtful cases it is well to consult a physician, as to the proper age and time for weaning.

BRINGING UP CHILDREN BY HAND.

THE difficulty of bringing up children "by hand," has been pointed out by medical writers, and is generally admitted by mothers.

"I am convinced," remarks Dr. Merriman, "that the attempt to bring up children by hand proves fatal, in London, to at least seven out of eight of these miserable sufferers; and this happens, whether the child has never taken the breast, or having been suckled for three or four weeks only, is then weaned. In the country, the mortality among dry-nursed children is not quite so great as in London, but it is abundantly greater than is generally imagined."

I am satisfied that if the mortality in our country is not equal to what it is in London, it is at least so great, and the injury to the constitution of those who do live, is such that it becomes the duty of parents, when the mother, from any cause, is not able to nurse her infant, to spare no pains to get a wet nurse, provided it can be done without depriving some other little one of the nourishment he may need as much as their own child. The writer feels called upon to say a few words to parents who may lose their children before they are six months old, from any cause, save the bad quality of the mother's milk; or who may have still-born children at or near full time, and are abundantly able to nurse a child. From the best evidence we have, in regard to the danger to children in bringing them up by hand, it is safe, perhaps, to calculate that, in our country, a new born infant stands at least twice the chance to die when fed, that it does when nursed. Therefore, by consenting to nurse the child of a neighbor, or even stranger, you have within your reach the ability, in one case out of two, of saving the life of some anxious mother's child, on the one hand; or by neglecting so to do, of permitting it to perish while you have the ability to rescue it. I am aware that to nurse the child of another, will be attended with labor, and anxiety; but all this will be more than compensated for, by the consciousness of having performed a good and noble act, and having done your duty as a philanthropist and Christian, under circumstances in which you have been providentially placed towards a fellow being.

COW'S MILK.

It not unfrequently happens, when the mother is not able to nurse her child, that it is impossible for the parents to obtain a wet nurse, and there remains no resource but to bring it up by hand. If it is very important to select a proper wet nurse, as it certainly is, when we obtain one, it is even more important to select proper nourishment for the child when we are obliged to feed it. As neither goat's nor ass's milk, which is often used in Europe, is accessible in our country, cow's milk is generally used; and it is true beyond question, perhaps, that this is the best food we can select until the child is at least six months old. In case of sickness other articles may sometimes be required to take the place of milk, for a temporary period; but a physician who is acquainted with all the circumstances, in a given case, is alone qualified to judge when this is necessary, and what substitute should be chosen. But there are many points to be attended to in the selection and use of cow's milk, which it is very important, for the welfare of the child, should not be neglected. In the first place it is very important that the milk should be taken from a single cow, and not a mixture from several. Then it is important for a young infant that the cow should not have been giving milk less than two or three weeks, or more than three or four months, if it can well be avoided. Cow's milk should be slightly alkaline, but it sometimes occurs, especially when the cow has been milked several months, that it is slightly acid, in which case it is very apt to disagree with children. Then in selecting a cow from which to obtain milk, for an infant, it is always well to test the milk by the means of blue litmus-paper. Hold the end of a narrow strip of this paper in fresh milk, for a short time, and if it changes it to a red color, the milk is acid, and not suitable to use for a young child, but another cow should be selected. Good milk will change red litmus-paper to blue, after some minutes contact. Litmus-paper can be found at the druggists. If milk which is being used disagrees with a child, or causes disturbance of the stomach and bowels, it should be rejected and the milk from another cow tried, but test the milk, as above directed, before trying it. For an infant it is important to use the milk which is first drawn, as it is much weaker than the last which is obtained, and will not require diluting with water, which may impair its quality. The first-drawn milk need not be diluted, but should be sweetened a little by sugar of milk, or in case that is not at hand, a little white sugar. Milk which has been boiled is not as easily digested as unboiled milk, and it is generally better only to heat it to the right temperature for drinking, and it is best that this should be done in a water-bath —that is by setting the dish containing the milk into a vessel of boiling or hot water. It would be better still, were it generally practicable, to give milk directly from the cow, while still warm, if it does not seem to be displeasing to the infant.

As the child becomes two or three months old, it will not be necessary, or in fact best, if it is well, to confine it to the first drawn milk, but milk the whole together and feed from that. In case of delicate or sickly children, it is well to look to the cow's food, as it may affect the milk for good or evil. Ordinary fodder produces milk of ordinary quality. It is said that, "carrots produce the lightest milk, and the most easily digestible; the one, in fact, best suited for the milk of sick children. Beets, on the contrary, produce the most substantial and richest milk." (DR. DONNE.)

As has already been stated, the mortality among children brought up by hand is fearfully great; even when the utmost care is used, it is much greater than among those which are nursed. It is well for both parents and physicians to bear in mind that young children which are being reared by hand, when they become exhausted and feeble from derangement of the stomach and bowels, can often, in almost desperate cases, be rescued by a resort to woman's milk, even although it be continued but for three or four weeks, or until the stomach is able to digest the first portion of the milk from the cow. If a wet nurse is obtained it often happens that an infant which has been weaned, or never nursed, cannot be made to nurse; then it frequently occurs that it is impossible to obtain a wet nurse, even if the child would nurse. In either case, in cities and villages, where derangements of the bowels are most common, by a little labor and care the little sufferer may often be saved by a resort to woman's milk. There are many mothers who have more milk than their own child requires, and who have the ability of extracting, or "milking" it, from their own breasts, without difficulty; who, if application was made to them, would cheerfully furnish, for three or four weeks, one or two meals a day, to save the life of a neighbor's child. Three or four such mothers can readily furnish enough to sustain a child, without robbing their own children, even if they have not a very abundant supply. If the child is not too feeble it may be taken around to the residences of the ladies from whom it is to receive its different meals, as the open air will be of service. If it is not able to be taken out, the mothers who are to furnish nourishment, should visit it at different hours, when it is required, until it is able to be taken to them. Four meals a day will be plenty, and three will do very well; and the infant should receive no other nourishment, and this should be given immediately after it is drawn from the breast, while it is warm, so as not to require heating. No harm will result from the child's receiving its nourishment from three or four different nurses, if a little care is used in selecting mothers, for such purpose, whose own children are not under three or four weeks of age, unless the one to be fed is under that age; nor is it well that their children should be over six or eight months old, especially if the one requiring the food is very young. About the same care is requisite as in the selection of a wet nurse. The course indicated above, has been pursued, and the lives of children have been saved by it; and when no other nourishment can be found which agrees with the infant, in cases of cholera infantum, and bowel complaints, it is worthy of more attention than it has yet received.

FOOD PROPER FOR CHILDREN AFTER WEANING.

The principal food of children, until they are at least three or four years of age, should consist of bread and milk—milk boiled with rice, and sweetened moderately—plain rice pudding—roasted potatoes—plain puddings of tapioca, arrow-root or sago—soft boiled eggs, and simple meat broths, with crums of bread or cracker. It is generally not well to give children meat, until they are at least three or four years old; and, as a general rule, it is better during childhood and youth to discourage rather than encourage the inclination to eat meat, if the young person is strong and healthy without it. Children should never be allowed a great variety of food at the same meal, nor any which contains the least particle of pepper or any other spice, or condiment, except a moderate quantity of sugar or salt. Our cooks in this country, are the most terrible enemies our children have to encounter, and when we look at the food, of which the children of many thoughtless parents are permitted to eat, it is not surprising that so many die, or grow up poor puny dyspeptics. They are often permitted to live almost entirely on articles and substances, which should never enter the stomach of a child. A correspondent of the Poughkeepsie *Daily Democrat* says:

"While visiting a school in Montreal, he asked the teacher if there were any American children there. She said there were, and she could tell them by their pale faces, bright eyes, and nervousness. They learned quicker, but lost so many days during the term from sickness, that they did not get along so fast as those who were able to be present constantly. He also took occasion to examine their luncheon baskets, and found the American fare to be a piece of mince pie, the same of pound cake, two doughnuts, a pickle, and a cold sausage; while the English, Irish, and Scotch children had either two days old bread and butter, or bread and apple with nothing else."

Butter may be used with moderation when cold, but never in the form of rich gravies. Plain custard, and bread-pudding, moderately used, are not objectionable, and sweet, ripe fruits may be used with moderation; currants and cherries are more objectionable, especially for young children.

It is very important that they have their regular meals, and that they are never allowed to eat between meals. "Children," says Dr. Condie, "who have no regular times for their meals, in general eat too much, and when refused food, however often they may crave it, become fretful and discontented." "They eat all day long—and soon impair their digestive powers, and become sick and debilitated," remarks another writer.

As an entire chapter is devoted to the consideration of the use and abuse of the digestive organs, where the reader will find suggestions which are even more important to be heeded in the diet of children than in that of the adult, it is not necessary to consider this subject further in this connection.

EXERCISE, AIR AND LIGHT.

In the chapter in which these agencies for physical development are considered, their importance has been fully pointed out. It only remains, in this connection, to make a few specific suggestions in regard to their application in the case of infants and young children; for in the chapter on Education, the attention of the reader is called to their influence on the development and health of the young, during the years devoted to educational purposes.

During the first two or three months after birth, the infant should be handled but little, and should never be placed in the erect or sitting posture; nor jolted, nor tossed up and down, for the bones are soft and pliable, the joints are imperfectly developed, and the muscles are small and feeble, and such violent measures may do injury to its delicate structures, and cause serious disease or deformity. It should be allowed to lie quietly in its bed or cot, or carried in the arms in the horizontal position, or permitted to ride in the same position in a small carriage. Rocking is injurious, and may cause unpleasant nervous symptoms, and even disease of the brain, and should be avoided. Accustoming children to go to sleep in the arms, or on the lap of the nurse, or mother, is injurious to the health of the child, by its being confined in an uncomfortable position, rendered hot by the heat of the body, and. preventing sound sleep. Begetting a habit difficult to break, it renders the child exacting, and teaches it to subject the persons who attend it to its own will, and thus does it a moral injury. Children, especially delicate children, should always be required to go to sleep in their own bed, placed there while awake, and required to lie till sleep comes. This soon becomes a habit; it is better for the child, and saves the mother from an immense amount of drudgery, as well as loss of sleep, and exposure during the night. After the first two months the child should be allowed to lie on the bed, or on a soft cushion, spread upon the floor, and amuse itself, and use its limbs freely, which is far better than for it to be held in the arms of a nurse; also there is less danger of deformity. A child should not be encouraged nor allowed to sit up too soon, for curvature of the spine may result. Nor should an attempt be made to induce it to stand on the feet, or walk too soon, as crooked legs frequently result from such a course. It is better to retard rather than to hasten walking.

In warm weather, so soon as the infant's eyes become accustomed to light, so as to be able to bear the light of day, it should be carried into the open air; care should always be taken, during early childhood, not to expose the eyes to the direct rays of the sun. Even in winter, not more than four or five weeks should elapse, after its birth, before the infant should be taken into the open air, during pleasant weather. In cold weather children should be well protected by clothing, and should be out but a short time at once, as very young infants are easily chilled by severe cold. Until the child is able to walk it should be carried into the open air and light frequently, and spend as much time as practicable out doors. After this period, as Dr. Donné truly remarks, "It is not enough to give a child the outer air in the streets of a great city, to make him pass from his nursery into a parlor or shop, or to have him take a ride in a carriage; he must be allowed to play in the open air, during the greater part of the day." Dr. Hoffland, as quoted by the above author, says: "It ought, then, to be for us a sacred and unavoidable duty not to let pass a single day without procuring for the child so important and life-giving enjoyment." "Let the beginning of life," says Dr. Condie, "the first six years, perhaps, be devoted entirely to forming the body and the organs of sense, by exercise in the open air."

The above are not the words of enthusiasts but of careful observers—of scientific men—but how are they heeded by the American people? Daily as I witness the delicate, thin, pale-faced little children, which are confined most of their time in the parlors, sitting-rooms, and nurseries of the wealthy, and in fact, of all who are above want, in the goodly city where I reside, my heart sinks within me at the sad sight of innocent children perishing for the want of the necessaries of life—air, light, and out-door exercise. Notwithstanding the fearful mortality among the young children of the wealthy, and comfortable livers, in every city throughout our land, and the fact that a majority of those who do not die young, grow up delicate, nervous, sickly, vicious, and worthless, still no systematic effort is made, even by parents, to rescue these little ones from suffering and an untimely grave. We have meetings and societies formed, and are a very benevolent people—or claim to be—when the object is to benefit our fellow beings at a great distance—in India, or Africa, or the Islands of the sea, or a distant part of our own country. Or, coming nearer home, we can sometimes get up a little enthusiasm in the way of an effort to school, clothe, and feed, the ragged children of the poor in our own city; but where are our societies for liberating—not the slaves down South who have no lack of light, air, and exercise—the children of the rich and middling classes of society, from the miserable prisons, or large gloomy houses, within whose walls the little sufferers, by thousands, are gradually, but surely, being destroyed by being deprived of the life giving air, the glorious sunlight, and the free use of their limbs? The angels plead, through the bright eyes and sweet smiles of our little ones as they point their hands toward the door, for the exercise of that charity at home which shall save our babes and innocent children, from suffering and death, and we heed them not. We are moved to enthusiasm by a knowledge of the minor evils of heathendom, and of other sections of our own country, but blind, and deaf, to the monster abuses and crimes against the infantile portion of the community in our very midst; as though it were worse to cast an infant into the Ganges to die quickly—a not very painful death—than it is to deprive it of light, and air, and feed it with high-seasoned food; thus causing it to die by inches, amid untold suffering; or live on for a few years a sickly wretched existence, to perish by disease, or premature old age.

Search the wide world over and no object of benevolence can be found more needy, or more worthy, than the children in our cities whose parents are above actual want. The children of the poor show by their very looks, that they fare better as to food, air, light and exercise, than the children of the rich, except in rare instances of actual starvation. It is only by the liberality of the wealthy, or by concert of action among others, that proper play grounds can be furnished for the children in our cities; for, to the disgrace of humanity, even in our Western cities, with a few worthy exceptions, the miserly grasp of avarice, as manifested by the acts of land owners, the original layers out of our city plots, whose farms have been made mines of wealth to them by the hard labor of other men, has no more dedicated proper breathing places, or play grounds for children, than it has lungs or parks for adults. Almost every inch has been sold at the highest price it was possible to obtain, and it frequently happens that what remains is only left because the cry, give, give, has not been able to extort from the needy purchaser, the coveted dollar. There is now but little prospect, except for those who have already been unkindly shaved, to provide suitable play grounds and parks, at an extravagant cost, or go without them. Truly the injustice of man, not only to his fellow man, but even to innocent children, is enough to warm the blood of him who does not heed the command, "Fret not thyself because of evil doers; neither be thou envious against the workers of iniquity;" or who does not remember that "Riches certainly make themselves wings; they fly away," if not in the present, almost certainly in a coming generation.

The day will come when the men who shall donate proper play grounds for young children, and provide for their perpetual superintendance, in our cities, will be regarded as among the noblest benefactors of our race; as much more worthy of being held in respectful remembrance, than the builders of hospitals and asylums; as the preservation of the health and lives of thousands of children annually, is more important than simply providing extra comforts for a few sick or deformed adults. The one charity prevents untimely death, and prevents and eradicates disease and deformity; the other simply palliates the evils of humanity—a worthy object, but immeasurably less important; for the sick and deformed may perish through neglect, and the physical integrity of our race not be seriously impaired thereby; but if the vitality and vigor of childhood is impaired through neglect, not only innocent children suffer, but humanity is impaired at the fountain head, and innumerable generations yet to come, will suffer.

The importance of play grounds, in connection with schools, will be considered in the chapter on Education. I am now speaking of their importance for children between the first and seventh, or eighth years. When we bear in mind that in order for the proper development of children, and the preservation of their health, during this period, it is absolutely necessary that they should be in the open air, and light, all the time during the day, except during severe storms; and that this is as important for girls as it is for boys, we can begin to realize the importance of play grounds for the *young children* in our cities. In a suitable play ground, in an airy location, a single nurse or governess, can take better care, with less danger of accidents, of thirty children, and give them more agreeable exercise in pleasant company, than it is possible for thirty nurses to do in our streets at present. Better care, and greater safety, are not the only good which will result from such play grounds: for parents will know where their children are, and that they are not off in some unwholesome alley, or street, in uncertain company, on a visit to the friends of the attendant. Then again, it is impossible to find, as a general rule, a governess who will faithfully spend her whole day in the streets, and public parks; (where there are any) so that, at present, most of our children, where parents take the utmost care, are cheated out of no inconsiderable share of the needed out door recreation. Then, multitudes of parents do not realize the importance of having their children out doors all the time, and, consequently, make no efforts for such a result; and a large majority are neither able to provide proper attendants, nor spend their own time with their children constantly out doors; so rather than to turn the latter out, loose, and permit them to risk, neck, limb, and morals, they keep them in the house, and when, as a consequence, they become pale, delicate, nervous, and susceptible to disease, and die from croup, inflammation of the lungs, bowel complaint, or some epidemic or contagious disease, with greater frequency than healthy and strong children, it is regarded as "a dispensation of providence," and of course, no one is to blame. No one thinks of forming societies for the purpose of rescuing these poor children from suffering and death, or from moral pollution, if parents should prefer turning their children into the streets to the risk of destroying them by confinement—the Fejee Islanders, the Hottentots, the Burmese, the Chinese, and the inhabitants of numerous other heathen nations, are not all converted yet. African slavery is not abolished, and, say the acts of the present generation, "of what consequence are the health, lives, and morals of the children of our cities, compared with the conversion of the heathen, or the abolition of slavery, or tyranny, in some distant part of the world."

"But," says the reader, "what would you have done for our children which we do not do?" I will tell you in a few words: At best the air in our cities, even the out door air, is not of the purest quality and the sun's light is dim, therefore I would not have the child, at the age of which we are considering, deprived one moment of their influence during the day except when at meals.

I would have all parents, who are able, and who care for the welfare of their children, form societies, of suitable size, purchase a piece of ground in a good airy location, and fit it up as a play-ground for their little ones, employing a suitable governess or two, to take charge of them while on the ground. Having done this, let them send to this play-ground, immediately after breakfast all their children over one, and under seven or eight years of age; let them be sent for at dinner and back again immediately after, to remain there until they are sent for in the evening. I would have parents do this every day, without fail, except when they have the desire and disposition to be with their children out doors, themselves. I would have a small building on one corner of the ground, so that a fire may be kept there in cold weather to warm the children, when necessary; and so that if the younger ones get fatigued and sleepy, they may have a suitable place in which to rest, and sleep, a short time.

Or what would be better still, and not much more expensive, I would have parents who are able, obtain a suitable park, adorned by shade trees for very hot, and cheap buildings for cold and stormy weather, outside the city limits in the fresh air and undimmed sunshine; then let an omnibus, with a governess, gather up the little children in the morning, with their dinners, and take them without the city to their play-ground, to spend the day in healthy exercise, in breathing pure air, and receiving the much needed solar rays, and fresh milk from cows running in an adjoining pasture. At night let them be returned to their parents blessed by the invigorating influence of the natural elements. The children alone would not long be allowed to monopolize such a "fairy-land," but our sickly delicate mothers would soon, upon every possible occasion, accompany their little ones, and find health and happiness. A similar course to this is pursued by parents in some of the cities of Germany, with the most satisfactory results; and, if adopted, in our cities, would save thousands of children from suffering and death, every year. A little concert of action among parents, which would benefit the neglected social faculties, is all that is needed to make the children of our cities as healthy as those in the country. Why do we neglect such a simple life-preserving measure? It is safe to say that at least one half of the children who now die in our cities between the ages of one and seven years, would be preserved from death by this simple measure.

When benevolent parents have thus cared for their own children, I would like to see them look around, form societies, and obtain play grounds for the children of their poorer neighbors. Then I would like to see some of our ladies, who are imbued with the genuine missionary spirit, volunteer to act as matrons for such play grounds. They will not have to risk the dangers from the fevers and climate of India, or Africa; and if they do not gain the notoriety and eclat, which they might have obtained as foreign missionaries, they will at least have the consciousness of having done far more good than they could ever have done in foreign lands. When the physical and moral wants of the children of our own land, are provided for, I shall certainly be heart and hand in favor of extending our benevolent operations to other lands, for I verily believe heathendom is not as well off as it should be. Even now it is not so much my object to weaken the support, which distant objects of benevolence receive, as it is to point out, in strong and true colors, evils of far greater magnitude in our very midst; and to stir up, if possible, my countrymen to a sense of their duty to the greater sufferers nearer home. It is safe to say that the providing of suitable play grounds with their attendants, convenient to every family in our cities, or conveyances for carrying children out of cities during the day, as above suggested, where all, both rich and poor, may receive accommodations, aside from the physical and moral benefit which would result to them and future generations, it would save the lives of more mothers, by preventing our delicate women from being worn out by excessive labor, care, and anxiety for their children, than all the hospitals and asylums in our country, do, or can, save of the diseased, the halt, and blind; and certainly no one can question but that the preservation of the health and lives of the mothers of our land, is quite as important as that of the poor, deformed, and outcast portion of our population; not that I would have the latter neglected, or that I do not honor, to the extent they deserve, the labors of worthy philanthropists in such directions.

MORAL MANAGEMENT OF CHILDREN.

UPON this subject a volume might be written, but I propose simply to point out some of the abuses which can, and should be avoided by all. The child should early be taught to obey his parents; this is important for his safety and health, as well as for his moral welfare. Mildness, kindness, and firmness should characterize all the words and actions of the parent, while giving commands which it is expected the child will obey; and a parent should never be hasty in punishing for disobedience.

"Be careful," says Locke, "before punishing a child for obstinacy, that his fault really arises from willfulness, and not from childishness, or inability to do what you bid him. Inadvertency, forgetfulness, unsteadiness, and wandering of thought, are the natural faults of childhood; and, therefore, where they are not observed to be willful, are to be mentioned softly, and gained upon by time."

A child is full of life, and it is not always easy for him to stop immediately, while engaged in any pleasurable amusement or exercise, at the command of the parent; and, instead of repeating the command in a harsh, or perhaps angry tone, it is better to speak gently, or perhaps present some new object to attract his attention. If it becomes necessary to punish, a parent should never do it while angry, or in a harsh and revengeful spirit; for a bad example is set the child which will more than destroy all the good effect expected from the punishment.

"All attempts to prevent or soothe the fretfulness of an infant by cakes, sweet-meats, and confectionary, should be absolutely prohibited," for children soon learn to cry for such things, when they find that crying will bring them; and they are injured by eating these improper substances, and by eating at improper hours.

A child should never be hired to obey, but required to do it as a duty; and always required to do the bidding of his parents, and never allowed to feel that he can disobey with impunity even in the smallest matter. If a steady and firm course is thus pursued, obedience will become a habit, and a pleasure to the child; and he will come to love and respect his parents, which he can never do sincerely if he is not required to obey them. A little watchfulness, kindness and firmness, will generally save the necessity for punishing the child, and is much better, for the former cultivates and strengthens the habit of obedience, whereas the latter does little more than restrain for the time being. The utter impossibility of parents, who are not able to be with their children out doors continually, teaching them efficiently correct principles of obedience, and seeing that they conform to them, without destroying them by in-door confinement, is a strong argument in favor of such play grounds as I have advocated in this chapter, and shall again speak of in the chapter on Education. We, as a community, have most shamefully neglected our children during their play hours, as well as in undue confinement from play, until disobedience to parents, teachers, and civil officers, and even contempt for religious teachers, has become the rule in our cities and villages among those children which have not been nearly or quite destroyed by confinement. Nothing can be more destructive to the future happiness of the young, or to the best interests of the community, than this spirit of reckless disobedience which we witness around us.

It is but a step from disobedience to parental requirements and laws, to contempt for and even hatred of parents; and from thence to contempt for all laws, both civil and Divine. If we would prevent crime we must teach children while young to respect and obey parents, teachers, and civil officers; and this would cost the community far less than it now costs to punish crime, as will be shown in the next chapter.

Parents should remember that children soon learn to imitate the improper language and actions of others, and it is important that they not only be careful what example is set before them, but also that they do not encourage or countenance the manifestation of perverted passions in the child. This is often done thoughtlessly by parents and others; for instance, a child accidentally gets hurt, and to pacify him, a stick is given him, with which to strike the article of furniture by which, or the individual by whom he has been hurt, and thus if he is pacified, his combativeness is being cultivated, and the spirit of revenge is planted deep in his soul. The same is true of vanity, which is doing a worse work for our American people than any, or perhaps all other evils. This monster vice is the parent of innumerable other evils, at this day; for the scramble for money is generally to gratify love of approbation; the same is true of all the destructive fashions which are so prevalent; and of many of the pernicious habits, such as using tobacco, and alcohol.

The young commence the use of these poisons to gratify vanity, and soon find it necessary to continue to use them to relieve the unnatural cravings they cause. If there is any one passion in the child, which his present and eternal good requires should not be cultivated, and stimulated, it is certainly love of approbation; for when perverted, as it is with the American people, it tends, in a thousand directions, to destroy all happiness, by leading to never ending discontent, jealousy and strife; and, sooner or later, unless overcome, to the destruction of both soul and body. Yet parents, even thoughtless Christian parents, in many ways, cultivate, directly strengthen and develop, the inclination to vanity in their children, and thus do them an irreparable injury.

"A correspondent of the New York *Tribune*, writing from Saratoga Springs, speaks thus intelligently and mournfully of the blight which falls upon the American children, cursed in early years by the indiscretion and folly of vain—shall we not say wicked? parents: The passion for jewelry is instilled in the cradle. It is disgusting to see nurselings with rings and bracelets, and so on upwards through all gradations of age. It is especially American, and we must suppose this fashion is borrowed from the Indians. * * * Their little embryo minds and hearts are already poisoned with coquetry and love of show. They have beaux (an expression considered vulgar, and nowhere used in Europe,) receive calls, bouquets, make appointments; rivalry and envy in their ugliest shape early take possession of their souls. For years I have observed this disease all over the country, in all cities where I have seen society. Above all it is painful to one's feelings at the hotels and watering-places. When I see here in the evenings, in the parlors, rows of these little dolls and fops dressed, ribboned, jeweled, fanning themselves monkey-like, in imitation of the elder part of society, I feel an almost irresistible itching in the fingers to pinch their mammas. Nurseries seem not to exist in America. In this respect the manner of bringing up children is far superior all over the continent of Europe. There children are kept children as long as possible, and all care of parents and families is bestowed to watch over the tender blossoms, and preserve them from the heating, unwholesome influences of parties and motley company.

'"It was so once likewise in England, until the bad example given by the reigning Queen, who, in her fondness for her numerous progeny, originated, or at least made fashionable these juvenile parties, in which children fully equipped in all the freaks and oddities of grown-up persons, represent withered dwarfs. Should I follow the prevailing absurdity of classing virtues, qualities or oddities according to races, this description of infantine naturalness should be called Anglo Saxon or English. But it is a disease, and as such it may be human, or it may result from certain combinations of social life, extending beyond the contracted and exclusive assignment of certain attributes, to certain races. One thing is certain, that no such bejeweled, affected, distorted little creatures as are to be met in America, in streets, public and private parlors, at juvenile and grown-up parties, were called to Himself by the immortal teacher of simplicity, love and sincerity."'

WHY SO MUCH BEAUTY IN POLAND!—"Because," (says Bayard Taylor) "there girls do not jump from infancy to young ladyhood. They are not sent from the cradle to the parlor, to dress, or sit still and look pretty. No, they are treated as children should be. During childhood, which extends through a period of several years they are plainly and loosely dressed, and allowed to run, romp, and play in the open air. They are not loaded down, girded about and oppressed every way with countless frills and superabundant flounces, so as to be admired for their much clothing. Nor are they rendered delicate nor dyspeptic by continual stuffing with candies and sweet cakes, as are the majority of American children. Plain, simple food, free and various exercise, and abundance of sunshine during the whole period of childhood are the secrets of beauty in after life."

DRESS.

"The essentials in the clothing of children," remarks Willis, a writer of the last century, "are *lightness, simplicity* and *looseness.* By its being as light as is consistent with due warmth, it will neither encumber the child, nor cause any waste of its powers, in consequence of its simplicity, it will be readily and easily put on, so as to prevent many cries and tears; while by its looseness it will have full room for the growth and due and regular expansion of the entire frame; a matter of infinite importance for the securing of health and comfort in after life."

But "Fashion," as Dr. Dewees, in his work on Diseases of children, truly says; "has exerted a baneful influence over the best feelings of the mother, for she has become willing to sacrifice the health and well-being of her offspring to its shrine. The preposterous, and unsightly exposure of the arms of children cannot be too loudly reprehended, since it has neither convenience or beauty to recommend it; yet it is attended by the most serious, and manifest injury to the child."

A serious charge, truly; but, alas! we have abundant evidence that it is but too well founded, and applicable to, perhaps, a majority of our American mothers.

"To have," says Dr. Condie, "the neck, shoulders, and arms of a child nearly or quite bare, however warmly the rest of the body may be clad, is a sure means of endangering its comfort and health; violent attacks of croup or bronchitis, or even inflammation of the lungs, are often induced by this irrational custom; and it is not improbable that the foundation of pulmonary consumption is often thus laid during childhood. It is an important precaution, therefore, to have the dress worn by children, so constructed as to protect the neck, breast, and shoulders, and with sleeves long enough to reach the wrist."

Such is the testimony of medical writers, as to the danger to children, and young ladies, from wearing short sleeves and low-necked dresses; and there is, perhaps, not a physician in the whole land who does not bear testimony against this style of dressing children, as being destructive to health and life; and yet short sleeves and low-necked dresses, are as freely worn by the children of a majority of our parents, as they would be if they never were the cause of the death of the young. It almost seems that vanity as Dr. Dewees intimates, is a stronger passion at this day, in our country, than love of children, at least with a majority of our mothers.

It has been shown, by anatomical investigations, that there is the most intimate relation and sympathy, between the arms and the lungs and air passages, which accounts for the great danger of causing diseases of the latter organs, by exposure of the arms; and explains the reason why fomentations, or hot applications to the arms, will often relieve oppression and congestion of the chest more readily than the same applications to the chest itself, or to the lower extremities. The shoulders, upper portion of the chest, and lower portion of the neck, should never be exposed, for there is no part of the body, except, perhaps, the arms, which more require to be properly clad, in our variable climate, than these; and to expose them in children, is cruel in the extreme. It not only endangers their lives, but it is a mode of dress which, with the utmost care that can be used, is sure to cause deformity of the shoulders and chest, as will be shown in the chapter on the Fashions and Habits of of the Ladies.

The wearing of thin-soled, and thin shoes and stockings, is also a fruitful cause of disease and death, among children. Parents in this country do not realize the importance of keeping the legs and feet of their children and daughters warm and dry. There is the most intimate relation and spmpathy existing between the lower extremities and the abdominal and pelvic organs. Inflammation of the bowels, diarrhœa, and dysentery frequently result from exposure of the legs and feet in children, and suppression of the menses, and disease of the womb and ovaries, in young ladies. In no country, perhaps, in the world are the lower extremities so recklessly exposed as in the United States. Europeans, especially the English, wear good, substantial, and thick-soled shoes.

"Among the items," says D. H. Jacques, in his work on Physical Beauty, "particularized in the published accounts of the bridal outfit of the Princess Royal of England, on the occasion of her marriage with the Crown Prince of Prussia, is the following: 'Twelve dozen pairs of boots of useful and solid make; some of them intended for rough walking, being provided with treble soles, and small but projecting nails.'

"'Only think,' an American newspaper says, 'of some of our paper-soled, delicate-footed damsels, sporting, by way of novelty, hob-nailed, tripple-soled shoes! Does any one doubt, however, that such an innovation would do more to preserve the roses in fair cheeks than any style of hygiene which the faculty could recommend? We denounce often the fashions of England as monarchical—we think the Princess Royal might set us good republicans an example in the matter of *understanding*.'"

Our thin-soled shoes are not only very injurious to health, but they are very expensive, as it will take several pair, to do the service which one good, substantial pair of English shoes will do; and yet, the difference in the cost holds no proportion to the difference in service.

Since the introduction of hoops the lower extremities, and even the lower part of the body, are but poorly protected, by clothing, against the cold, and it is very important that not only good, thick woolen stockings should be worn, but also good, substantial and tight flannel, or, what is better, broad cloth drawers, extending to the shoes, should be worn by girls and ladies during cold weather. In no othef way can the lower extremities be properly clad, with the present style of dress, and danger to health and life avoided.

The wearing of flannel has been all the rage with many, and it has been earnestly recommended by physicians; and, I do not question its efficacy during the changeable weather of spring, and fall, and the cold weather of winter, but during the hot weather of summer it should be omitted. I question very much the propriety of wearing flannel next the skin, except on the extremities, but prefer its being worn over cotton, linen, or silk; as all the benefit so far as protection is concerned, is derived when it is thus worn, without its creating any unnatural irritation of the skin.

Miss Harriet Martineau, in speaking of "Dress and its victims," says:

"As for the children—how many have been swept off pathways, or foot-bridges, or steamboat decks by the pitiless crinoline, or hoops of some unconscious walking balloon! More children have been killed, however, by the extension of the absurd petticoat fashion to them. For many months past it has been a rare thing to see a child under the tunic age duly clothed. The petticoats are merely for show; and the actual clothing, from the waist downward, is nothing more than thin cotton drawers and socks, leaving a bare space between. For older boys there is a great improvement in dress—the tunic and loose trowsers being preferable in every way to the stiff manish tailed coat and tight trowsers of half a century ago. But the younger children are at present scarcely clothed at all below the arms; and the blue legs of childhood are a painful sight, whether in a beggar boy or a citizen's son. * * * In winters like ours to see children's legs covered with nothing better than thin cotton (thin, because the ornamentation is the vanity,) is in fact reading the sentence of death of many victims. Let it be remembered, too, that the neuralgic, rheumatic, and heart diseases thus brought on are of a hereditary character.

"What is to be done? Will any thing ever be done? or is feminine willfulness and slavishness to fashion to kill off hundreds and thousands of the race, as at present?"

CHAPTER VI.

AN IMPERFECT SYSTEM OF EDUCATION ONE OF THE MOST PRODUCTIVE OF THE CAUSES OF DISEASE, INSANITY AND DEFORMITY IN OUR COUNTRY.

IT requires no argument to show that the most important duty and use which men and women have to perform in this world, is to train and properly educate their children; and society has no higher duty to perform, and none more important, so far as the welfare and preservation of our race is concerned, than to look after and care for the rising generation.

The young of the animal kingdom, beneath man, are born into all the science, or receive by perception or instinct, all the knowledge which is necessary for their preservation and happiness, and are capable of but a very limited and imperfect improvement; but the young child, although more ignorant and helpless than the young of the brute creation, possesses the capacity for endless improvement, both intellectually and morally; and into the hands of parents, guardians, and society, is given the responsibility of training up the young immortal in the way he should go, that when he is old he need not depart from it. It becomes us, in view of the physical suffering, mental depravity and ignorance, which we so generally witness around us, even among the young to inquire how we are discharging our duty to the rising generation; and no time could be more suitable than the present when the selfish pursuits of men have received a check, and the attention of the community is so generally turned to the subject of christianity. True religion has relation to life, and the life of religion is to do good from the love of the good and the true. We have a right to expect that men and women will more earnestly desire to know their duty, and strive to do it in all the relations of life. But before we can understand how a child should be trained and educated, it is necessary that we have some knowledge of the being we are to educate. First, then, man has, while he lives here, a natural body, which is given him that he may live in this world a life of usefulness, and in due time, that his spirit, which is within the physical body, and gives life to it, may be prepared for a better world. Now the fact that man has a physical body, is almost entirely ignored in our present system of education and juvenile training, and most fearful are the consequences to our race. A more fatal mistake could scarcely be made; better, far better, that the intellect should be neglected; but we will let this rest for the present. Man, spiritually, *may be* divided into the will, which is the seat of the loves, and the understanding, which is the seat of the intellectual and rational faculties. We will leave to phrenologists and metaphysicians to subdivide these two great departments of man's spiritual nature, as they may see fit.

Man is but a receptacle of life, and we should ever bear in mind that he does not possess life of himself, for by so doing, we shall be able to perceive more clearly a most important law of both physical and mental development, namely, that the capacity to receive will depend upon the use which is made of that which has already been received.

The child, then, which is to be educated, possesses not only intellectual faculties, which require to be cultivated, but also affections, which supply, as it were, the motive power to the intellect. It must be evident to every one, upon reflection, that it is of immeasurably more importance, that the affections of the child should be properly guided and educated, than it is that the intellect should be stored with the knowledges taught in the schools, for the affections compose the very substance of man's spirit, and upon their right development depends man's happiness here and hereafter. Yet this all important department of man's spirit is neglected almost entirely, in our present system of education. This is by far the most pernicious and destructive mistake which could be made. It is bad enough to neglect or destroy the body, but it is worse to neglect or destroy the spirit within the body. By simply cultivating the intellect, we may store the memory with knowledges which have no relation to life and which, so far from making the individual better, happier, or more useful in his day or generation, will leave him egotistical, cold, selfish and miserly of his intellectual treasures. The great aim, in the acquisition of all knowledge, should be to lead the possessor to a true life; and use should be the leading motive for the acquisition of knowledge, that we may be able to live in accordance with natural and spiritual laws, and be more useful to our fellow men.

Let us ever bear in mind the important facts that the child has a physical body, as well as a spiritual organization; and that it has affections, as well as intellectual faculties, which require to be educated or trained, even more than the latter; and yet, by observation we can but see, that our present school system not only neglects these important departments of a true education, but it also does violence to both the physical and affectional portions of the child's nature, to an extent that renders our public schools even worse than none, if they cannot be improved; that is, unless we can regard a cultivated intellect—with morals depraved—a diseased and suffering body, which will transmit a delicate organization to children, and result in a destruction of the race, as greater blessings than physical health, an uneducated intellect, and a degree of true living, and moral goodness, which is not incompatible with health and life. It is far from my aim, or desire, to tear down or destroy our schools and institutions of learning—for I well know that the hope of the world lies not in that direction—but, to stir up my countrymen to the importance of adding to, and of perfecting our present imperfect system, and of making it what I have reason to think it may be, and faith to believe it will be,—the salvation of our country, both physically and morally. If man were but a machine, and not free to *will* to do good or evil, but would of necessity do and live according to the teachings he might receive in our schools and churches, our present system of education would not be so deficient.

The physical body, intellectual faculties, and affections, are all parts of one whole, and it is all important, in order that we may realize the highest state of development of which the young person is capable, that each department of his being should be developed in harmony with the rest. A premature development of a part is at the expense of the whole. Of the three great departments of the child's being, I have named, there is far less danger of doing harm by striving to develop the body, and neglecting the faculties of the mind, than there is in prematurely developing the latter, especially the intellect, and neglecting the body, from the fact that the body is the organism, and, as it were, the basis, through and from which we have all the manifestations of mind in this world. If the body is imperfectly developed, deformed, or diseased, through neglect, want of proper training, or violence done to it, it is impossible for the mind ever to reach the stage of highest development of which it would have been capable in a well developed body.

If the proper development of the physical organism does not take place during the days of childhood and early youth, the chance is in a great measure lost forever; and a comparatively puny and delicate body, and a life-time of suffering and disappointed hopes are almost inevitable. Whereas, if the intellect is neglected during the same period, but a healthy body secured, even although the young man or woman may not know his or her letters at the age of eighteen or twenty years, with industry and perseverance a good practical education can be obtained. If we strive to prematurely develop the intellect of a child by undue mental application, an unnatural flow of blood is directed to the brain, to supply the unnatural activity and consequent waste which is going on in this organ; therefore the rest of the body suffers. Nor is this all, for all premature development of a part is necessarily but an imperfect development of even such part; for this reason, we rarely ever hear of our precocious children in after life as distinguished men or women. How much more important then is the physical education of the child, than the intellectual; and we have but to look around us at the puny, pale-faced, deformed children in our streets, to see how fearfully this most important department of education is neglected. I say *most* important, from the fact, that the moral education, which is perhaps the most important of all, is so intimately connected with the physical, as I shall endeavor to show, that the latter cannot be neglected, without almost destroying all good and noble affections, or at least, in a great measure preventing their development.

But the effects which result from our present system of education are not confined simply to the impairment of physical health, comparative mental imbecility, and perverted affections, according to the testimony of careful observers. The following I have taken from the New York *Evangelist.*

MODERN EDUCATION AND INSANITY.

"Dr. Ray, superintendent and physician of the 'Butler Hospital for the Insane in Rhode Island,' in his recently published annual report, affirms that much of the present mental infirmity and insanity, has its origin in the modern character of education. That is to say that 'the amount of lessons and task work imposed upon the young while at school' very often lays the foundation of mental weakness or aberration. This is a grave allegation, and coming from such an authority, it is entitled to calm and candid consideration. Dr. Ray makes his allegation in the following terms:

" 'To know what amount of work may be safely put upon the youthful brain, having reference to age, constitution, and endowment, would seem to be a matter of paramount importance, to be determined by all the light derivable from experiment and observation; but practically it is made subordinate to another and very different question, viz: how much will satisfy the public,—that public which mistakes the glitter of display for solid acquirement, and measures the skill of the teacher by the rapidity with which the pupil is pushed forward. The radical fault is the same which characterizes our movements in other departments of effort. We grudge the time a sound education necessarily requires, and are impatient to turn the acquisitions of the pupil to some practical account. Discipline and development may be theoretically recognized as legetimate objects of education, but practically they are regarded as subordinate to that which predominates over all others, viz: the means of distinction which it gives—the medals, prizes, honors. These are to be obtained if possible, and obtained quickly. Here, as everywhere else, speed is the only test of merit. Lesson is piled upon lesson, the hours of study are increased and the active, irritable brain of youth is habitually forced to the utmost power of effort.

" 'The effects of this system of over-studying is a disturbed or diminished nervous energy. It rarely comes immediately in the shape of insanity, for that is not a disease of childhood or early youth. The more immediate effects upon the nervous system, are unaccountable restlessness, disturbed and deficient sleep, loss of appetite, epilepsy, chorea, and especially a kind of irritability and exhaustion, which leads the van of a host of other ills, bodily and mental, that seriously impair the efficiency and comfort of the individual.' "

On the above the *Commercial Advertiser* makes the following judicious comments:

" Conductors of public education are not alone to blame in this matter. Parents and guardians share in the responsibility. They are far too apt to rank a school, public or private, according to the rapidity with which the pupil's powers of acquisition are made available in the progress of education. The pale complexion, the sunken eye, the ever present headache, and even the hectic flush are unheeded if the boy or the girl 'gets on rapidly with his or her learning;' or if heeded, the only remedy is postponed, or but partially applied. But this suffering of mind and body under a constant and excessive pressure is rarely attributed to its true cause, the forcing system pursued in that school. And the pressure does not cease with school hours. The boy brings home his books, or the girl hers, and with an ambition stimulated to the utmost by the system of marks, prizes, and exhibitions, continues the close application, during evening often till a late hour into the night, and with aching eyes and wearied brain, goes from his or her task to the greatly needed rest. But the brain is in no condition for sleep after such occupation, and the result is that the mind becomes jaded and dispirited, and the child enters upon the duties of the day, with little of that buoyancy which comes only from nature's sweet restorer."

It would seem that both parents and teachers ought to take warning from such testimony as the above. It is well known that insanity is rapidly increasing in our country, which is undoubtedly, owing in a great measure to the incessant mental excitement to which our people are subject. As like begets like, a tendency to excitable brains is transmitted to children; and this is a reason why the American children cannot safely be crowded as rapidly as those of less excitable nations without increasing the tendency to insanity.

MORAL EDUCATION AND ITS NEGLECT.

The intellect of the child is educated or developed by being taught truths by others, and by his learning, or storing the memory with various items of knowledge derived from the senses. As the child comes to years of discretion, by reflecting on the treasures thus stored up, the reasoning faculties are developed. But the affections of the child are educated or developed, first, by the manifestations of the affections which he witnesses in the acts of others, especially of parents, teachers, and playfellows; second, by his acting out himself the truths and knowledges he may possess; or else acting according to his hereditary inclinations. The intellect then, is developed by learning, and being taught; the affections by doing, and seeing done. Of course the child's ability to do, will depend in a great measure upon his possessing a knowledge of how to do; and the true use of knowledge is to teach him how to act and live. Truths and knowledges only become living when we carry them out into act, or when we have an earnest desire to do so, which may unite them with our affections. Until such time they are dead, being alone, and form no substantial part of our spiritual organism. Learning and doing, in a true education, must go hand in hand.

At least there must be a sincere desire to obtain knowledge for the sake of use hereafter, if not at present, in order for such knowledge to be abiding. Every one must be aware how much more impressive teaching is when the lessons taught are acted out in the life of the teacher, for they then reach the affections.

I well remember, while a very young child, following my father through a field, as he was crossing a rill, he accidentally stepped upon a little frog, and crushed him; he felt him beneath his foot, turned saw what he had done, and gave a single expression of regret. I do not remember the words, or even a word he used; but the act taught me a lesson which eternity cannot efface—that my father would not cause unncessary suffering, or do harm to the least of God's creatures; and that I should do likewise—and I am able to see clearly that the influence of that simple act over my subsequent life has been very great. I remember it distinctly as though it were but yesterday; while of the hundreds of sermons and lectures which I heard before, and even for years after that incident, scarcely a distinct vestige can I recall at this day. How different would have been the effect upon his son, if my father had said, in a thoughtless and petulant manner, "I am glad of it; served you right; you might have kept out of the way; there is one frog less in the world."

Truths of science are to the spirit of man, what water is to man's natural body; they relieve intellectual thirst. But as the latter, although a medium through which the body may be nourished, of itself gives no substance to the famishing organs, so simply educating the understanding gives no substance to the spirit of man; and the affections must famish or seek food elsewhere. We would certainly think a parent very unwise who should furnish his child for nourishment simply water, and allow, or even require him to go without or seek more substantial food, to supply substance to his body, elsewhere, as he can pick it up in the streets, alleys, and about the markets, at the risk of getting improper food, or perhaps even poisonous substances. Every one would pronounce such a parent unworthy the name of "father;" and if he were to build a splendid house, and employ accomplished waiters, and even dispense his water from golden goblets, when one-half the extra expense would supply substantial food, as well as drink, I rather suspect that we should all, without any hesitation, pronounce the man a monomaniac. And yet, we may inquire if he would not be doing better towards supplying natural nourishment for his child, than the parents of our cities are doing towards educating, or supplying spiritual nourishment for their children. We have built splendid school-houses and churches, and employed accomplished teachers and preachers, with all the necessary ornamental and useful appliances to tempt the desire for knowledge, and are able to quench the intellectual thirst even until our children are satiated, and become precocious prodigies, so far as the intellect is concerned. But how is it with the nobler part, the affections of the children? What are we doing towards educating the hearts of our children? —towards supplying food as well as drink for their indwelling spirits? Very little, almost literally nothing. Our children are famishing for bread, and we do not heed their cry; or, if we do, we give them little better than stones on which to feed their hungry souls. It is rare that a child has a natural appetite for natural substances which are poisonous to the physical body; but our children all inherit from their parents an inclination to do evil, therefore we all know that without proper example, and constant watchful care, they will almost necessarily act in accordance with their hereditary inclinations, instead of acting in harmony with the truths stored up in the memory; for such truths, as we have seen, are lifeless until they are united with the affections, or carried out into act by the child; or he sees them carried into life by others. So that we may inquire if the parent who is satisfied with simply teaching his child that which is right and allows him to run at large for living examples, and to act out his hereditary inclinations unrestrained, is not even more foolish and culpable than the one who provides his child only with water for nourishment?

Let no reader for a moment suppose that the writer desires to withdraw children, or remove them one moment, from parental society and influence, when the parent is able to devote that time and care to his child which his good requires. It is the duty of every parent and it should be his pleasure to spend every moment he can, consistently with the due performance of other necessary duties, with his child. But the child needs constant care during every hour of the day, especially while at play; he needs instruction also, and parents usually are not able to bestow all their time upon their children, nor are they always qualified to teach them, and it is with reference to such care as parents are not able to bestow that I am now speaking. The importance and even necessity of employing teachers is generally recognized; and we certainly spare no pains in our efforts to enlighten the understandings of our children; but, alas! of what avail is it, when we allow them to run in the streets, in crowds, and to act out their natural inclinations unrestrained, stimulated on by vicious associates, who set them the example of cheating, swearing, lying, fighting, stealing, and many other evil habits; and when, not unfrequently, such examples are set them by adult men and women? Or when we retain them at home, in our yards, without any associates with whom to develop their affections, to be influenced by the example of servants, who are often annoyed by their presence, and are not over amiable; or perhaps, are heedless, indifferent, or vicious? Have we a right to expect them to be swayed by the truths which are dormant in their memory, rather than by the living examples, which are in harmony with their hereditary inclinations? Experience certainly shows that we have not; that "evil communications will (even) corrupt *good* manners." And what are the examples of life, which the child witnesses at home, when he is kept from running at large, and kept from the society of servants? Are parents always able, amid the cares and perplexities of business, and daily duties to which most parents are too much confined, to set their children such an example of patient forbearance, kindness, and cheerfulness, during every hour of the day, as they desire them to follow? Are they able at all times to watch and see that in their amusements and sports, they always act and do right towards each other? Can parents allow their children always to have proper associates at home, with whom to develop good and kindly affections? and, if they can do this, are they willing to constantly hear the noise, and witness the confusion which must inevitably result from their engaging in proper sports—even necessary amusements? If parents have the virtue to perform and the patience to endure all this, they cannot confine their children, either boys or girls, to their houses, offices, stores or shops, any considerable portion of the time, without preventing the development of and destroying their physical bodies. So that in the present state of society in the cities and villages, especially of our country, where good behaviour among children in the streets is not enforced by police regulations and the watchful care of civil officers, and under our present system of education, the parent's choice lies between confining his children from the light of the sun, air, and active exercise, to an extent entirely incompatible with life and health, and thereby seeing his little ones, slowly but surely going to premature graves, or unnecessarily cut off by the diseases of childhood; or, on the other hand, turning them into the streets to see them morally polluted and destroyed; and even physically destroyed by the vices and follies of after-life. A terrible alternative indeed, and one which has caused me more mental anxiety than any other I have ever encountered in the path of life, and when I reflect that, even in a city of seventy thousand inhabitants, there are not parents enough who seem to care for the present and eternal welfare of their own children, to say nothing of the children of their neighbors, to establish even one school for the physical and moral education of the children of that city, I am sometimes led to inquire what claims we have for being considered a civilized and Christian community; while we are permitting even our own children to perish without systematic effort to save them: yea, more, as I shall hereafter show, in not a few ways hurrying them on to destruction. Vain boasting and empty pretentions are nothing; we are what we are, and it is well for us to occasionally examine our true characters, and see whether we are discharging our duties as philanthropists and Christians, or are being ourselves destroyed by selfishness, sensualism and vanity. Do you suspect that I have drawn an over-dark picture? Does not all experience show that the population of our cities is only preserved from destruction, by a constant influx from the rural districts? What right have we to permit our cities to remain, for the want of a proper system of education, one great charnel house for the country, when, as it can be shown, it is entirely unnecessary! A farmer who can have his children with him in his fields, in the open air and light, away from vicious associates, and, as soon as they are old enough to work, can keep them employed at active labor, can, if he is disposed, do something like justice towards giving his boys, and even his girls, if he will take them into the fields or garden, a proper physical and moral education; and during years gone by, they have done this to a considerable extent; but at present, vanity, that vampire upon American society, which, together with its obsequious servant, love of money, is doing so much towards destroying the population of our cities, is carrying devastation and ruin through our rural districts, as I shall point out in future chapters. The female portion of the population, in such sections, possess far less vigor of constitution, and physical strength, than was possessed by their grandmothers; and this is true, not only in the United States, but it seems by the testimony of English writers, that the same is true in England, where of course change of climate cannot be accused, as the cause of the difference. The causes of this degeneracy, both there and here, will be found in the violation of the laws of our being.

Play is to the child what labor, business and amusements are to the adult—the school for developing the physical body and affections, the most important departments of man's nature, as we have seen. I am fully aware that, in this age, intellect is regarded by perhaps the great mass of men, and even women, as first. And if a man is a candidate for an important office of trust under our government, or in our monied institutions, or even for a clerkship in a mercantile establishment, the questions are not, generally, is he good, honest and upright—but is he smart, learned, and can he talk well. And this respect which has been, and is being paid to superior intellect and learning, instead of goodness and integrity, has brought our government to the verge of destruction; many of our railroads and banking institutions to bankruptcy, and multitudes of our merchants to poverty. It is strange that a merchant should be so blind as not to see, that a man who will deceive and take advantage of the ignorance of a customer, will surely not hesitate, when opportunity offers, to take advantage of his employer.

The day has been, when more regard was paid to the heart than to intellect. No one would think of comparing George Washington, so far as intellect, scientific attainments, fashionable polish, and even oratorical powers, are concerned, with Aaron Burr. Both alike have completed their course, and have gone to their own. Burr, with all his intellect, scientific attainments, polish and eloquence, died in obscurity; neglected and despised for his many vices. His intellectual lamp went out in moral darkness, and his name can hardly be mentioned before our children. How different with Washington—a true and good man, who lived a life of usefulness, guided by strict integrity, with affections ever burning for the good of his country—he died the death of the righteous, and left behind him a name which will endure while time lasts, and an example which every parent delights to hold up for his child to imitate. Our nation is now reaping the natural fruits of a system of education which regards the intellect as more important than the affections, and therefore neglects the latter. And what are those fruits, that we need to covet them? Political corruption in high places, unbounded vanity, financial dishonesty, infidelity, and physical degeneracy, prevailing to an extent unheard of in the annals of history. Children and men may learn truths in our school-rooms and churches, but they are dormant until carried out into act, and thereby united with the affections, as we have seen. With the adult, the real man is built up, for good or evil, as he carries the truths in his understanding into life, or perverts them, in the external acts of his daily life—in all the affairs of business, labor, family relations, social intercourse and amusements, and works of benevolence. Man's physical body can be sustained in vigor by performing the active duties of adult life, aided, when necessary, by proper gymnastic exercises although, as will be shown in another chapter, amusements are far more important for the adult than is generally supposed. But the child is not prepared for the duties of active life, and the play ground is his school for the affections, and also for his physical body. And, if we will but stop a moment and reflect, it seems to me that we can but see, that proper teachers here are far more important than are our present teachers in our school houses; especially for children under twelve years of age; and even for those many years older.

For it is here that the child, or young person, outside of the family relations, receives his or her first practical lessons of life, for good or evil. It is here that practical lessons can be given, and the child stimulated by example, and the truths taught can be united with the affections and carried out into act, and thereby become immeasurably more abiding than when simply taught in the school-room or church. How important, then, that in all his little games and plays, the child should be taught to be kind and truthful, and required to act, strictly, honestly and justly. To avoid deceiving, cheating, stealing, lying and back-biting or slandering his play-fellows. Also, to restrain his angry passions, and to be kind and cheerful, even under disappointment and defeat; or to avoid boasting and self-glorification when triumphant. Also, to strive to assist and cheer the weak, by gentle words and kind acts, instead of teasing and making sport of them. How all-important, then, are out-door teachers, who shall teach and take charge of the children while at play; watch their every act and word, and see that no improper acts are done, or words uttered, and bestow that attention to the moral education of the young which it is impossible for parents who are engaged in the active duties of city life, constantly to bestow.

Here is an unoccupied field for missionary labor—if our civil government, which is so liberal in providing for intellectual education, will not take it in charge—far more important than can be found on the distant plains of India, or the burning sands ot Africa, or the isles of the sea. Not that I would have the latter neglected, but the future of the world depends much upon the success of Christianity in OUR country, and the evil man will sink immeasurably lower here than in pagan lands. What! so zealous to Christianize the poor, ignorant, and therefore comparatively irresponsible Hottentot or New Zealander, and yet neglecting our own children in our streets, unnecessarily permitting them to perish, not only spiritually, but even physically, almost en masse! Strange infatuation! most wonderful neglect of duty!

THE IMPORTANCE OF PHYSICAL EDUCATION.

As yet I have only considered the subject of education in detail, so far as the child's heart is concerned; it remains to take a more deliberate view of the short-comings of our present system of education, in regard to the physical development and organization of the natural bodies of children. Here we shall find, as I have already intimated, that our children are subject not only to the most dreadful neglect, but also the most destructive abuses. Our nation has, without much doubt, sank lower, in regard to physical education, than almost any nation on the earth.

Before proceeding to a consideration of the subject, I have thought best to notice hastily an article, entitled, "The Hypocrisy of Gymnastics," recently published in the "Scalpel;" extracts from which have been extensively published in the newspapers throughout the country. The following extracts, although containing a shade of truth, are calculated to do great harm.

The writer says:

"It has filled us with horror to see a proposal to add a gymnasium to every public school in this city. A boy, until he is fourteen or even more wants no exercise besides the plays he gets up with his associates in the open air; he will exercise from his natural impulse, and in the most rational and natural manner; so you need only give him a dry piece of ground, and a place to swim in in summer, and plenty of ice and snow in winter, and then leave him alone with his mates.

"Boys from eight to twelve years of age, who work in the gymnasium regularly (a bad habit,) often develop their muscles to a hideously ugly degree. Instead of the soft, plump, juicy outline of youth, we have the skinny, overworked, hard and dry outline of an old man, induced by over exertion at an age which does not demand violent exercise of any kind; besides this, we think such processes are apt to retard the growing of boys, and will ultimately destroy their carriage and figure when they become men. Our readers may have observed the same thing in the dissected appearance of the legs of some of our juvenile dancers."

The first paragraph in the above looks very plausible upon the surface, and the more so for the reason that it accords exactly—all except in the conditions named—with past and present habits; especially so far as leaving children alone with their mates; which, at a single sweep, leaves parents free from all anxiety in regard to their children's associates and secret habits. That children should have a "Dry piece of ground and a place to swim in in the summer, and plenty of ice and snow in winter," a plenty of open air and sunlight, and space for active games, will, perhaps, be questioned by no one; but is it true that children in New York, or any city in our land, have these favorable conditions? Is it true that children now actually get all the exercise they really need in order to develop substantial bodies? Are not boys and girls and particularly girls, in our cities, perishing for the want of play grounds, open air, light, and, especially, exercise? But supposing, as in country places, to a great extent actually occurs, children have all the conditions named above, does it follow that it is best to leave them without any instruction to educate the muscles of the body in their own way? and without any restraint over their passions? Is it true that children will always exercise, from "natural impulse," "in the most *rational* and natural manner," either physically, intellectually or morally? If this is true, why do we not teach a child to read, and then place before him all manner of books, and let him exercise his intellect in his own way? We do not do this, simply because we have every reason to suppose that our child will spend his time in reading novels, and books which will not develop his intellect in an orderly and useful manner. Allow children to associate without restraint, and how long is it before lying, swearing, and fighting, are confirmed habits, and secret vice is practiced by a majority of them? Allow children to exercise their muscles without instruction, or restraint, and how long will it be, especially in our cities, before they will spend a large share of their time in playing marbles, pins, and other games, which incline to a bad position of the body; and which, although they may develop certain muscles of the fore-arm "to a hideously ugly degree," will cause deformity and general debility of the body as a whole. We witness such results around us on every hand. The advocates for the introduction of calisthenic and gymnastic exercises into our schools desire to prevent and remedy such deformity, and develop a symmetrical, healthy and substantial body; and to produce such a result, teachers who shall instruct the children in such exercises, and in proper plays, and restrain the outbursts of passion, are at least as important as our present teachers. All such exercises, of course, should be in the open air when possible. A company of children will enjoy proper calisthenic, and gymnastic exercises, as much as they will many other sports, and even more, for they will see a use resulting from them. Physical exercises, when the hand of true science guides must ever be for development, and never be carried to the extent of retarding the growth of the child. We want "The soft, plump, juicy outline of youth," instead of "The skinny, overworked, hard and dry outline of an old man, induced by over-exertion at an age which does not demand violent exercise of any kind." Excessive work, or play, or exercise of any kind, especially when only a portion of the muscles of the body are brought into activity, will prevent the development of the body and cause deformity and premature old age. To prevent such a result, the direction and restraint of a qualified teacher is indispensable for the young, when parents cannot perform the duty of teachers themselves.

The publication of such an article as the one we are reviewing, by a medical man, in a medical journal, at this day of our country's need, may well fill the hearts of parents with "horror," as they behold their children suffering and dying for the want of systematic exercise, or physical training.

I have already hastily called the attention of the reader to the importance—even to the mind—of a well developed and healthy body. Rosseau says:

"The body must be healthy to obey the soul; a good servant must be strong; the weaker the body the more it encumbers and weakens the soul." He still further remarks: "If you wish to develop the mind of a pupil, develop the power which that mind has to govern, exercise his body, make him healthy and strong, that you may make him prudent and reasonable."

Both Aristotle and Plato required that children should be trained in the bodily exercises of the gymnasium for several years before entering upon their studies, and that such exercises should be continued in connection with their intellectual pursuits. The latter says:

"The excess of corporeal exercises may render us wild and unmanageable, but the excess of arts, sciences and music, makes us too trifling and effeminate; only the right combination of both makes the soul circumspect and manly."

Never were truer words spoken, and none more important to be heeded by the degenerate sons and daughters of this generation. Rothstein truly remarks, that "we employ a scientific horseman to train a valuable horse, but let the development of the *human* body go." Such is the wisdom, or rather folly, of this day, especially in the United States, a land claiming superior civilization and Christianity; and we are now receiving the just penalties which inevitably follow such neglect of our physical bodies. The careful and intelligent observer can but see, in the palefaced, delicate, nervous, distorted and deformed children growing up around us, abundant evidence that we cannot violate the laws of God, as manifested in creation, with impunity. Cleveland in his Essay on the Classical Education of boys, says:

"It is melancholy, indeed, in our institutions of learning, especially our Colleges, to see so many puny-looking young men; hollow chests, round shoulders, and bending body, are characteristics of our students, and premature old age or consumption carries off but too many of our most gifted men."

But yesterday I saw a student from one of the most flourishing Colleges of our country, where congregate from five to eight hundred students. I inquired of him what attention was paid to physical education; although such a question was almost superfluous, for I could have told by the physical appearance of the student then before me. He said that they had no gymnasium; no systematic physical training; some of the students worked some, and they sometimes played ball, and that it was no uncommon occurrence for students to break down, and be obliged to leave on account of ill health.

I inquired what attention was paid to the education of the affections; he replied—"We are taught to keep them in abeyance while pursuing our studies." A teacher might as well attempt to stop the pulsations of the heart as to attempt to prevent the affections flowing forth, either in innocent and useful, or vicious and pernicious acts.

When such a heartless philosophy governs the actions of our teachers, and they are thus reckless as to the physical and moral welfare of their students, and good seed is not sown, and good affections are neither stimulated by example, nor strengthened by being permitted to flow forth in proper recreations and amusements, under the direction of *living* teachers, is it strange that rank weeds spring forth, in such neglected mental fields as are found in the mental atmosphere of students, who are away from under the social sympathies and restraints of the home-circle? Is it a matter of wonder, that habits of idleness, dissipation and profligacy, are so frequently formed within the very walls of our Colleges; and that parents, in return for the healthy, virtuous, temperate, prudent, and industrious boy they have, under many sacrifices, sent to a literary institution, so frequently receive back a feeble, broken down, vicious, intemperate, indolent spendthrift? Students in such institutions are inclined to become listless and indolent, therefore they should be required, as a matter of duty —and this requirement should be imperative—to spend several hours during the middle of the day, in a regular course of active, systematic, physical training, and active amusements; such as will sustain the body and mind in health, and satisfy the demands of both for recreation. Let them thus spend a large portion of their time during the day, and they will be compelled to spend their evenings at their studies, instead of amid scenes of dissipation and folly.

I have often noticed the grass growing green and thrifty in the small yard which lies in front of one of the Detroit union schools. Not long since I inquired of one of the teachers how it happened that the grass was so green. He very promptly replied, "because we do not allow the children to go on to it, or tread it down." What! in the small yards which surround our public schools, which are not generally even a quarter large enough for necessary recreation and exercise, the children required to keep upon the narrow walks, and not even allowed to step upon the grass? As though a few square rods of green grass were of more consequence than the physical and moral development, health and lives of the hundreds of children who congregate there for instruction! O, shades of Aristotle and Plato! Are the parents of our cities in a Rip-Van-Winkle sleep, or are they blind, or perhaps mad, and consequently reckless in regard to the consequences to their little ones.

Hufeland advises "to let the child, until the seventh year, pass the greater part of the time in bodily movements and gymnastic games of every kind, and mostly in the open air, for that is most healthy." Yet, in our country, parents do not hesitate to send their children even at the age of four or five years, to school, where they are required to sit still six hours a day on hard benches. To confine a child under twelve years of age, to the school room six hours a day, is an outrage which should not be tolerated a day. Two or three hours at most is the extent for which such young children should be confined; nor can they be confined a longer time without injury. In the healthy air of the country, where they have a chance for active out-door play in the fields, when out of school, they may stand it for a few months in the year; but not almost the year round, and they should never be thus confined, even in the country, for a single day. Parents often send their young children to school to get rid of them, and to know where they are, and will even complain if the teacher does not keep the poor restless little creatures there the full period of six hours a day. Yes, parents who are loudest in their complaints and denunciations, if the lecturer or clergyman happens to detain them, by the length of his discourse, more than one hour and a half, once or twice a week, do not hesitate, and that apparently without the least compunctions of conscience, to require their poor little children to sit upon hard benches, four times as long, for five days out of the seven; and will even complain if they have not the privilege of doing it on Saturday.

I know, by observation, that adult men and women will complain bitterly, if they are required to sit six hours a day and listen to lectures, with an intermission of five minutes at the end of every hour. Nor can they stand such confinement, without taking particular pains to counteract its effects by active out door or gymnastic exercises. What right have we, then, to suppose that delicate young children, who are growing, and, more than at any other period of life, need exercise, air and light, can withstand such confinement with impunity; and, more especially, when little or no attention is paid to their physical education, out of the hours of imprisonment in the often crowded and imperfectly ventilated and lighted school room? Is it strange that under such treatment, our children fade and die young, or live to grow up delicate, nervous, dyspeptic or consumptive, men or women? To every one who understands the laws of physical development, it is not strange.

"Children," says Dr. Condie in his work on Diseases of Children, "are frequently confined to the school room for many hours daily, when not occupied in any useful pursuit; which time, without detracting from that necessary for the cultivation of the mind, might with great propriety, be devoted to those bodily exercises and recreations, which tend to develop the strength, and promote the regular and energetic action of every organ of the frame—the brain and nervous system included."

" Sir Walter Scott," says a writer in the Atlantic Monthly, "gave it as his deliberate opinion in conversation with Basil Hall, that five and a half hours form the limit of *healthful* mental labor for a mature person. 'This I reckon very good work for a man,' he said—adding, 'I can very seldom reach six hours a day; and I reckon that what is written after five or six hours' hard mental labor is not good for much.' This he said in the fullness of his magnificent strength, and when he was producing with astonishing rapidity, those pages of delight over which every new generation still hangs enchanted."

If five and a half hours is the extent to which the adult can be confined to steady mental labor with safety, it must be manifest to all, that the young man or woman between twelve and twenty cannot safely be confined to close study and recitation, a longer period than four hours daily.

"To suppose the youthful brain," says Dr. Ray, of the Providence Insane Hospital, in a recent report, "to be capable of an amount of work which is considered an ample allowance to an adult brain, is simply absurd, and the attempt to carry this fully into effect, must necessarily be dangerous to the health and efficacy of the organ."

Yet in defiance of the laws of both the physical and mental constitutions of the young, it is no uncommon thing—in fact it is almost universal—for teachers and parents to confine the young and immature, of both sexes, six hours a day in school, and then to stimulate them to excessive study, not only in school, but also out of school hours, by offering rewards and presents to those who shall excel in mental attainments. Thus is the brain over excited, and the body impaired or destroyed, and even if the individual lives to middle or old age, it is but to be a mental dwarf, in a prematurely broken down body. But all this is not the worst which results from this system of giving prizes in schools, for the most infernal passions are developed by it. The child is not thus taught to strive to obtain knowledge and to develop both body and mind in harmony by due exercise of every organ and faculty of both, in order that he may be useful to his fellow man, and do good, but he is practically taught to strive to store up knowledge, as the miser heaps his gold, that he may excel others, out-shine them, glory over them, or to gratify his vanity.

If he is disappointed and others excel him, jealousy, envy, and hatred result—the natural fruits. Even Sabbath school superintendents and teachers are, I am sorry to say, sometimes found engaged in this work of destruction.

The necessary requisites for physical development and preservation are, a due supply of proper food and drink, wholesome air, light and exercise. Although an imperfect development may take place when these requisites are but imperfectly supplied, still we can never have a robust and healthy organization under such circumstances. Without a due supply of food and drink, the body languishes, or dies for the want of nourishment. If the food or drink is improper or poisonous, it causes disease and even death. Without air man can live but a few moments. If the air contains an excess of poisonous gases, or exhalations, or lacks a due supply of oxygen, debility, disease and death may ensue; according to the extent of the change from healthy air. Without the aid of light, vegetable development will not go on to maturity; and animals and men can only sustain a sickly and imperfect organization, from the fact that they feed upon food which has been already organized, in the vegetable or animal kingdom. Without a due supply of light the skin becomes pale and bloodless, the flesh soft, the bones, especially in children, are imperfectly developed, and are flexible and yielding, instead of compact and solid; curvatures of the spine and deformity of other bones ensue; the teeth decay, from the lack of healthy structure, and even the very blood becomes changed, loses its red globules, becomes watery, and possesses less vitality than healthy blood; and the whole system becomes much more liable to contract diseases of almost every kind. The effects, or consequences, which result from a lack of exercise, are very similar to those which we find ensuing from a want of light. With the child but an imperfect organization takes place, the adult becomes and remains puny, the structures of the body soft and liable to disease. If the mind of an individual deprived of exercise is unduly excited, or even excited to the extent a well developed person might bear with impunity, the individual becomes liable to a variety of mental and nervous diseases. It is the harmonious development of both body and mind, in all their parts, which gives health and life in their highest manifestations—a noble, robust, well formed man or woman.

Exercise is not only indispensable for the development and preservation of the body as a whole, but also, it is equally important for the growth and strength of each organ and member of the body; for even every muscle will grow strong by proper exercise, or weak, delicate and emaciated for the want of it. In the development of the vocal organs of the accomplished speaker or singer, or of the arm of the blacksmith, the leg of the professional dancer, and of the general muscular system of the circus actor, we can see what wonders can be accomplished by the systematic training of parts, or the whole of the muscular system. Even all the senses are quickened by their legitimate use, and the organs through which they are manifested grow strong and vigorous from being used, whereas, if not used, they slowly but surely lose their ability to perform the functions for which they were intended. In some of the fish which swim in the dark waters of the Mammoth Cave there is scarcely a vestige of an eye left; and in most, or all of them, this organ is very imperfect. Almost every nation on earth has had, and does have, its manly sports and games of strength and skill; which, although the players are not generally guided by the hand of science, still do much toward developing the human body, and sustaining symmetry of form. But among many of the nations of antiquity physical exercises were taught, and among some of the nations of Europe to-day, they are taught as a science, and the gymnasium is a necessary part of a school or a college. In no nation is this more important than in the United States; for, after the days of childhood are over, it is almost literally all work, or idleness, and no play; for we here see little attention paid to those athletic games which have saved other nations from destruction. Active physical labor is almost our only dependence for both physical development and preservation, after the child is a few years old. Yet, this is generally entirely insufficient to develop and preserve symmetry of form, as but a portion of the muscles, in almost any occupation are brought into energetic action, therefore, while those grow strong from use, others, from want of exercise, grow small and feeble. For this reason we find our laboring men, even our active farmers, often grow round shouldered, one sided, or otherwise deformed, and sooner or later diseased.

All this may be, and should be avoided by a frequent resort to gymnastic exercises, or active games, which will bring into action the muscles and parts of the body not used during labor. It is wonderful how much can be accomplished towards rejuvenating the deformed, delicate and diseased bodies of even adult men and women, by systematic training in the gymnasium. I can hardly believe my own senses, on witnessing the feats of strength and activity of men who, during years gone by, have visited my office for that relief from debility and disease, which they have now found from the active exercises of these truly important institutions. If the nervous, dyspeptic, delicate and deformed men and women of our cities would but spend a couple of hours daily in the gymnasium, the doctors would find fewer patients, and sextons would have more leisure for decorating our cemeteries.

Although our cities abound with delicate and feeble children, who need physical training far more than they do intellectual, still there is rarely a gymnasium in connexion with our public schools, nor even a yard, of sufficient dimensions for a playground, which the children are allowed to use. Nor is there, generally, the least systematic attention paid in our public schools, to this most important part of a true education. Our schools, in this respect, are far behind many of those on the continent of Europe.

Mr. Sedgwick in his address delivered before the Alumni of Columbia College, says:

"From the time that the boy, whose fortune it is to be educated, is immured in school, till the period when he is again to be immured in the lawyer's office, the counting-room, the dissecting-room, and from that time again until he enters upon the profession of his life, no systematic attention whatever is paid to the subject of physical education. All the health—all the exercise that he gets, he gets by nature or by chance. No regular opportunity is provided for it—no authoritative encouragement is given to it, no stimulus, no prize; all the ambition, all the zeal, all the ardor of his young, ignorant and unreflecting nature is concentrated on the vigil and the midnight lamp. Severe labor, long terms, short vacations, crowded rooms, late hours, bad air—what is the natural result?

"What can be the result? Well has it been said, that the mind perishes as the body dwindles. Not for the pale crowd of sickly dyspeptics whom our colleges annually turn out, are the great prizes of life. There have indeed been Pascals and Byrons and Channings who, despite frail and miserable health, have achieved immortal things; but these are only exceptions which prove a great general rule.

"It is the man of robust and enduring constitution, of elastic nerve, of comprehensive digestion, who does the great work of life. It is Scott with his manly form. It is Brougham with his superhuman powers of physical endurance. It is Franklin, at the age of seventy, camping out on his way to arouse the Canadas, as our hardiest boys of twenty now camp out in the Adirondacks or on the Miramichi. It is Napoleon, sleeping four hours, and on horseback twenty. It is Washington, with his splendid frame and physical strength. These are the men who make the names which the world will not let die. Miserable is the philosophy and the practice which fails to recognise the importance of the animal part of our complicated structure.

"What is there in our system to raise or develop such men? How is it possible for them to be produced by it? I mean our system of *education*. Among the classes which do not so much boast of their intellectual training, the physical man is indeed infinitely better cared for. If you seek among our people for bodily strength, look at the great turn-outs of our firemen. Look at our crack volunteer regiments exchanging national courtesies with our sister states. Among them you shall indeed find that sturdy vigor, that bodily strength and agility, without which all mental culture is but a preparation for disappointment and mortification."

The writer of an excellent article in the *North American Review* on "Gymnastics as a part of Education," says:

"O for a touch of the Olympic games, rather than this pallid effeminacy! O for a return of the simple Persian elements, of telling the truth and hurling the javelin, instead of the bloodless cheeks, and fleshless limbs, and throbbing brains of our first scholars in Harvard, Yale, or Princeton! But there is a medium, doubtless, between the ancient and modern discipline, by which we might secure the benefit and exclude the vices of both. And until some measure of this kind is adopted, we must continue to have our hearts agonized by the spectacle of brilliant scholars, dragging out a miserable existence, in unstrung and dilapidated systems, the mind, with all its tastes, faculties, and energies, tuned like an angel's harp, and performing all its fearful and wonderful operations to a charm, while its earthly companion, seconds its high functions in the feeblest manner, and jars and grates with its crazy aches and ills, in harsh discords amid the sublime concert of intellectual and spiritual harmonies.

"It needs to be rung into the ear of every educator, as with the peal of a trumpet that the body cannot be neglected with impunity; that in its effeminated capacities the morbid and monstrous passions will hold their saturnalia; and that only in its vigorous exercise and expansions, as well as in the development, culture, and equipment of the intellect, and the enriching and purifying of the heart, can the world have 'assurance of a man.' No school or college with any pretensions to be level with the spirit of the age ought to proceed upon the old system of drugging the intellect to satiety with knowledge, and leaving the physical and moral powers comparatively uncared for, since only as all the capacities are harmoniously unfolded, can any one of them attain its maximum of strength, usefulness and happiness. The ancient philosophers can yet teach us many a lesson of high wisdom: but they can give us no more significant symbol of the fine balance of their systems than the lovely walks of the gymnasium, the arena of active sports for innumerable youths, musical with voices of Socrates, Plato, and Aristotle."

D. H. Jacques, in his excellent work on "Physical Perfection," published recently by Fowler and Wells, says:

"The neglect of bodily exercise, which is compulsory in the school-boy and school-girl, becomes finally habitual; and men and women whose occupations do not necessitate their exercise, voluntarily allow many of the muscles of their bodies to fall into almost total disuse. And even those engaged in pursuits which call for considerable physical exertion, are generally well developed and strong only in particular parts. The blacksmith wields his sledge with as little difficulty as the child handles his painted toy, but ten to one, he cannot run a quarter of a mile without putting himself out of breath, or climb a rope to the ridge-pole of his shop without feeling the effects of his exploits for a week. So the farmer manages his heavy plow and follows it all day with ease, but talk to him of walking twenty-five miles a day (not to say forty;) climbing the precipitous sides of the Black Mountain, dining on its summit, and sleeping at night by a log fire, on a bed of fragrant boughs at its base; or swimming across a river a mile wide (easy feats for any tolerably healthy man with a good physical education,) and he will open eyes and mouth with astonishment. As to female pedestrianism (or any kind of out-door exercise, in fact,) the tradition of it has long since died out among us. In short, the lack of physical education shows itself in both sexes and in all ages and classes of people.

"The only school, so far as we know, where anything like an effectual system of physical education is carried out, is the National Military Academy at West Point. The pupils of that institution are graduated with broad shoulders, full chests, finely developed frames, and an erect and graceful carriage. In fact, they are generally among the finest specimens of manhood that we have had the pleasure of seeing. They go forth, as some one has happily said, 'fully armed and equipped with better than shield and spear for life's great struggle, even with the panoply of a vigorous sheathing of muscle upon a rock-like groundwork of bone, operated by untrembling nerves and steadily-beating pulse.' In the other professions, activity and vigor are generally supposed to be of no special utility. Our colleges with all the learning and wisdom brought to bear upon their management, manifest no clearer recognition of the body and its wants than the common school. The forcing system, commenced in the latter is continued in the former."

Ling, a celebrated Swedish philanthropist, invented a system of physical exercises founded upon scientific principles, the aim of which was to develop equally and perfectly the whole human form; and also to remedy deformity and disease. The advantages resulting from his method of training were so manifest that he became very celebrated, and was knighted, and appointed at the head of a public institution for preparing teachers to propagate it. His system of physical training was introduced years ago into all the military academies, universities, colleges, town and country schools of Sweden; and it has been carried into several other European nations, under the authority of their governments. But in the United States, even in this young-fogy country, it seems almost impossible to arouse our citizens to the importance of such a system of education, which every one can but know is much more needed here, especially for girls, than in the old world. A writer in the *Atlantic Monthly* says:

"It is beyond question, that far more out-door exercise is habitually taken by the female population of almost all European countries than by our own. In the first place, the peasant women of all other countries (a class non-existent here) are trained to active labor from childhood; and what traveler has not seen, on foreign mountain paths, long rows of maidens ascending and descending the difficult ways, bearing heavy burdens on their heads, and winning by the exercise such a superb symmetry and grace of figure as were a new wonder of the world to Cisatlantic eyes? Among the higher classes, physical exercises take the place of these things. Miss Beecher glowingly describes a Russian female seminary in which nine hundred girls of the noblest families were being trained by Ling's system of calisthenics, and her informant declared that she never beheld such an array of girlish health and beauty."

And this even in Russia, while in the United States we are neglecting the physical training of our children, notwithstanding our race is perishing from such neglect. In regard to our girls, the author of the work on Physical Perfection says:

"They are expected to be ladies, instead of children, and to avoid all those vigorous exercises which their natural instincts would lead them to engage in. Pale cheeks, indigestion, headache, nervous debility, and crooked spines, are among the inevitable results. Give us the romp, or tom-boy, with her vigorous limbs and her rosy or nut-brown cheeks, rather than the delicate little lady of ten summers. It is among the former, depend upon it, that the young men of the rising generation will look for their wives."

When will our parents, teachers and the superintendents of public instruction, arouse from this fatal slumber, to a sense of their duty to the children of our land? When will our churches arouse, and let their voices be heard in favor of the physical and moral education of our children? Nor is scarcely any attention paid by parents at home to the physical education of their children. They are either allowed to run wild in the streets, or confined in the house, when out of school, secluded from air and light; or in small, often unwholesome yards, without proper instruction, or companions to stimulate them on to physical activity; and yet parents expect their children to be healthy and strong, and are even so short-sighted as to suppose that their little boys and girls will grow up robust, possessing the physical requisites for performing the active duties of adult life, when thus trained. Strange infatuation! A short lived dream! Sad reality beyond!

"The London *Guardian*," says the *N. Y. Independent*, "gives a gratifying account of the new gymnasium at Oxford. The institution is the result of the efforts of a townsman, Mr. M'Laren. There appears to be little fear that modern Oxford should turn out many specimens of the class of students, once not uncommon, whose minds were exclusively developed at the expense of their bodies. The tide has, in fact, set rather strongly the other way. Your readers will be glad to hear of the movement—for so it may be called—which has been going on in favor of a scientific system of gymnastics—or physical education, as it is becoming the fashion to term it—of which the most zealous university reformer cannot but approve. Mr. M'Laren has spared no pains in visiting all the English and continental institutions of a similar kind, and has adopted all the latest improvements, besides inventing several of his own. It is not surprising that the number of his pupils should have so rapidly increased under this new impulse, that the cause really bids fair to become a recognized part of an Oxford education. It will be interesting to have a sight of the photographs taken for the purpose of measuring the effect of the course on different men. Here you will see a picture taken by the truth-telling sun of a poor emaciated student's chest, or rather the place where the chest ought to have been, his head drooping, his shoulders forward, and not a vestige of muscle to be seen. Lift it up, and the next is the same person at the end of the course. You can trace his features, but it is a man. His head is erect, his chest thrown out, his muscle developed, perhaps he has just won the 'belt.' It is clear that these results could not be attained by a chance application of exercise—they are the fruits of no inconsiderable amount of skillful treatment. The gymnasium of Oxford is, in fact, no longer an experiment, but an institution."

I am happy to see that some of our Colleges are encouraging, or at least, some of the American students are giving some attention to physical exercise, and that the good effects begin to attract attention. The New Haven *Palladium* says:

"For the benefit of those old fogies who may think that a fondness for boating and splendid physical training may unfit a man for the highest intellectual culture, we may say that the crew of the Yale College boat club comprise men not less distinguished among their fellows for scholarship and literary ability than for skill and muscle. Mr. Watkins graduates with one of the highest honors of his class, and his Greek oration at the Commencement yesterday, is spoken of with high praise. Mr.

Twitchell bears off one of the six Townsend premiums for English composition, which are among the most enviable honors of the college course. We find the name of Mr. Owen among those to whom prizes for composition and declamation were awarded; Mr. Colton stands very well in scholarship, and the college records will show that the others will not graduate without honors."

PROPOSED CHANGE IN OUR SCHOOLS.

It seems to me that it must be evident to every one who has his eyes open to the effects of our present system of education and training, upon both the physical and moral development of the children of our cities and country, that a reform is not only necessary, but indispensable. That we must pay more attention to the physical and moral training of our children, and not crowd the intellect of the child with studies which are only suitable for the adult, at the same time that we are not only neglecting both their physical and moral education, but also doing violence continually to both the body and the affections, or the heart.

How shall such a reform be brought about? We are already spending our money freely for the support of our schools, which are little better than prisons and the rack for our little children, as their delicate pale faces and slender bodies abundantly demonstrate. We are now spending tens of thousands of dollars towards building splendid houses, to make room to confine all the little children in our cities six hours a day to hard benches; thereby we are making ample provision for the destruction of the rising generation. Let us see what could be done with even less money, towards a harmonious and true education, which would preserve multitudes of our little ones from an untimely grave, or an adult life of debility and suffering; or of dissipation and crime. I think I speak within bounds, when I say, as a medical man, (and nine-tenths, if not every one, of the most intelligent and observing physicians of our land will bear witness to the truth of my statement,) that no child between the years of four or five and twelve can be safely confined in the school-room at diligent study and recitation, more than two hours a day—one hour in the forenoon and one in the afternoon; and that, if the rest of the time is devoted to physical and moral training in the open air, thereby developing a strong and healthy body, in which can dwell a vigorous mind, the child would actually learn more in the two hours, than he now does even in the six long—and I well remember how tedious—hours required by our present system. I also think I am safe in asserting positively, that no young person between the ages of twelve and twenty, the period of life during which the child becomes a man or woman, and both the human body and spirit undergo the most important change which takes place during life—can be confined with safety in the school-room more than three, or at most four hours a day; and that, if they do not acquire any more, or even quite so much, intellectual knowledge, the physical development and strength, and moral instruction, which would be received from proper out-door exercises and teachings, would far overbalance any defect in intellectual acquisitions; and leave the young person with a capacity for future intellectual attainments, such as the boy or girl can never have under our present system; for the intellects of our children are stunted by precocious development, like the pear engrafted upon the quince.

We are in the habit of sending our children to school quite too young. No child should ever be sent to school before the age of seven years, as nothing in the end is gained by it, but much is lost. The celebrated Dr. Spurzheim says:

"Experience has demonstrated that of any number of children of equal intellectual power, those who receive no particular care in childhood, and who do not learn to read and write until the constitution begins to be consolidated, but who enjoy the benefit of a good physical education, very soon surpass in their studies those who commence earlier, and read numerous books when very young. The mind ought never to be cultivated at the expense of the body; and physical education ought to precede that of the intellect, and then proceed simultaneously with it, without cultivating one faculty to the neglect of others; for health is the base, and instruction the ornament of education."

"A child," says a writer in *Blackwood's Magazine*, "three years old, with a book in its hands is a fearful sight. It is too often the death-warrant, such as the condemned criminal stupidly looks at—fatal, yet beyond his comprehension."

Our ablest men and women are those who are longest in arriving at maturity, as a general rule. Parents and teachers are too anxious to crowd the intellects of children, to be able to make them show off, without reflecting that comparative mental imbecility must inevitably result from this course. If children could have all necessary exercise, recreation and amusements, at school, in the open air, during daylight, and not be confined in-doors more than two or three hours during the day, they would need neither vacations, nor Saturdays for recreation and contamination; and they would be, physically and mentally, satisfied to spend their evenings at home, and would have the physical strength and energy, and might be required with safety, to spend a reasonable share of their evenings at their studies; so that they would be able to accomplish as much, intellectually, with perfect safety, as they do at present with the destruction of health and the hazard of life. Upon the supposition that one-half of the children in our cities, who are attending our public schools, are under twelve years, if they were required to spend but two hours a day in the school-room, and the older half but three or four hours, the average would be three hours or less, so that, by varying the hours of attendance, it will be seen that our present school houses would accommodate about twice the number of pupils they can under our present system. Now, to meet the wants of the increasing number of scholars in our growing cities, who are and will be seeking accommodation in our public schools, instead of building more school houses, let us purchase or rent, in the vicinity of our present houses, play grounds, and erect proper gymnastic fixtures in the open air and sun, for pleasant weather, and in cheap buildings for stormy and very cold weather. This will not cost anything like as much as it will to build houses, such as we are now building, to accommodate the same number of children. Having done this, let us keep the young children two-thirds of the time they are now in school, out-doors, and the older children one-half, or at least one-third of the time. This, in our large schools, will materially relieve the teachers in-doors, even if the same number of recitations are heard; as the time now spent in restraining the natural restlessness and playfulness of the children, will be saved, so that one or more of the teachers can be spared to teach the children out-doors how to use their muscles, limbs and body, so as to develop a symmetrical form; or correct any tendency of a part to deformity or disease, by bringing into activity the weak muscles and relaxing the strong, thereby saving them from being afflicted with round shoulders, distorted spines, narrow chests, and small waists; also from the multitude of diseases to which these deformities predispose. And, if the teachers in our school-rooms were all to qualify themselves for teaching the children out-doors, in necessary physical exercises and graces, and should alternate in out-door exercise and teaching, the poor, anxious, elongated countenances, which we so frequently witness among our teachers, would soon give way before the bright rays of the sun, fresh air, and regular, active, systematic exercise; and we should soon see in our school-rooms men and women physically worthy of being the teachers of our children—strong, robust, natural-colored and healthy; and all this without adding one cent to the expense we are now paying for the education of the children of our cities. In the city of London they are forming societies for the purpose of providing play-grounds, not only for children, but also for adults.

BENEFITS WHICH WOULD RESULT FROM THE CHANGE.

I NOW propose to consider some of the innumerable advantages which would result from the proposed change in our schools.

Such a change will tend to cultivate a love for active social recreation and amusements among our children, girls as well as boys, which will tend to keep the heart warm and kindly, instead of selfish, vain and penurious when the child becomes an adult.

I have made the following selections from different parts of an excellent editorial article in the Presbyterian *Quarterly Review*, for March, 1856. The entire article is well worthy of being re-published in every religious paper of our country: the writer says:

"The nation is morbid—physically, mentally and morally—and something must be done for its health and social life." After alluding to the evidences that our people are physically deteriorating, and making quotations from the New York *Times* and also from Miss Catherine Beecher's book to the same effect, he goes on to say: "We must express our sincere belief and regret that the statements as to the deteriorating physical condition, both of the men and women of the country, are true. The main causes seem to us to have been over-work, over-anxiety and want of exercise." In regard to exercise, the writer says: "Exercise will not and cannot be taken profitably as a mere matter of duty. A solitary walk or ride is a very imperfect method of reaching the object in view. See how boys take exercise. They need a large quantity of it, and they invent a thousand active sports. What genuine boy ever thought of the necessity of exercise in playing ball or skating, with half a hundred of his fellows? This is nature's own prompting; the duty of exercise is to be laid aside, and some pleasurable motive is to excite it.

"The Grecian games," says the writer, "have not been looked at sufficiently in the light of a grand contrivance of that wonderful people for promoting the health, agility and beauty of their people." After giving a sketch of these games, he says: "At such immense pains was Greece to train her free citizens to health and vigor! Where are our Olympic games: And where is our substitute for them? Exercise in the American mind, seems to be connected with vice, and only allowable when business or labor, to make money, requires it. It is a Herculean task to get a little exercise, and public sentiment puts down everything like amusements that lead to it." After noting the prejudice which exists against students, clergymen and others engaging in certain amusements and games, he exclaims: "It will not do, fellow citizens. These things must be altered. The stamina of the country will give way under it. A healthful development of chest, flesh and muscle, is becoming more and more rare.

Americans are becoming remarkable for their irritable nerves and excitable brains." After noticing the lack of amusements and the improper kinds of amusements now in vogue, and the consequences which follow, the writer says: "Now we stand between the living and the dead, and ask if there is no remedy for these things? Is this the outcome of our puritanism? Is this young and mighty nation to fall by its own inward moral corruption, and are the strong, the wise and the good to stand looking calmly on until they perish in the ruins?" The writer subsequently responds: "No; we are wrong in America. The conscience of the country is murdering the choicest men in it. It refuses to allow the conditions that are essential to health and social happiness; it brings its purest and best to premature graves or insane hospitals, and it drives multitudes who would be sober and respectable men, under any tolerable system of social life, into extravagance and dissipation. In formally making over social enjoyment to the worldly and wicked in America, we greatly err; it is a thing that never was done for any length of time in any country; for even in Scotland, among Presbyterianism of the strictest forms, there is far more social life and organized society than among us. For our part we lay this matter upon the conscience of the church, and upon the good sense of the American people. We have told them the evils of the present system as plainly as we could find language to do it with; and if they will not listen to us we cannot help it.

The following sensible remarks from the same article should be heeded by all:

"We suppose that the playful and social tendencies in man were implanted as a relief from the more grave and intense duties of life, and that the attempt to treat him as a being who does not possess these faculties, or does not need them, is to be wiser than God, and that the result will always be the same, that the attempt to improve the divine teaching and institutions will show itself sooner or later to be not only a failure, but one fraught with the most dangerous consequences. We need hardly remark, that any attempt to make that which should be a mere recreation the main business of life, must necessarily result in folly and misery. The man of pleasure is proverbially a miserable and vicious man."

The article from which the above extracts are taken, is a notice of a Memoir of the Rev. Sidney Smith, and is thirty-eight pages in length. I do not know that it can be obtained in a form separate from the journal in which it is published. The general circulation of this article, in a tract form, among professed Christians, would, in my opinion, do more for the salvation of our country, than all the tracts, to the unconverted, which have been published by the American Tract Society for the last ten years; for, let the professedly Christian portion of the community be converted to the importance of doing their duty, others seeing their good works would glorify our Father in Heaven. But while they are destroying their own children by their neglect and improper treatment of them, as must be manifest to every observer, and are countenancing, and even requiring a neglect of "the conditions that are essential to life and social happiness," to an extent that "is murdering the choicest men" of our country, what right have they to expect that their appeals to the non-religious portion of the community will be heeded? What right have we to expect that their converts, when made, will be any better than they are? And if the men and women of our churches are training their children for premature graves, and are freely, as I shall hereafter show, following practices and habits, to some of which allusion has been made in the extracts above, which are slowly but surely destroying our race physically, have we any assurance that they are not being also destroyed spiritually? Do obedience to the Divine commands, and a life which leads to Heaven, tend to destroy men, women and children, and even races physically? No! "If ye be willing and obedient ye shall eat the good of the land." "The righteous shall inherit the land, and dwell therein forever." "For evil doers shall be cut off."

I am told by one of our citizens, who is a native of Scotland, and has recently visited his native land, that in that country they have schools to which quite young children are sent, not to be confined to hard benches, nor to sit still and study, but to play in the open air, under the watchful care of a matron, and to be amused and instructed by the aid of pictures, etc.

If we only had proper play grounds and gymnasiums in connection with our schools, under the care of proper out-door teachers, where the parents of our city could send and leave their little children over two or three years of age, knowing that they would be carefully watched and cared for, and have suitable exercise and amusements in the open air and light of the sun, with proper, or well-behaved play-fellows, what a relief would it be, especially to mothers who are worn out with constant care, anxiety and watchfulness, in taking care of their little, and even older children. Many a mother, from this cause alone, is hurried to a premature grave, leaving her children to the care of others. And with what a light heart might fathers go to their daily labors, if they knew that the physical and moral training of their boys and girls were thus cared for while they were absent, instead of their running wild in the streets, or being cooped up in the house or yard, deprived of those indispensable requisites for developing healthy bodies, light, air, and cheerful exercise. And how much better would it be for society if not a child was allowed to make the streets his home, or if children were not allowed to congregate in our alleys, back yards, vacant lots, and outskirts of the city, to teach each other, unrestrained, all sorts of evil habits, or to lead one another on in doing wrong. But the attention of the reader has been specially called to this subject in the chapter on Children.

At present, we have not a few children in our cities, whose parents are vicious and dishonest, and not only teach them to lie, cheat, beg, steal, swear and fight, but also set them the example in all these evil habits; so that such children do these things, scarcely knowing them to be wrong, and are therefore comparatively innocent; yet good and virtuous citizens are compelled either to shut up their children, or to let them run in the streets in contact with such, whose example will almost necessarily be much more potent than home teachings. Nor is this all; it is much more injurious for a child who has been taught better, to do these evil acts, than it is for the ignorant; therefore, the children of the Christian portion of the community suffer far greater injury than others.

"Charity begins at home," is a common adage; whether it is true or not I do not propose to inquire at present. But I certainly must inquire whether it is not the duty of parents who have the intelligence and wealth to aid others, to first establish schools which shall save their own children from almost inevitable physical or moral destruction—from sinking lower than it is possible for the outcast children of our cities to sink—before laboring and spending their money to establish ragged and industrial schools for the children of the poor; and, especially, schools which will destroy their physical bodies as they are destroying those of the children of the wealthy. My earnest advice to every parent is; take care of your own children first, for they are suffering far more than a majority of the vagrants in our streets; and if you do not change your course, time will almost certainly demonstrate the truth of this remark to your entire satisfaction, but it will then be too late to save your beloved children. There exists as I have already said, no object of benevolence beneath the sun so needy and worthy, as the children of the rich and middling classes in our cities.

It has already been shown that it need not cost our cities any more, or even as much, to furnish all the children within their limits proper amusements, and physical and moral training, than does our present school system. I now propose to show that we should, indirectly, save thousands of dollars in money by educating our children thus for a life of usefulness and virtue. Notwithstanding we are a professedly religious community, we can, without any hesitation, neglect the poor children of our cities, allow them to grow up surrounded by evil example and teachings, under the most perverse circumstances, trained, perhaps even by parents, to petty thefts and crimes, until they are ten or fifteen years of age, and have had little or no better teachings or example, during their entire lives, when we can cheerfully spend our money to fee, and can find officers to detect them in their crimes against this society which has so unjustly neglected their moral training. We can pay prosecuting attorneys, judges and juries, for convicting them; we can build workhouses, jails and prisons, to confine them; and we can, without any scruples of conscience, disgrace and confine these poor, outcast, neglected children, who have not yet arrived at years of rationality, in such houses and prisons, often with old offenders, to be taught how to accomplish more desperate crimes. No lack of money to do all this, even when by the aid of a proper school system, which would have respect to our children as physical and moral beings, as well as intellectual, and would not cost as much as we at present pay for the schools of our cities; a large portion of the immense sums paid for the support of officers, jails and prisons, could be dispensed with, for the want of criminals upon whom to exercise our benevolent faculties. Yes, even the professed followers of the Lord, who has taught us to train up children in the way they should go, and to do good to all, can freely spend their money to build splendid churches, and fine houses, at an extravagant cost, and dress in purple and fine linen, and fare sumptuously every day, at the very moment when Lazarus, in the form of the neglected children of our cities, lies at our gates full of physical and moral sores! I have no objection to the building of nice churches if we can afford it; that is, if we can do it without neglecting other duties. Large houses are but little better than prisons, in which our women and children are now being destroyed by thousands, by being deprived the necessaries of life—air, light, and active out-door, or even in-door exercise. Extravagance in dress, and useless display, it would seem, are untimely and unbecoming in the followers of Him who taught, that it is our duty to love our neighbors as ourselves; when even our neighbor's children are clad in rags, and their physical and moral training remain uncared for; when less than one-half of the money and time spent in useless display and extravagance, would supply their wants, and train up the children in our midst for an active life of usefulness, virtue and happiness, instead of permitting, and even almost driving them into habits of idleness, vice, dissipation and crime, and consequent violation of the laws of physical health, resulting in a premature death, or a life of suffering in this world, and unhappiness, perchance, in the world to come.

Another important advantage which would result to the child from a system of physical and moral training such as has been named, would be the cultivation of habits of obedience. Until the child's rational faculties are developed, the will of the parent, teacher or guardian, should guide him; and nothing is more destructive to both the natural and moral life of the child, than to allow him to act out his natural and hereditary inclinations unrestrained. The child is not only injured thereby, but he soon comes to cease to reverence his parents and teachers, and treats them with contempt; and he soon begins to exalt himself above others, and becomes jealous and contentious. Every day's observation, even aside from man's nature, satisfies me, that few things are more essential for the future well-being of our children, and our own happiness, than that with a steady hand, we teach our children the duty of obedience, and require them to obey and respect our commands. I have never known a disobedient child to become a kind and affectionate husband, wife or even parent. Above almost every thing else, both boys and girls should be taught that they have before them a life of usefulness —of active labor; and that they are not to be drones in the world, eating up the proceeds of other men's labors; and that all useful labor is honorable. No man or woman can enjoy health of body or mind, or be happy, or permit those around to be, who does not occupy some field of useful labor.

How important, then, is a well cultivated mind in a well developed and healthy body. Children, while young, should be taught to engage in active, athletic plays or sports, for the purpose of developing their bodies, against the time they are able to perform active, useful labor. Having before them lives of industry, children, as soon as old enough, should be made to work; and it is very desirable that, as far as possible, the employment should be such as will bring into activity all parts of the body, or all the muscles. As this can only be imperfectly done, the child, or young person, should have seasons of active play, which will not only relieve the natural desire for recreation, but also give the necessary exercise to the parts of the body not used during labor; that a healthy, harmonious development of the whole organization may be the result.

While active labor is almost indispensable for physical development, it is as important that the young and growing organism should not be over taxed, by excessive labor, as it is that it should not be dwarfed by idleness. Industrious habits should be cultivated as a matter of duty, and conscience.

The physical and mental training, as has been shown, should go on hand in hand, and the young boy or girl thus educated, will grow up with a well developed body and cultivated mind, prepared, physically, and above all morally, to play well his or her part in the drama of active life. The child thus trained escapes many of the temptations, and consequent vices, which are the inheritance of the idle; and has physical, intellectual, and moral stamina, unknown to our hot-house plants. Such should be the training of the young, and in harmony with it should be the habits of the middle aged and the old.

How different from all this is the present method of bringing up children, especially girls. Children, to-day, are not allowed to be children, and to engage in active sports, such as are indispensable for properly developing the physical organism. They will soil their clothes, and will not always look trim. Then girls will not be genteel, and feminine, if they are allowed to run and play, jump and dance, and act out the overflowing life which is seeking to be manifested in the body. As for work, do mothers in fashionable society, generally set their daughters to work? No: Idleness and uselessness and consequent delicacy, ill-health, and premature old age and death, are strangely preferred for their daughters, to an active life of industry and usefulness, which will develop and sustain healthy and substantial bodies, and give long life. Is there no need of a reformation—of a LIVING Christianity, which shall ultimate itself in life? Such only can save our American people from physical destruction. Can our raco be saved? Time will tell the story, and a future historian will write it out.

NEGLECT OF ORATORY AND ELOCUTION.

THE consequences of such neglect are so various and pernicious, both to the student and the community, that this subject is worthy of a separate chapter. To the student a loss of health, usefulness and life, and never ending mortification.

The position which students are apt to occupy during their studies cramps and compresses their lungs and vocal organs, and prevents their vigorous action, and healthy development, and the results are round shoulders, a "caved in chest," premature decay, and death from consumption, dyspepsia, or some other disease. The active laborer by the general activity of all the organs, or of most of them, creates a demand for pure blood; and even without any special effort, compels the lungs to act vigorously to supply the demand, and the health of the respiratory organs is thus preserved. But this is not the case with the student, if he neglects, as most students do, to devote a large share of the time during the day to active physical exercise. But he may, by a vigorous use of the lungs in reading or speaking, purify and send to debilitated organs and parts an increased supply of pure blood, and thus do much not only to sustain the lungs in health, but also other parts of the body. The breathing, whispering, and vocal exercises which are indispensable for properly developing the vocal organs, and for giving purity, volume, and control over the voice, are admirably calculated to develop the lungs and chest, and to prevent any tendency to deformity or disease. Vigorous and eloquent speaking not only exercises the lungs, chest and vocal organs of the throat, but when accompanied by proper expression and gestures it brings into activity almost every muscle of the body. Such exercises may well constitute no inconsiderable share of the physical training, especially of students who are intending to become public speakers. With the vocal organs properly educated, and trained, a man can talk all day as easily as one whose muscles are trained can labor all day. And if our clergymen were thus trained, we should hear no more of the "clergyman's sore throat or bronchitis," as it is called, but (more properly Laryngitis), and many a talented, and useful, and otherwise accomplished pastor, would live to serve his parish to old age.

But when such training is almost entirely neglected during the student's life, as at present, and the clergyman neglects the active use of the vocal organs during six days out of seven, and on the seventh day preaches two or three times, is it strange that his organs of speech fail him, and that his parish feels obliged to send him off to Italy, Palestine, or to some other remote spot, in search of that health of the vocal organs which he has sacrificed by his own neglect and abuse, and which can only be regained by regular systematic persevering training. Would a man thus trained as to his general muscular system from childhood, be able to perform the duties, more satisfactorily, of a wood chopper, hod carrier, mower, or ditcher, if he were only to labor one day out of seven, even though he were to labor but two or three hours on that day. Let our clergymen and sedentary men who are so fool-hardy as to neglect active physical exercise, try either of these vocations, for two or three hours only, one day out of seven, and labor with the same energy a laboring man can bear with impunity, and they will soon find that debility, rheumatism, and other diseases will soon trouble them as do the clerical diseases clergymen; and especially, will such a result follow, if when they get well warmed up, or into a fine perspiration, they will pour a pail of cold water over their shoulders, as many public speakers do a glass of cold water over their vocal organs under similar circumstances. But let them commence cautiously and labor six days out of the seven, and in a few months they will be able to do a fair day's work, with far greater impunity than they could labor even a single hour at the commencement. So in regard to speaking. When I commenced lecturing, it fatigued my vocal organs excessively to lecture a single hour. I had very little control over my voice, it was feeble and high-toned; but although over forty years of age, at the time, with the aid of a very few lessons from a competent teacher, and daily practice, I soon became able to speak in a much lower tone of voice with more volume and force for several hours a day with impunity. I have referred to my own case as an encouragement to others, and to inculcate the idea that we are never too old to learn to improve and mend our bad habits, or develop our physical organizations.

If our public speakers wish to be cured of these chronic throat difficulties so as to be able to continue their avocations, there is but one course to be pursued, and that is the one dictated by physiology and common sense; medicine alone cannot cure so as to enable the individual to continue speaking; change of climate cannot do it. Medicine and change of climate may benefit, or may palliate for a time, but they can no more radically cure when a man continues to abuse his vocal organs, than they will cure a man of the effects of drunkenness while he continues to drink to excess.

To prevent or cure this disease let public speakers, if practicable, take lessons in Elocution from a competent teacher; commence with breathing and whispering exercises, moderately of course at first and only for a short time, but gradually increase both in force and duration. Add reading, and, as the irritation of the throat abates and the lungs and vocal organs gain strength, declamation; gradually increase until able to speak and read several hours a day. If speakers never fail to thus exercise the organs of the chest and throat at least one or two hours every day, they will be able to do all the public speaking they wish with impunity; nor is this the only benefit which will be derived, for the whole system will receive renewed vigor and life by being supplied with purer blood, resulting from the proper exercise of the respiratory organs.

If no teacher of Elocution is at hand, let the reader who may desire to preserve from disease, or restore his vocal organs if already suffering—providing the disease is not too acute—commence immediately such exercises as he may understand; or if he has no knowledge on the subject, let him stand up erect with his shoulders thrown back with the hands upon the hips, and fill his chest with air to its utmost capacity, then allow it to escape as slowly as he can with a slight audible sound until he has expelled all the air he is able to from the lungs. This will develop the chest, and give gentle exercise to the larynx, and accustom the individual to control the escape of air from the lungs which is very important in reading, speaking, or singing.

This exercise should be repeated many times a day; it, like the following exercises, may cause a little dizziness at first, but it will soon cease to do this, as the vessels of the brain become accustomed to an active circulation of blood.

After having practiced the above exercise for some days, let him alternate it with expulsive breathing. Fill the lungs as above, then contract the larynx, or upper portion of the windpipe, partially so as to prevent the too rapid escape of air, and gently force all the air he can out of the lungs. This exercises the organs of the throat far more than the first, and requires to be used with moderation at the commencement, if the parts exercised are diseased. After having practiced the above methods of breathing for some days, finish by filling the lungs and forcing the air out as rapidly as possible without contracting the larynx at all. This should not be repeated more than once or twice upon the same occasion.

After having continued the above exercises for some time, add to them the following; fill the chest, and expel the air forcibly while pronouncing two or three words in a distinct whisper, and thus read a line or two.

It is always well, before commencing the regular exercises of reading and speaking, to practice all of the above exercises for a few moments, so as to equalize the circulation, and allay any irritation which may exist in the throat or air passages; after which read or declaim half an hour or an hour. By going through with such exercises not less than twice a day, gradually increasing them in force and duration, the individual will soon be able to speak with ease, comfort and pleasure; and disease, unless it is too acute or far progressed, will gradually disappear, for the cause will be removed.

No public speaker, nor any one else, should ever shave, especially beneath the chin. There is no doubt, but that Miss Harriet Martineau speaks the truth when she says:

"Those who have the sense and courage to wear the natural comforter, which gives warmth without pressure—the beard—improve their chances for a sound throat, a clear head, and a long life."

IMPORTANCE OF ELOCUTION AND ORATORY.

Cannot the student who is intending to devote his life to public teaching or speaking well afford to neglect, if necessary, many of the studies which are pursued at our schools and colleges for the purpose of obtaining proper elocutionary training? When a good reader or speaker will draw crowded houses, attracted simply to hear other men's thoughts—which may be so familiar as to be contained even in our school books—read or recited, is it not time that our legal, and theological, and in fact all other students, begin to inquire if it is not quite as important that they be able to tell what they know, as it is that they acquire knowledge.

This subject has been considered thus far principally in its relation to the physical development, and health of the student and his vocal organs; but there are considerations beyond these which require our attention.

In order for the full development of any of the faculties of the mind, or organs of the body which partake of voluntary action, they require proper training or educating. This is true in regard to the intellectual faculties; it is true in regard to the affections, and also in regard to the organs of the body. The cultivation of the intellect has placed civilized nations at the head of our race, intellectually speaking. The cultivation of good affections has placed Christians at the head of the race, morally speaking. The writer has endeavored to show that if we would attain a high development of the human body we must cultivate the body; and this is true of every organ of which it is composed. So if we would excel in the use of any organ of the body, that organ must be trained to the use. Let the man who doubts the truth of this proposition, take the blacksmith's hammer and attempt to make a horse nail for the first time; a very simple operation, surely, and requiring no great amount of mechanical skill; still he will find that he has got to learn how to do it, and have a lengthy practice, before he can excel as a nail-maker. It is certainly true that one man may learn to make a nail more readily than another, from a natural capacity, still there are no competent natural nail-makers, any more than there are competent "natural bone-setters."

It is only by the aid of proper instruction, and long-continued persevering practice, that a man becomes a good writer, painter, or watchmaker; or a good artist, or mechanic of any kind. If we hear of a justly celebrated singer, we take it for granted that the individual is acquainted with all the best rules and principles of music, and has not only received proper instruction, but has also devoted years to careful daily practice; and there is no approach to perfection short of such an education. No one, at this day, for a moment thinks of relying upon a natural gift without instruction, or systematic practice, with the expectation of excelling as a musician.

Yet strange as it may seem, we often hear of individuals and writers talking of natural orators, and even speaking contemptuously of established principles and rules of oratory; as though a man can excel in the use of his vocal organs in speaking and reading without proper instruction, and without persevering systematic practice. It is true that one man may excel another without instruction, but there can be no approach to perfection, without understanding, and applying all the principles of elocution and oratory; and the best so called "natural orator" will be improved as much as the poorest, by a thorough education. True art does not, and should not, destroy all individual peculiarities, and natural characteristics, but guides and develops them in an orderly manner.

What can be more important, among the branches usually taught in our schools and colleges, than to teach the young how to read and speak well and gracefully, yet how little attention is paid to this department of education. The student stands up, in the presence of a room full of others, and reads a few lines once or twice a day, without the least pains being taken to develop his voice or vocal organs, or to properly cultivate either. After having practiced reading for a time he is required to commit a chapter of prose or poetry to memory once or twice a month, and without the least preparatory instruction, and generally without practice he is required to exhibit himself upon the stand to be stared at, and criticised, not only by his teachers, but also by his fellow students, and perhaps strangers. Is it strange that such a performance does the trembling victim little good? How different would be the result, if the student were to receive proper instruction in regard to the proper use of his vocal organs, and his voice; also in regard to walking, standing, gestures, etc., before being required to exhibit his oratorical powers publicly. Would any teacher of music require a pupil to stand up, and sing before the public with such slight preparation, before receiving proper instruction, and without long continued private practice? Certainly not; and yet it requires even more instruction and practice to qualify a man as a public speaker, than it does to qualify him as a singer, for he has not only to modify and train his voice and vocal organs, but also his whole being; his eyes, his face, his body, his hands, and even lower extremities, for they all speak in true eloquence.

The results of this neglect are to be seen on every hand, and are no credit to our schools and colleges. Young men are graduated in the latter who intend to devote their lives to public speaking, in the Pulpit or at the Bar, who have not the slightest practical idea of what constitutes good reading, to say nothing of good speaking. Occasionally a man, after having been mortified by his inability to read and speak well, and his consequent want of success in the profession he has chosen, sets himself earnestly about remedying the defects of his education, by applying to a competent teacher for that instruction which, above all other, he should have received during his school and collegiate days; and presently we hear of a man distinguished at the Bar, or in the Pulpit, as an orator. It is safe to say that few ever attain much deserved distinction, as public speakers, who have not taken private lessons in reading and speaking, and diligently practiced according to such instruction in private.

There is no department of education where a man so much requires a competent teacher as in the one of which we are now speaking; and where he requires him while young. Every one is aware how much more easy and graceful a man is, who has been accustomed to polite society from his childhood, than it is possible for one to become who has only had the benefit of such society after arriving at adult age. The adult man may certainly improve wonderfully, but he can never attain that excellence which he might have attained by earlier instruction. There is a flexibility of the body, and the different organs, during childhood, which does not exist to the same extent during adult life; for this reason it is all important that Elocution and Oratory should be taught to students while young.

In the opinion of the writer, a teacher of physical exercises is by far the most essential teacher in every literary institution, and next to him in importance is a teacher of Elocution and Oratory. Better, far better, to neglect entirely, if necessary, Latin, Greek and the higher mathematics, and in fact three-fourths of the studies now taught, than to neglect these. Health, cheerfulness, life and usefulness lie in one direction—disease, suffering, disappointed hopes and a premature death in the other.

CHAPTER VII.

FASHIONS AND HABITS OF THE LADIES, AND THE CAUSES OF ILL HEALTH AND MORTALITY AMONG THEM

THE use of Alcoholic drinks and Tobacco, to the credit of the ladies be it said, is almost entirely confined to the male sex. I have never seen a woman suffering from delirium tremens, and I have seen but comparatively few women drunk. Would that the ladies of our country were as free from all other violations of natural laws as they are from the use of alcoholic drinks; then, indeed, for the sake of the favorable opinion of the sex, which every gentleman desires to retain, would it give me pleasure to cheer them on with pleasant words of approbation; but alas! the observation of many years, while engaged in the active duties of a profession which has for its end the amelioration of the sufferings of fallen humanity, compels me, as I value the welfare of the ladies of our country, and even the perpetuity of our race, to speak earnest words of admonition, caution and advice, and duty forbids that it should be done in the soft language of semi-adulation. I know that I shall receive the thanks of every noble right-minded woman, for plainly pointing out those evils and habits which are so rapidly sapping the physical constitutions of the ladies of our country—the mothers and daughters of our race—and causing an amount of suffering and disease which can only be witnessed with the deepest sympathy for the sufferers, and solicitude for the welfare of the American people. I am sorry to be compelled to state, that which will be corroborated by every physician of our country, that to the habits and fashions of our ladies we must look, if we would view the most fruitful of the causes of the degeneracy of our race in the United States, if such degeneracy actually exists.

To be satisfied that this is true, we have but to go into our streets and compare the relative strength and vigor of the foreign men and women with the American males and females; and we all know that the emigrant women are much stronger, compared with the men, than are our American ladies, compared with the American men. Miss Catherine Beecher, in her work on Domestic Economy, says:

"One of the greatest difficulties peculiar to American women is a delicacy of constitution which renders them early victims to disease and decay; and the fact that their youthfulness and beauty are of shorter duration than those of any other nations, is one which always attracts the attention of foreigners, while medical men and philanthropists are constantly giving fearful monitions as to the extent and alarming increase of this evil. Investigations make it evident that a large proportion of young ladies from the wealthier classes have the incipient stages of curvature of the spine, one of the most sure and fruitful causes of future disease and decay. A large portion of the young ladies in our boarding schools are affected in this way, or have other indications of disease and debility. An English mother at thirty or thirty-five, is in the full bloom of perfected womanhood; as fresh and healthful as her daughters. But where are the American mothers who can reach this period unfaded and unworn?"

"The more I traveled," says Miss Beecher, "and the more I resided in health establishments, the more the conviction was pressed on my attention that there was a terrible decay of female health all over the land, and that this evil was bringing with it an incredible extent of individual, domestic and social suffering, that was increasing in a most alarming ratio. At last certain developments led me to take decided measures to obtain some reliable statistics on the subject."

She obtained statistics from about two hundred different places, in almost all the free States, and she could learn of but very few strictly healthy women in any place. In regard to country places she says:

"But the thing which has pained and surprised me the most, is the result of inquiries among the country towns and industrial classes in our country. I had supposed that there would be a great contrast between the statements gained from persons from such places, and those furnished from the wealthy circles, especially from cities. But such has not been the case. It will be seen that the larger portion of the accounts inserted in the preceding pages are from country towns, while a large portion of the worst accounts were taken from the industrial classes."

I hazard nothing in saying that the ladies in every city, village and rural district throughout our broad land, are not as robust, strong and healthy, when compared with the gentlemen in the same localities, as they should be, and as females are in other nations. I simply state that which we all know, or can see to be true. Here then we have positive evidence that the chief causes of our physical suffering and diseases are to be sought in the habits and lives of the female portion of our community, for the climate affects men as well as women, and yet we find that the latter are deteriorating more rapidly, even in a single generation, than the men. So that we are compelled to cease accusing our climate of the mischief, or at least to a great extent, and to charge it to those who have been called the better half of creation; and respectfully to ask them to mend their ways, that our race be not destroyed by the just visitations of the Lord, in the penalties which follow the violation of His laws. Bayard Taylor in his letters from Northern Europe, speaking of the ladies of Sweden, says:

"Their clothing is of a healthy, substantial character, and the women consult comfort rather than ornament. I have not seen a low-necked dress or a thin shoe north of Stockholm. The damsel who trips at day-break is shod like a mountaineer. Yet a sensible man would sooner take such a woman to wife than any delicate Cinderella of the ball-room. I protest I lose all patience when I think of the habits of our American, especially our country girls. If ever the Saxon race does deteriorate on the American side of the Atlantic, as some ethnologists anticipate, it will be wholly their fault."

I intend, in this chapter, to point out the causes of the present debility, suffering and disease among the ladies of our country, and to press home to their consciences the importance of their shunning these evils. Can any duty be more sacred to those who are to be the mothers of the next generation, than that they shun those evil habits which are undermining their own constitutions, causing disease, suffering and premature death, and thus impairing the integrity of our race? Has any man or woman a moral or religious right to destroy his or her own constitution, and cause deformity, disease and premature death by using tobacco, whisky, neglecting proper recreation and amusements, habits of idleness, shunning the light and air, improper exposure of the feet and neck, or by tight dressing? And if any one is doing this, is it not the first act of a good and true life to cease to do these evils?

The writer of an excellent article on Saints and their Bodies, in the March number of the *Atlantic Monthly*, says:

"Guarantee us against physical degeneracy, and we can risk all other perils—financial crises, slavery, Romanism, Mormonism, border ruffians, and New York assassins; domestic malice, foreign levy, nothing can daunt us. Guarantee us health, and Mrs. Stowe cannot frighten us with all the prophecies of Dred; but when her sister Catherine informs us that in all the vast female acquaintance of the Beecher family there are not a dozen healthy women, we confess ourselves a little tempted to despair of the republic."

Miss Beecher, in her letters to the people, says:

"In Mrs. Gleason's article have been indicated *certain deformities and internal displacements* which have resulted from general debility of constitution, brought on both mature women and young girls by over-excited brains, by want of pure air, simple diet, and exercise, and by the abominations of fashionable dress. But the terrible sufferings that are sometimes thus induced can never be conceived of, or at all appreciated from any use of language."

Again she says:

"In regard to this, and in reference to cases that have come to my personal knowledge, I can truly say that, if I must choose for a friend or child, on the one hand the horrible torments inflicted by savage Indians or cruel inquisitors on their victims; or on the other the protracted agonies that I have seen and known to be endured as the result of such deformities and displacements, I should choose the former as a merciful exchange. And yet this is the fate which is coming to meet the young as well as the mature in every direction. And tender parents are unconsciously leading their lovely and hapless daughters to this horrible doom. This it is that has pressed like lead upon my heart and burned like fire in my bones, as for more than two years of debility, anxiety and infirmity, I have been striving to bring this subject to the attention of the American people. There is no excitement of the imagination in what is here indicated. If the facts and details *could* be presented, they would send a groan of terror and horror all over the land. For it is not one class, or one section, that is endangered. In every part of the country the evil is progressing."

When one of the most intelligent ladies of our land is compelled to use language like the above, is it not time that the members of the Medical Profession, to whom all the facts to which she alludes are well known, should raise their voice of warning to save, if possible, almost the entire female portion of our population from self-destruction?

TIGHT DRESSING.

First and foremost, among the causes of the ill health, deformity and suffering among the American ladies, stands the habit of tight dressing or of compressing the chest and waist; a habit which cannot plead even the paltry excuse of sensual gratification; but is the offspring of the love of approbation or love of the world.

That this dreadful practice has done more, within the last century, than war, pestilence and famine, toward the physical deterioration of civilized man I verily believe. More than this, I believe it is doing more injury to our race to-day, than intemperance in all its horrid forms. The drunkard may make himself unhappy, and those around him, and finally go down to his grave prematurely; and, as a result of his sins or habits, his children may sometimes inherit a strong taste for alcoholic drinks, or be foolish, but such instances are rare. In a great measure, the evil consequences of his drunkenness, so far as the perpetuity of the race is concerned, are confined to the victim himself. As a general rule, the members of his family will be found nearly as robust, in physical appearance, as their neighbors. Not so with the victims of tight dressing: the sins of the mother are visited upon the children until the race becomes extinct. This habit not only carries the mother down to a premature grave, but it destroys the unborn. It does seem to me that if the ladies of our land could only see the terrible consequences which follow this practice, not only upon themselves, but also to the children with whom they may yet be blessed, that if their hearts are not made of adamant, they would relent and never permit a tight dress to approach their persons again.

But I am often told that this practice is passing out of fashion, and that the ladies do not dress as tight now as formerly.

I would that I had some evidence of the truth of this assertion. I have only to say that if it was ever more prevalent than now, or carried to a greater extreme, it is no wonder our race is physically where it is, and that so many children die. If any one questions but that tight dressing is carried to a *greater* extreme to-day than ever before, let him compare the present forms of our ladies with a natural form, or the unperverted form of a little girl. Let him view the caricatures of the female form which are scattered over the length and breadth of our land in the Fashion plates of our popular Magazines, neither one of which should any father, who has daughters, ever permit to enter his doors, if he has any regard for the health and lives of the fair ones under his charge. These are your model forms, and I ask if it is possible for a woman to live at all with a greater perversion of the body?

This habit grows upon the individual like the drunkard's thirst for whisky, and it soon becomes a necessity and requires to be steadily increased. The muscles of the body were intended to sustain it erect, but the very moment a lady applies a tight dress, it takes off the action of the muscles; and in accordance with a well known law of the muscular system, when they cease to be used they grow small and feeble. Now if in addition to tight dresses, whalebones or boards are used, this only the more effectually destroys the action of the muscles. The longer tight dressing has been continued, the more feeble and delicate these natural supports, and the person feels the necessity continually of increasing the tightness of the dress, to sustain the body erect. It is for this reason that no lady ever feels that she dresses too tight, any more than the rum drinker feels that he drinks too much, unless she suddenly increases the force applied. She may even destroy life without actually feeling that she dresses tight; in fact, feeling all the time that she dresses just tight enough to make her feel right, that is to give her proper support.

Slight but constant compression followed every day, is producing such distorted forms as we have represented in the fashion-plates of our popular periodicals, which claim to be taken from actual living beings. If we should by direct force, bring a natural chest and waist into such a shape, we would destroy life by the violence which we should do to the internal organs. But a few years ago, especially in country places, when ladies wore tight dresses only upon particular occasions, it was no uncommon occurrence for them to faint away, or have hysteric fits in the church or ball-room, from the sudden application of compression; but such occurrences are rare now, although the ladies are doing immeasurably more harm by their tight dressing now than then; for tight dresses are worn, not only at church and at parties, but also every day of the week, as well by the maid-servant in the kitchen as by the lady in the parlor. The Chinese prevent the development of the feet of their daughters by gently bandaging them, and the use of well-fitted shoes constantly worn, and never by direct force. The latter, if applied, would cause mortification and death of the feet. The greatest possible distortion of the human chest and waist may be caused without ever using a particle of force, simply by pinning or hooking or even buttoning the garments around the body; and thousands are thus destroying themselves without ever suspecting the cause of their failing health. Does the reader ask how it is done? I will tell you.

The chest above the lower ribs expands about an inch in its circumference during inhalation. If when the air in her lungs is expelled a lady simply pins, hooks, laces or buttons her garments snug around her chest, without using any force, the chest cannot expand, when she draws in her breath, into about one inch as much as before her dress was fastened, and she feels a slight degree of tightness for a short time, when her breathing becomes very good, except upon active exertion. The air is not all expelled from the air cells after exhalation, but a large quantity remains, and, when owing to tight dresses the walls of the chest cannot expand—as the lungs must do the best they can under the circumstances—a portion of the air which ordinarily remains after exhalation is forced out, so that the air cells continue to act, but receive less air, and are diminished in size. Now, when the walls of the chest and air cells become accustomed to their present state of contraction, by the time the lady is ready to have another dress made, there will be no difficulty in making it about one inch smaller, and yet pinning it when the air is expelled from the lungs without using any force; and thus step by step the chest may, in a short time, be brought into the contracted form we witness in our streets, and which are represented in the caricatures of a true or natural human form, which appear in our popular periodicals. Of course by the aid of laces which are daily tightened, this mischief can be accomplished more readily and rapidly.

You can hardly astonish a majority of our ladies more than to tell them that they dress too tight. They know that ladies do sometimes dress or lace too tight, and will often refer to such and such ladies as examples, and the ladies to whom they refer, will perhaps point right back to them as striking examples, for none of them, uninstructed, realize that they dress tight. I have never found a lady who, upon the first accusation, acknowledged that she dressed tight. I have found those who admitted that they had formerly dressed too tight, when I have called their attention to their deformed waists, but generally they will, with apparent sincerity, assert that they were born so, and that their present is only their natural form. A young lady from the country, a few years ago, came into my office to consult me in regard to a supposed tumor in the region of the stomach. Upon examination I found one of the most contracted waists I have ever seen, caused by tight dressing. She had followed the habit a long time until the ribs had become fixed to their unnatural position, when, the very moment she loosened her dress, the much abused liver, stomach and spleen, pressed out the yielding abdominal walls, immediately below the breast bone, and between the cartilages of the ribs, presenting the appearance of a tumor, which of course was very tender to the touch. I frankly explained to her the character of the tumor, and told her that it was caused by tight dressing. In amazement she caught hold of her dress to show me how loose it was, and exclaimed: "Why! you don't think I dress tight, do you?" From that time to this, I have not often tried to make a lady acknowledge her dress was tight. But I do say without any hesitation, that the instances in which the ladies of our country do not dress too tight are the rare exceptions to the general rule; so rare that few can be found at any age, and I doubt if ten ladies, American born, between the ages of fourteen and twenty-five or thirty, can be found in the city of Detroit, or in any other city in the United States, who are not at present distorting their forms, laying the foundation for future disease, and slowly, but surely destroying their health, and shortening their lives from wearing tight dresses. It is all important for the preservation of health and life that there should be a chance for the full action of the lungs, unrestrained by the clothing. How many of the ladies of our land can draw in a full breath without heaving up the shoulders? It is doubtful if one in a thousand, when she shall read this, can even fairly begin to expand her chest within her present dress.

In healthy respiration the thorax, or chest, expands freely in every direction, but more freely around the central and lower portions. If we examine the human skeleton we shall find that special provision has been made for this freedom of motion around the waist, by having the lower ribs terminate in longer cartilages, or elastic gristly structures, instead of bone, which connect the ends of the ribs with the breast bone or sternum. The cartilage connecting the upper rib with the sternum is less than an inch long, but this structure as we descend from rib to rib, will be found to grow longer until those from the lower ribs, with the exception of the floating ribs which are not thus connected with the breast bone, are several inches long.

Almost every lady may be made to convict herself, in two minutes conversation, of tight dressing; and that, too, by giving in almost voluntarily, testimony which cannot be gainsaid. Say to the next lady you meet, if you please, "Madame, do you wear tight dresses?" She will be very sure to say, "No." "Is the dress you have on comfortable?" "Certainly, very comfortable," she will reply. "You feel better in it than in a loose dress, do you?' "Yes," she will be very sure to reply, "I feel much better in this dress than I do in a loose dress; for I feel the want of support in a loose dress; I feel all gone"—very much like the rumdrinker when without his accustomed dram. Here you have the testimony. Why does she feel better in her tight dress than she does in a loose dress? Simply because she has dressed tight, and her dress is tight, and she has taken off, or destroyed the natural action of the muscles, and substituted cotton, linen, and perhaps whalebone. Every gentleman who has not made a fool of himself by apeing the ladies, understands very well that he is just as comfortable in a loose dress, and much better supported than he would be in a tight dress. Then, when a lady feels that she is not properly supported, and does not feel comfortable in a loose dress, she has positive evidence that she not only dresses too tight, but that she has to a greater or less degree destroyed the natural activity of the muscles, and therefore rendered them incapable of supporting the body erect, and that deformity and disease must surely follow soon, unless she ceases this evil practice.

Deformity is the inevitable result of tight dressing. The muscles of the trunk, chest and abdomen, extending up and down the spine, between the ribs, and from the ribs to the hips, or bones of the pelvis, were intended to sustain the body erect. They extend in almost a straight line, with but a slight graceful curve, from the upper part of the chest to the hips, and upon the two sides of the body you will perceive they are nearly parallel. Here, then, the shoulders and head are well supported; there is plenty of breadth for the shoulder blades, or scapula, to rest upon on the posterior, or back region of the chest. Now, if instead of this noble form of God's image—a well formed woman—the ribs are drawn in, by dressing, to one half or two thirds the natural size of the body, not only are the muscles rendered feeble and delicate, but instead of being parallel upon the two sides of the body, as nature intended, they are drawn from their true direction into the form of an hour glass; of course they can give the chest, shoulders and head, but a feeble support; and the result is, the shoulders begin to stoop, the shoulder blades begin to stand out, and you have the peculiar rainbow form of the spine, with more or less depression beneath the collar bones, or clavicles, which is so common among the ladies of fashion to-day. Lateral, or sideway curvatures of the spine are also common, especially when tight dresses have been applied to girls before the bones have obtained proper solidity. Scarcely a good and noble formed woman, of erect and dignified carriage, is to be found among the fashionable ladies of our country. Deformity! deformity! is the rule — symmetry of form, and consequent beauty, the rare exceptions to that rule—and this deformity has been in a great measure, caused by tight dressing.

If deformity alone resulted from tight dressing, it would be bad enough; but, alas! this is not the worst of the consequences which follow this absurd practice. The Chinese females may compress their feet, and prevent their development, and yet no serious consequences to the general health follow, as the feet are not vital organs; the rest of the body may live after the loss of one or both feet. The aborigines of our country may compress their heads at a given point, and the brain will expand in other directions, and no serious injury result to the race. We may not admire their taste, when in their self-conceit, they imagine themselves wiser than their Creator, and set themselves about marring the truly beautiful form of God's image, but no serious consequences follow to the race. Children of such parents continue to be born with well developed feet and heads, and no deformity nor disease is inherited by posterity as a consequence of the folly of the parents; simply because these deformities do not seriously interfere with the functions of any organ or organs, which are indispensable to the health and life of the organism as a whole. Not so with the habit we are now considering; for if we judge as to the degree of the evil, when this practice is ignorantly indulged in, or as to the sin when it is knowingly practiced, by the physical consequences which follow to our race, it is certainly one of the most fearful and deadly evils and sins in existence—compared to it, intemperance sinks into insignificance. It may be thought that simply compressing the chest is a very simple act, and no great evil, but the swallowing of ten grains of strychnine, or the placing two or three drops of prussic acid upon the tongue, are much more simple acts, but when either is done with a knowledge that it will cause disease and premature death, as simple as the act is, it becomes one of a fearful character—it becomes self-murder.

But let us examine why it is that such fearful consequences follow tight dressing; and also take a particular view of some of the effects which do result from this practice. In the first place let us examine some of the organs which are affected, compressed or pressed out of place by this habit; and first we will notice the organs within the chest.

We have within the chest, above the diaphragm or midriff, the lungs and heart. The lungs are composed of air cells, bronchia, or air tubes, leading to the air cells, and cellular tissue, together with nerves and blood vessels.

The heart is a double organ, as it were, having two sets of

cavities, (the right auricle and ventricle, and the left auricle and ventricle,) each of which performs a similar function, or office. The blood returning towards the heart in the veins from every portion of the body, enters the right auricle, which contracts and forces it into the right ventricle; this contracts and forces it into the pulmonary artery, through the branches of which it flows, in more and more minute vessels, until it enters the minute capillary or hair like vessels, in the very walls of the air cells; and after passing through these, it returns through the pulmonary veins to the left auricle, through which it passes to the left ventricle, by the contraction of which it is forced into the aorta. The blood is prevented from returning in the opposite direction, in its passage through the heart, by valves. The blood flows through the aorta, or large artery which extends from the left ventricle, through its subdivisions, to every part of the body, until it enters the capillary vessels, which are so perfectly distributed at every part that the prick of a needle will wound more or less of these minute vessels; having passed through these, which unite and form the veins, it returns again to the right side of the heart to be sent to the lungs. During the passage of the blood through the lungs, changes, all important for the life and health of the whole body, take place. When the blood enters the lungs through the pulmonary artery and its branches, it is dark, purple, venous blood, similar to that which flows from the arm when a patient is bled. In the lungs it comes sufficiently in contact with external air, to allow oxygen to be absorbed from the atmosphere, and carbonic acid to be given off.

The blood thus purified by the separation of this poisonous gas, and vivified, or made alive, by the reception of its precious load of oxygen, becomes of a rich crimson color, when it is prepared to return to the left side of the heart to be sent to every part of the body, carrying with it the new nutritive material, which was received into the veins from the digestive organs before the blood was sent to the lungs, and also a supply of oxygen. The latter, when it arrives in the minute capillary vessels, finds in every part of the body particles of matter which are worn out, and require to be removed. It lays hold of such particles and decomposes, or oxydizes, or, as it were, burns them up, thereby furnishing heat to the entire organism. New particles of matter take the place of the old, in the various structures, and the blood by the loss of its oxygen and new material, and by the reception of the products of combustion, and worn out particles—carbonic acid, various saline, and other substances—becomes again of a dark color, and returns through the veins to the right side of the heart. The various earthy, saline, watery, and other particles, which are no longer needed in the circulation, are cast out of the system by the kidneys, liver, skin and bowels.

The reader will now be able to perceive the important part which the heart and lungs play in the animal economy. So important are the changes in the blood, which are produced by respiration, that if the latter ceases for the short space of five minutes, the patient can rarely be restored.

What must be the effect of compressing the chest, of binding down by the aid of corsets, hooks or pins in dresses, the ribs, and thus preventing that freedom of motion which nature intended by the long cartilages to which I have referred? Bear in mind that the lungs and heart fill the entire cavity of the chest, so that strictly speaking there is no cavity, even when the chest is fully distended. Such compression, of course, lessens the capacity of the lungs to receive air, which is so essential to health and life; the changes which should take place in the blood, in its passage through the lungs, are but imperfectly effected; now if the compression has been suddenly applied, the blood is rendered so impure that the minute capillary vessels of the lungs refuse in a great measure, to return the blood to the left side of the heart, and the heart and large vessels are also compressed, so that they cannot act efficiently, and the individual becomes faint, from the want of a due supply of blood in the brain. In other instances, the obstruction to a return of blood in the veins, causes congestion of the brain, flushed face, and even convulsions. But when the compression has been applied more gradually, the effects are not so manifest, still not the less certain. It has been already stated, that if the blood is not changed in the lungs, it ceases to be circulated in the blood vessels; if it is only partially purified in the lungs, it is imperfectly circulated, and distant parts of the body first feel the effects of the imperfect circulation, the extremities become cold. Dark, impure blood, instead of scarlet, life-giving blood, flows to the delicate structures of the brain and spinal marrow, or cord, causing disease and derangement of the functions of these organs. The obstruction to the circulation of the blood, together with its impurity, causes congestion of the brain and its spinal elongation, and the victim begins to be troubled with headache, neuralgia, spinal-irritation, and the protean forms of nervous diseases, hysterics and the like.

If this evil habit is continued for any considerable length of time, these diseases become fixed, so that it is very difficult to remove them, and a lifetime of suffering often results. Nor does the mischief end here; the lower portions of the lungs become more or less inactive from the obstruction to the flow of blood through them, the central portions have a double duty to perform, and become liable to irritation and inflammation; the free action of the upper portions is prevented, and they become congested; which together with the impure state of the blood, gives rise to deposits of a tuberculous matter, and the individual finally dies from the consumption. Palpitation of the heart, and pain through the side and shoulders, almost inevitably result from tight dressing.

Nor are the lungs, heart, and the organs I have already named alone affected. The diaphragm or midriff, plays an important part during respiration, and when the lower portion of the ribs, to which this organ is attached, are thus contracted, it is impossible for it to discharge its duty. The liver, stomach, and spleen lie immediately beneath the ribs, in a great measure within the concavity of the diaphragm; these organs are more or less compressed and crowded out of place, and of course can but imperfectly perform their functions. The liver is a very broad and solid organ, extending fully two-thirds of the distance across the abdomen beneath the lower ribs; the stomach and spleen extending the rest of the way in a healthy and natural body, but, in the fashionable forms of our young ladies to-day, the entire waist is not as broad between the ribs, as the liver in its transverse diameter; and yet, into this narrow space are crowded, or jammed, the liver, stomach, and spleen, of course more or less distorted and displaced. Is it strange that almost all the ladies have great tenderness and soreness at the pit of the stomach; or that they have neuralgia, weakness, and other diseases of this organ, when they thus wantonly abuse this portion of the body? The kidneys cannot escape injury from this compression; the bowels are crowded downwards, pressing down upon the bladder, and other important organs within the pelvis, or hip bones, causing prolapsus, congestion, inflammation and ulceration of the womb, and the various other forms of female diseases, which are so prevalent at present, and which make the lives of so many of our fashionable females almost unendurable; and to which Miss Beecher alludes in the earnest language which I have quoted from her pen.

Nor do the internal organs alone suffer from the bad practice under consideration; the breasts become irritated and indurated from the pressure of dresses, stays, whalebones, and the like, and the foundation is laid for future inflammation and abscesses, which so frequently trouble nursing females. And it is not improbable that even cancer of the breast often has its origin from this cause, or from the indurations caused by lacing, assuming a malignant character.

I have given but a hasty sketch of the terrible consequences which follow in the wake of this violation of nature's laws. It is utterly impossible for a lady with her waist deformed according to the representation of our fashion plates, to enjoy good, or even tolerable health, for any considerable length of time. It is true that active, out-door exercise may do something towards counteracting the bad effects of tight dressing, but sooner or later, deformity and disease result, if the practice is continued. The active, out-door habits of the English ladies save them from the rapid and early sacrifice of health and life which we witness here. Mary Lamb writes to Miss Wordsworth, (both ladies being over fifty years of age) "You say you can walk fifteen miles with ease; that is exactly my stint, and more fatigues me." She speaks compassionately of a certain delicate lady who could walk "only four or five miles every third or fourth day keeping very quiet between."

That the English ladies are beginning to feel the effects of this destructive practice, is beyond doubt, for the Englishwoman's Review says: "It is allowed by all, that the appearance of the English peasant, in the present day, is very different to what it was fifty years ago; the robust, healthy, hardy-looking country-woman or girl, is as rare now as the pale, delicate, nervous female of our times would have been a century ago." And we are informed that even the children in the English schools are not as robust as formerly; thus, there as here, are the consequences of this dreadful practice visited upon the rising generation, who have, above all dispute, to suffer the physical consequences which result from the sins of their parents.

It has been my aim to show that the habit of tight dressing is almost universal, although perhaps generally unknown to the victims themselves; that the heaving up of the shoulders, instead of expanding around the waist, during inspiration, and a feeling of goneness, or want of support, or weakness, when in a loose dress, or when without any dress, are positive signs of suffering from the bad effects of tight dressing; for such symptoms only occur when the natural action of the muscles has been destroyed by compression, or stays, except in rare cases of disease. I know full well, that few, if any ladies can be found, in fashionable society, in our land, who, upon observation, will not find that these positive signs of dressing too tight, exist with themselves. That many of our ladies have followed this practice ignorantly, without being aware, either that they dressed so tight as to impair health and shorten life, or of the fearful consequences which follow this violation of the laws of God, is beyond question; but this fact will not save them from suffering, disease, and premature death, and even from destroying our race, if they continue it.

Believing that many of our ladies are conscientious and true women, and desire to know what is right for the sake of doing accordingly, I will take the liberty of making a few suggestions to such. Never, as you value health, life, our race, and a conscience void of offence before God and man, depend upon hooking, pinning, or fastening your garments around the waist for their support, for you can do neither without doing injury. Use shoulder strap waists, or suspenders; let them be placed distinctly upon the shoulders near the neck, and never allow them to rest upon the external points of the shoulders, or on the arms, as is so common at present. Who has not been pained by seeing little girls walking our streets, throwing up their arms to keep on their dresses? This method of dressing children and young ladies is one of the most sure means of causing deformity of the chest and shoulders. The constant compression thus caused, even though but slight, will be very sure to cause more or less distortion of the undeveloped and growing form of a child; and beyond all question, it is a fruitful cause of the uncouth round shoulders which we now so frequently witness among young girls and ladies. If there is a portion of the body which, above all others, needs to be properly protected from the cold, and atmospherical changes, it is the upper portion of the chest and shoulders; and this is especially true during the days of childhood and youth; therefore, avoid low necked dresses. Never fasten your garments so tight around the waist but that you can draw in a full breath, whether sitting or standing, without the least restraint. Take particular pains to expand the chest by frequently drawing in a full breath. Such a course together with active out door exercise, will do much towards restoring your natural form and health.

If you desire a beautiful form, one which shall be worthy of being admired, remember that it must be as the God of beauty has created it,—natural. The least appearance of an unnatural contraction about the waist, even in the external garments, is a departure from symmetry of form, and sacrifices all ease, gracefulness, harmony, and beauty, and substitutes stiffness and awkwardness; and is as painful to behold as is a tight jacket on the body of a criminal.

The following sensible remarks on the subject of female dress, have been extracted from the writings of Miss Harriet Martineau:

"The variety, the cheapness, the manageableness of clothes in our day, compared with any former time, ought to render us obedient in an unequalled degree to the main conditions of good dress. Instead of this, we see trains of funerals every year carrying to the grave the victims of folly and ignorance in dress.

"If we consider the female dress of 1859 under any of the remaining conditions, what can we say of it? Does the costume, as a whole, follow the outline of the form? Does it fit accurately and easily? Is the weight made to hang from the shoulders? Are the garments of to-day convenient and agreeable in use? Is the mode modest and graceful? So far from it, that all these conditions are conspicuously violated by those who think they dress well. Here and there we may meet a sensible woman, or a girl who has no money to spend in new clothes, whose appearance is pleasing—in a straw bonnet that covers the head, in a neat gown which hangs gracefully and easily from the natural waist, and which does not sweep up the dirt: but the spectacle is now rare; for bad taste in the higher classes spreads very rapidly downward, corrupting the morals as it goes. The modern dress perverts the form very disagreeably.

"Compare the figure of the Graces of Raffelle, or the Ven de Medici, with the smallest and most praised waist in a factory, and observe the difference. Before the glass, the owner of the latter sees the smallness in front, and fancies it beautiful; but it is disgusting to others. It is as stiff as the stem of a tree, and spoils the form and movement more than the armor of ancient knights ever did; and we know what is going on within. The ribs are pressed out of their places, down upon the soft organs within, or overlapping one another: the heart is compressed, so that the circulation is irregular; the stomach and liver are compressed, so that they cannot act properly: and then parts which can not be squeezed are thrust out of their places, and grave ailments are the consequence. At the very best, the complexion loses more than the figure can be supposed to gain. It is painful to see what is endured by some young women in shops and factories, as elsewhere. They can not stoop for two minutes over their work without gasping and being blue, or red, or white in the face. They can not go up stairs without stopping to take breath every few steps. Their arms are half-numb, and their hands red or chilblained; and they must walk as if they were all of a piece, without the benefit and grace of joints in the spine and limbs. A lady had the curiosity to feel what made a girl whom she knew, so like a wooden figure, and found a complete palisade extending round the body. On her remonstrating, the girl pleaded that she had 'only six-and-twenty whalebones!'

"Any visitor of a range of factories will be sure to find that girls are dropping in fainting fits, here and there, however pure the air and proper the temperature; and here and there may be seen a vexed and disgusted proprietor, seeking the ware-house-woman, or some matron, to whom he gives a pair of large scissors, with directions to cut open the stays of some silly woman who had fainted. Occasional inquests afford a direct warning of the fatal effects which may follow the practice of tight lacing; but slow and painful disease is much more common; and the register exhibits, not the stays, but the malady created by the stays as the cause of death. That such cases are common, any physician who practices among the working classes will testify.

"The prodigious weight of the modern petticoat, and the difficulty of getting it all into the waistband, creates a necessity for compressing and loading the waist in a way most injurious to health. Under a rational method of dress, the waist should suffer neither weight nor pressure—nothing more than the girdle which brings the garment into form and folds. As to the convenience of the hooped skirts, only ask the women themselves, who are always in danger from fire, or wind, or water, or carriage wheels, or rails, or pails, or nails, or, in short, everything they encounter."

But it is not tight dressing alone which is doing so much towards destroying the health and lives of our females. Other habits of fashionable life are scarcely less pernicious. Almost the entire training of even young girls as well as of young ladies, is in open violation of nature's laws; and education, we have seen, is not much behind, for every effort is made to educate the intellect, but the affections—the essential part of woman—are left comparatively uncultivated—barren, or to grow up to rank weeds, stimulated by the false ideas of real life found in novels, or the light literature of the day, and bitter fruits, in after life, are the consequences. All this is wrong. The life of Heaven is a life of active usefulness, and all true life on earth is a life of usefulness to our fellow creatures, and all genuine happiness must flow from such a life.

As our young ladies grow up to ten or fifteen years of age, they, instead of active out-door sports, must be required to spend six hours a day in the school-room, and to thrum on the piano one or two hours more, and to walk genteelly in the streets. No chance for active play, and as for work, do parents require their daughters to work? O, no! Work is not fashionable; cooking, washing, attending fires, and the like, are vulgar employments in the eyes of this generation; and young ladies—even those expecting, or perhaps hoping, to become wives and mothers—are to know nothing about active work, or such employments. They may spend their time over a little embroidery, but no active employment is permitted—their hands will not look delicate. No opportunity to develop, by active work, the physical organism. Nor is this all—although light and air are indispensable for physical development, beauty and health, still these young ladies are rarely allowed to enjoy them, except with a veil or parasol over their faces, for fear they will get tanned, and will not look delicate. Yes, even fathers and mothers, who have sense enough to perceive that the bloodless plant of the cellar is not as beautiful as the fresh, robust, and natural colored vegetable that grows in the sun, are afraid their daughters will get tanned, or become natural colored, and will not look pale-faced. And these young ladies are allowed to stay, or perhaps, kept in the house, not so much as required, or permitted, to attend or cultivate the garden. There must be blinds on the windows, and they are kept closed so as to keep both young ladies and furniture delicate. Well, these young ladies grow up delicate enough to suit their anxious parents, with little or no employ ment except sewing—the very worst work they could do—perhaps they are not even allowed to do that, or at least any kind of necessary or useful sewing; so they have a plenty of time to build air-castles. At last they begin to dream of getting married, all of which is, or rather would be, right, if they had been brought up properly and were really fit to be married. In this age of dissipation among young men, the latter are not all rich, or even in comfortable circumstances to do more than support themselves; and even if they are rich, they sometimes have some ideas of home comforts free from the annoyances of servants and nurses, for idleness brings sickness.

So those who are not rich count the cost, and perhaps conclude that they cannot afford to support a wife in the style she will expect, or in idleness, so they never propose, and for every young man who never marries, one young lady must live an old maid, and has not a chance to marry; which, under the circumstances, is perhaps very fortunate for all parties. I saw a statement in our newspapers not long since, that in the State of Massachusetts, during, if I recollect right, the year 1856, more than one-half of the marriages occurred among the Irish—they being almost the only class, it seems, that can afford to get married. Dr. Cushman, Principal of the Mount Vernon Ladies' School at Boston, says:

"In the family, the knowledge of domestic affairs is coming to be regarded as vulgar. Habits of indolence and extravagance in the one sex are at once deterring the other from entering into the married state, and aggravating the evils of licentiousness and prodigality among them."

If all this is true in Massachusetts, that old Know-Nothing State, where native Americanism has been so rampant, let me ask members of that party, to look forward barely one generation —say thirty years—and in the light of such facts tell us who are to rule America? For if more marriages occur among the Irish than among Americans, I need not inquire among which class the most children will be born, for the reader has but to take a walk into "Cork Town" to be satisfied on that point.

IDLENESS, AMONG THE LADIES.

Few causes more speedily destroy races or individuals, both physically and spiritually, than habits of indolence. When active useful labor comes to be regarded as vulgar and degrading, among the inhabitants of any country, that nation is in its decline, for effeminacy and corruption follow as necessary consequences.

The men of our nation are generally industrious, and young men are usually taught, and understand that they must labor in some field or other, and this does much towards preventing, notwithstanding their other bad habits, the rapid deterioration among them which we witness among the ladies. But the indolent habits, which prevail among the young ladies to such an extent, entirely fail to develop strong, robust organizations, consequently we can have no corresponding standard of health among the next generation of the mothers of our land, as we shall witness among the fathers, with all their vices.

Could a more insane—I might, perhaps, more correctly say, infernal—idea ever have gained dominion over the minds of the inhabitants of any land, than that active, useful labor, such as is necessary to develop strength of body and mind, is unbecoming for the young ladies who are to be the mothers of the next generation? It destroys the body by preventing that activity which is necessary to give muscle, bone and nerve, and subjects the individual to an increased liability to innumerable diseases. It prevents a healthy development of, and tends to destroy, the soul. One of the noblest and highest affections of the human spirit is a desire to serve, and a love of thus doing good to others; for this is the very delight of heaven; and how important, not only for this life, but also for the next, that every child should be taught, both by precept and example, this great truth. It would almost seem that the present sentiments in regard to labor, which prevail among our young ladies, constitute one of the strong delusions which we are told that men are, for certain reasons, sometimes permitted to believe.

What can be more beautiful and cheering than to see a

daughter with active hands, guided by knowledge and a willing heart, engaged in attending to the affairs of the household, cooking and preparing food for the family, washing and scrubbing floors and wearing apparel, cultivating useful vegetables in the garden, and ornamenting the grounds by rearing flowers, and thus contributing her share towards the support and enjoyment of the household? What can be more noble in a young lady than a disposition to be thus useful? and what more honorable than to allow such heavenly affections to flow through the hands into every act, instead of their being perverted and centering upon herself, leading her to imagine that the main object of life in this world is simply her own gratification?

The cultivation of industrious habits, from the love of doing good to others, leads to cheerfulness, contentment, mutual co-operation, peace, and a life of usefulness in this world, and Heaven in the next; whereas, idleness leads to selfishness, strife, jealousy, vanity, envy, separation from others, and consequent unhappines in both worlds. Does any one question which of the two would be the best qualified to discharge the duties of a wife or mother, the industrious or indolent young woman?

But some of the young ladies, fashionably brought up, do get married. Such a one, although entirely unfitted, either physically or intellectually, owing to her false bringing up, to have the care of children, may become a mother; but she runs many risks, and is subject to many annoyances from which her more robust but less fashionable neighbors are exempt. Her children are necessarily feeble, for it is a law of nature that like begets like, therefore they require unusual care. Now this young wife and mother, entirely unaccustomed to hard labor, is aroused and stimulated on by the wants of her, perhaps, suffering child. Maternal love—one of the strongest and most noble of the affections of a true women—prompts her to an amount of physical exertion and mental anxiety, for which she is entirely unprepared; her health slowly fails under this load of care, she becomes nervous, peevish and unhappy. Her huaband, perhaps not fully realizing the delicacy, and want of capacity for endurance of the wife he has chosen, begins to regard her peevishness as a manifestation of a bad disposition, and becomes morose and neglectful himself, and thinks she might control herself if she would, which only makes his poor suffering wife, unhappy and discontented, and mutual unhappiness results. Years roll on—family and cares increase, with perhaps, loss of the delicate children, bringing sadness and sorrow to the poor mother, until at last she is worn out, and dies, leaving her delicate and imperfectly organized children to the care of her husband and strangers. The husband, after a time, finding that he cannot bestow that care upon his children which they need, and that hired help does not supply a mother's place, finally seeks another wife, and perhaps one as poorly prepared for the duties of a mother and housekeeper as the first; and she has to commence with the care of a family at once, and, of course, if equally feeble or delicate, she is sooner worn out than the first wife.

Such is a just and fair picture of the results of the practice of tight dressing, and the cruel and wicked methods of bringing up ladies, as frequently practiced in fashionable society to day. All this is wrong and in direct violation of nature's laws—and nature's laws are the laws of God. We need and must have an entire change to save our race from destruction. No half-way reformation will answer. The lungs must be left entirely free, and tight dressing must be unknown except in history. Good, substantial, warm, thick-soled shoes, such as are worn by the ladies of other nations, must take the place of paper soles; heavy skirts must never re-appear; improper and indelicate exposure of the upper part of the chest must cease. Young girls and ladies must be allowed and required to play at active games in the open air and sun; and nor allowed to remain in the house, and not confined in school more than three or four hours a day, at most; and as soon as they are old enough, they should be made to work; and young ladies should not be allowed to do much sewing, but should be kept diligently, a considerable portion of their time, at active work, washing, baking, ironing, scrubbing floors, and cooking, and at least several hours a day at work in the garden, or taking other active exercise in the open air. All useful labor is honorable, and should be so regarded. Ladies must also cease the use of those enervating drinks, tea and coffee, and also the various stimulating condiments in use, such as cloves, cinnamon, mustard, pepper, nutmeg and the like, for the use of such substances prematurely wears out and destroys their already delicate organization.

Thus change, and there is hope for our race; we may gradually return, in the course of a few generations, to a state of physical development equal to that of the most robust foreigners; yes, even to a beauty of form and a state of health far superior to any race now on earth.

But go on as we are now going, and the American people will gradually be destroyed; for it is manifestly a law of Divine Providence, that when races of men become so wicked and evil as to be almost entirely under the sway of particular evil passions, as many of our American people are at present under the sway of vanity or perverted love of approbation, their evils, in being ultimated, destroy them; and this is certainly a merciful provision, for if parents for a long series of generations, were to give way to the love of approbation as their ruling love, this passion would grow stronger every generation, so that insanity, and an entire loss of mental freedom would inevitably result.

It has often seemed to me, that no young lady with a deformed, or small waist, with delicate hands, with a bloodless and semi-transparent skin, which is so much admired, should even think of marrying; for it is just as impossible, especially without an entire change of life and habits, for her to transmit the name of her husband to posterity, as it is for the Ethiopian to change his skin or the leopard his spots. As a general rule she will never see her children's children; in the first place, because she will not live to see their time, and in the second place, that generation will generally be wanting, or die in infancy. By marrying such a young lady only brings suffering upon herself, and becomes the mother of children but for them to die young.

There is but one view of the case which reconciles, to the lover of humanity, the permitting such imperfectly developed young ladies to marry; and that is the hope which perhaps we may all indulge, that when our Heavenly Father removes so many of their little ones during infancy, they are placed in the care of guardian angels, to become angels of Heaven themselves; and life to them may be a blessing, they never having ultimated on earth the evil dispositions inherited from their parents.

The young woman who, with a knowledge of the consequences which follow tight dressing, and habits of indolence, still persists in such habits, is physically and morally unworthy to take upon herself the endearing names of wife and mother, and should never think of marrying; and wo to the man who takes to his bosom such a bundle of selfishness. Call her a wife who is willing to sacrifice health and life, not only her own, but also of unknown generations, to the gratification of her vanity? She is unworthy; but I trust there are but few such. Not a few of the fashionable young ladies of our country, have so far destroyed their physical bodies, that they can never perpetuate the race, and multitudes are rushing on in their wake. To the hardy foreigners who are flocking to our shores, we shall be compelled to look for the mothers of coming generations if our American ladies do not speedily reform. This is lamentable, but it is true, and it is high time our American people were aroused to the importance of such a reformation. The time has been when these pernicious fashions were in a great measure confined to our cities and villages, and country girls grew up comparatively healthy, but the fashion plates of certain periodicals, which no parent should ever permit to enter his house, have polluted the minds, and already done much towards dragging country lasses down to the level of those of our cities physically; and since the spinning wheel and loom have disappeared, idleness has taken the place of active industry, and this forlorn hope of our country is about destroyed.

As I have already stated, no woman, distorted into the form represented in the fashion plates of our popular periodicals, can live and enjoy good health for any considerable length of time. She must die a lingering death, and her race must perish with her. Strange as it may seem, not an effort, to my knowledge, has ever been made to restrain the publication and sale of these plates, which are doing many times more towards destroying our

American people than all the grog shops and obscene publications in our land. The rumseller who would sell whisky to little girls and young ladies, would certainly be regarded as an abandoned character; but how is it with the publishers and booksellers, who, for the love of money, will not spare even young girls? You fathers and brothers who have been striving for the enactment and enforcement of laws against simply selling alcoholic drinks, and have, at the same time, disregarded the traffic in these caricatures of the human form, and have allowed them to be sent to your daughters and sisters, without ever even petitioning our Legislature for the passage of a law to suppress this murderous traffic, you are straining at a gnat and swallowing a camel.

But I am occasionally told by the ladies, as an excuse for their bad habits, that the gentlemen like to see them looking delicate, with small waists, and colorless lifeless skin. If there are any such foolish young men or bachelors among the readers of this volume, I have a few words to say to them. The time will come, gentlemen, yes, it will surely come to some of you, as you will some day sit by the sick bed of a suffering wife, who will be realizing the inevitable consequences of violating nature's laws, tortured night and day by neuralgia, and other nervous diseases and female disorders, or slowly wasting away with consumption, constantly enduring untold agony, and a source of constant care, watchfulness and mental anxiety, instead of being, as she might have been, a help-meet for you, able and willing to endure and sustain her share of the burdens, cares, responsibilities and pleasures of married life; I say the time will come, when, if you shall love your wife, as I trust you may, you would be willing to give all the wealth you may possess if you could but see her in the possession of a good well formed, robust, healthy body. Beware, then, how you encourage them in the idea, which, it is to be feared, most ladies have formed, that the gentlemen prefer delicate ladies; beware that their death be not chargeable on you.

Your sorrows and regrets at having encouraged this cruel method of training the young lady who is to become your wife, will not end with her sufferings and death, for these delicate ladies will not be the mothers of robust children; then, as you sit by the sick bed of your innocent little ones, one after another, and see their sufferings and convulsions, and hear their piteous cries, at last, closing their eyes in death, you will begin to realize the fearful consequences, which, by your folly in encouraging this disposition of the ladies to look delicate, and to mar God's image by tight dressing, you will have brought, not only upon yourself, the wife of your bosom, and your little ones, but also upon your race. Beware then! for so true as God's laws are just, and change not, so true is it that the evil doer shall not go unpunished. Is it not a fearful crime, and one which every man should shun, to lure on young ladies to self-destruction by the violation of natural laws?

I have but barely glanced at the consequences which follow, not only to the victim, but also, ultimately to the gentlemen. A young lady with small waist and delicate skin lacks, as we have seen, the first requisites for the physical comfort and happiness of herself and her future husband—she lacks substance, strength, health and life. The indolent young lady lacks the mental capacity and development necessary for the happiness of herself and her future husband—she lacks contentment and cheerfulness, as well as strength and health, and she can never without a change of habits, duly sympathize with her husband, and sustain his hands amid the cares of life; but often will it occur, when he may be bowed down by care, labor, and perhaps business perplexities, and feels himself called upon to strain every nerve, and devote almost every hour of his time to sustain his reputation, and discharge his honest obligations, that his sensibilities will be stung by reproaches of neglect and a want of sociability; if not in words, at least in act; and he will find at last, when he least suspects, that, while he has been laboring night and day to provide for the comfort and happiness of his wife, she has been dwelling, for the want of something better to do, on his shortcomings, until she perhaps views him as one of the worst of men; thus, often, the prospects of the married couple for happiness are destroyed, or materially lessened, before the first anniversary of their wedding day. How important, then, in a young lady, are industrious habits, and work for her hands to do?

Permit me to inquire, should a gentleman be matrimonially inclined, if it is not of far more consequence for him to know whether a servant girl is kept to do the work in the kitchen, a gardener to attend the garden, and whether the baker and washerwoman visit regularly the house of his intended, when the daughter or daughters are abundantly able to do all the work, than it is to know that the young lady he is thinking of choosing as a companion for life, understands French and Italian music?

It is well known that active labor is discarded by multitudes of our fashionable young ladies, and yet neither proper physical recreation, nor gymnastic exercises are substituted for it. We have had a gymnasium in the city of Detroit to which ladies were admitted, and an effort was made by the proprietor to keep up a class; still, in a short time, it dwindled away until the rooms were empty, even during the most debilitating season of the year, when exercise and recreation is so much needed to sustain the body in health. There are few, if any young ladies in our cities who would not be perfectly astonished at the idea of walking ten or fifteen miles a day, who require a carriage if they have to travel a good deal less than half that distance, and who are rarely seen walking even a mile from their residences. Is it strange that our young ladies possess so little stamina, and that so few of them can reach even thirty years in the enjoyment of good health, and that so many of the married ladies are so soon worn out by the cares of a condition of life for which they are so totally unprepared by previous habits? How cruel in parents to thus bring up their daughters without active employments, recreations and amusements?

Is there no need of reformation in our country? We have had revivals of religion within the last few years which have prevailed in almost every portion of our land; which have for the time, rejoiced the hearts of many; but where do we witness their fruits? I must confess that my heart has been made sad as I have witnessed the pale faces, and distorted forms, going to and from our churches on the Sabbath day; for I had hoped to see some brighter prospects opening up for the future of our race, especially among the ladies; but what are the facts? I will not state my own convictions, but will ask the reader if he has any evidence that tight dressing and habits of idleness, are not as prevalent now as they were years ago. And if low-necked dresses and thin shoes are not as freely worn by our ladies, and if the fumes of tobacco and the juice of the filthy weed do not as freely flow forth from the lips of gentlemen now, as formerly? I certainly hope there are those who have ceased these evil practices, but at best the work of reformation has but barely begun.

Awake, then, ye philanthropists and Christians, to a sense of these terrible evils which are destroying our American people. Let the pulpit no longer keep silence; for if these evils are but the sin of ignorance, as I would charitably hope they generally are, there is a want of a correct knowledge; but if knowingly they are practiced, has the self-murderer any promise of the life of heaven?

A year or two ago I had occasion to give a much needed lecture to the wife of one of the most popular clergymen then in Michigan, on tight dressing. After I had finished I turned to the clergyman, and said: "Sir, I should think you would feel it a duty to preach at least every other sermon against tight dressing, until the ladies of your congregation cease this practice." In perfect astonishment he exclaimed: "What, I preach against tight dressing? I don't know what I have to do with the subject, or how I should get at it." I replied to him: "What, you sir, a minister of the gospel, with a knowledge of the fact, or at least the testimony of the medical profession almost to a man, that the ladies of our land, and even of your own congregation, are not only destroying their own health and lives by this practice, but are even destroying our race, and you have nothing to do with it? Will you be so kind, sir, as to tell me if you have anything to do with any of the actual sins of the people, or are you here a watchman on the walls of Zion to cry peace, peace, when there is no peace; when even ignorant members of your congregation are rushing on to physical destruction, and when others, perchance, are knowingly violating natural laws and thereby destroying both soul and body?" I received no reply—I expected none.

We have had enough of such fashionable preaching as simply pleases the understanding, and treats of the evils of the world only in a general, superficial manner; which neither enlightens the understanding, nor stirs the conscience, as to the individual, actual sins so prevalent in external life at this day. Repentance and reformation must precede regeneration. A repentance and reformation which shall be ultimated in life, from the heart, can alone lead us in the straight and narrow way that leads to life, or heaven.

In the present fallen state of man, we need line upon line, and precept upon precept, here a little and there a little.

Let every lover of humanity, by precept and example, use his or her utmost exertions to revolutionize the present method of training young ladies and girls, both as to dress and as to labor. Away with your indolent, and consequently unhealthy and unhappy women and girls. Give them active labor about the house and in the open air, to develop red blood, muscle and bone—an organization worthy of God's image, and worthy to be the dwelling place of a wife and mother—a helpmate for man, when he shall put away his filthy habits, and stand forth in the true dignity of a free man.

CHAPTER VIII.

NEGLECT OF AMUSEMENTS.

THE Lord has formed in the spirit of man a faculty which phrenologists denominate mirthfulness. We see manifestations of this propensity even in the animal kingdom; in the playfulness of the young kitten or puppy, in the gambols of the lamb, calf, colt, and other young animals. The manifestations of the continued activity of this faculty do not cease with the youth of the animal, and this fact should teach the cold, calculating, selfish men of this day, an important lesson. I am satisfied that in instrumentalities for moral improvement, in few things are the American people lacking more than in proper recreations, and amusements. The young child, even before he can lisp his parent's name, will respond to the playfulness of his little brother or sister with a hearty good will; and we can perceive, in the ceaseless playfulness of childhood and youth, that this is one of the strong traits in the character of man. To me it is evident, that this faculty has been implanted in the human soul for a great and good purpose. It seems to me that it must be manifest to every one who, without prejudice, reflects upon this subject, that the coming together of neighbors and friends, to join in cheerful, joyous, and innocent amusements, which agreeably exercise both body and mind, or joining their voices in sweet and cheerful songs, is calculated to make men better, by drawing out and cultivating kindly and neighborly affections and thus strengthening the bonds of neighborly love. Has not our Creator manifestly intended amusements to be among the most important of the instrumentalities for developing and keeping alive the good and kindly affections which he has implanted within us? Does not all observations show that when men and women neglect social amusements, there is, to say the least, a great tendency to become cold, and hard-faced towards each other, also calculating, selfish, and evil, and to engage in deceiving, cheating, and backbiting each other.

Cheerfulness and contentment are all important for both health and happiness. If there is cheerfulness in the heart it will, according to the laws of development which we have been considering, die or fade away, if we do not allow it, at suitable seasons, to come forth into act. The physician finds amusements among the most important auxiliaries to aid in the restoration from disease of body or mind, and they are also among the most useful instrumentalities to prevent disease, and especially insanity, which is so rapidly increasing in our country. The mind of man is composed of various faculties, both intellectual and affectional; and one of these faculties, of either department, can no more be long exercised to the neglect of the others without causing mental derangement, than can one organ or member of the body be thus exercised, to the neglect of others, without causing disease and deformity. In such active amusements as bring energetic physical exercise, such as ball-playing, running, dancing, and the like, almost every muscle and organ of the body is brought into active use, and pleasantly exercised, far more so than in any one kind of ordinary labor; and for this reason such amusements are found more useful in either curing, counteracting a tendency to, or preventing disease, than common labor--when considering simply the physical man. So in regard to the faculties of the mind, in such active amusements as have been named, and many others that will occur to the reader, there is scarcely an intellectual or affectional faculty, which will not be brought into play *or exercised*; and, if worthy motives prompt, legitimately exercised. The perceptive faculties—form, size, weight, number, time, etc.,—the intellectual faculties—comparison, causality, ideality—the affections, benevolence, love of approbation, hope, combativeness kindness, conscientiousness, and even veneration, all have a legitimate chance for exercise, and with more uniformity, perhaps, than during ordinary labor of any kind. Mirthfulness, then, seems to be to the spirit of man, a kind of balance-wheel, as it were, and when duly exercised, tends to preserve a healthy action in every other faculty; and, by being allowed to manifest itself in the form of active cheerful amusements, it contributes, perhaps, more than any other faculty, towards preserving health, and preventing, and even curing diseases of the body.

The importance of amusements is far from being properly recognized at present, although a few intelligent men, even among the clergy, are beginning to throw out hints upon this subject. Henry Ward Beecher, in his Lectures to young men, says:

"The necessity of amusement, is admitted on all hands. There is an appetite of the eye, of the ear, and of every sense, for which God has provided the material. Gayety of every degree, this side of puerile levity, is wholesome to the body, to the mind and to the morals. Nature is a vast repository of manly enjoyments. The magnitude of God's works is not less admirable than its exhilarating beauty. The rudest forms have something of beauty; the ruggedest strength is graced with some charm; the very pins, and rivets, and clasps of nature, are attractive by qualities of beauty, more than is necessary for mere utility."

Rev. James L. Corning, Pastor of the Westminster Presbyterian Church of Buffalo, N. Y., in a recent work on the "Christian Law of Amusement," published by Phinney & Co., of Buffalo, which I can cheerfully recommend to the attention of the reader, says:

"We infer that mirthful recreation is not only lawful for, but it is morally obligatory upon, every rational being. It not only does not conflict with religion, but it is one of its *great demands.* It is not only permitted to a Christian man to divert himself, but it is his most solemn duty—solemn duty, I say—for there are some people who are dying for the want of recreation, but who never can be got to obey the imperative demands of their nature except they hear the very thunders of Sinai rattling over their heads, and the voice of the Most High commanding them out of their frozen propriety and austere behaviour. There are many Christian men and women worn out by dyspepsia and chronic melancholy, who could actually be trebled in value to the church and the world if they could be persuaded to devote an hour every day to mirthful sport, just as scrupulously as they devote a given period to reflection and prayer."

Nor does there apparently exist in the minds of many, a distinct idea between the proper use and abuse of amusements; or what constitutes an abuse. Let us examine this point hastily, for it is all important to have correct principles to guide us, that we may avoid excess on the one hand, or the denouncing of good and useful amusements on the other; both of these extremes being alike destructive to both spiritual and physical health and happiness.

In the chapter on the use and abuse of the digestive organs, and in the little work on Marriage, and its Violations, the writer has endeavored to show that use is the only legitimate object for gratifying our appetites, and passions; and that, whenever we fail to have a worthy motive, and seek simply sensual gratification alone, we pervert our appetites and passions from their true end, and thus debase both soul and body. If instead of eating and drinking to live, and being governed, both as to quantity and quality, by a desire to give health and strength, we have first in view the gratification of appetite, we become gluttons, and drunkards. If we seek the acquisition of wealth without regard to making a worthy use of it, we become misers. So the end in view makes the acquisition of knowledge a blessing or curse to ourselves; and others are benefited or injured by the use we make of it when acquired. So in regard to amusements; if we seek them simply as selfish and sensual gratifications without regard to any good use to be accomplished by them, we pervert them from their legitimate end; and are almost sure to carry to excess such as are proper, and to seek such as are improper and unlawful to both our spiritual and physical being. But we have a good end in view when we seek our mental and physical health, in such amusements as best tend to promote a healthy state of mind and body; and the very object we have in view, or the motive which prompts us to act, will tend to restrain us from excess, and from such amusements as are injurious to health, or destructive to morals. We have a good end in view when we engage in innocent amusements which will interest, amuse, or in any way benefit others; and especially when we engage in such as will benefit our own families, and immediate neighbors; when we permit and take part in such amusements with our own families as will make home attractive to our children, and cause them to love us, and feel that we desire to make them happy. If we will but let our children have proper recreations at home, and superintend, and join hands with them, we can teach them the true use and abuse of amusements, and by example lead them to enjoy the one, and shun the other; and it is as much our duty to restrain and direct our children in regard to their amusements, as it is in regard to their eating and drinking; and, when they arrive at a suitable age to understand, to instruct them in regard to what end, or motives, should prompt them to seek amusement; so that they may be guided by reason to seek the quality and extent of amusements they need. Then they will not feel it a hardship, to be deprived of the privilege of abusing this faculty, and parents can, with a better show of reason, require them to avoid carrying them to excess, or seeking them in improper places and company.

The most important and useful amusements are, of course, such as exercise freely and harmoniously the faculties of the mind and organs of the body at the same time. Among these may be named athletic sports and games in the open air, running, sliding, skating, riding, etc., during day-light, for both gentlemen and ladies. Among in-door amusements none is so appropriate, so far as I am able to judge, as dancing. I do not mean the miserable shuffling of this day, when delicacy and laziness are fashionable, but the regular "cut down," of a quarter, or half century ago. Waltzing is objectionable, as whirling around rapidly is an unnatural and injurious form of exercise. If there were no other objections to this form of dancing, it should not be practiced or countenanced. Dancing is an orderly form of recreation; it is to music, and is graceful, and tends to improve the manners; and where the two sexes join in amusements, it is even in the polka, far less objectionable than the various plays, attended by kissing, which are often countenanced by those who discard dancing. But let no one for a moment suppose that I am an advocate for midnight revels, or of the ball-room adjoining the bar-room; or of midnight, or until broad day-light dances; or even of our fashionable parties of folly and extravagance, where vanity sits enthroned. Our amusements should be with our own families, friends and neighbors, in our own parlors, or beneath our own vine and shade trees, or in the fields and groves, on the silvery lake, the gliding stream, or upon the mountain top, young and old, hand in hand. Our amusements should never be carried beyond ten or eleven o'clock at night, at farthest, that they need not encroach upon the hours required for rest. Frequent amusements are far more useful than occasional and long continued exercises. Our late suppers are destructive alike to health and morals, and should be discarded entirely. They are generally composed of high-seasoned stimulating dishes, tea, coffee, and often even fermented and alcoholic drinks, all of which excite the passions and appetites, and are a fruitful cause of vice and dissipation. No one should ever eat, even wholesome plain food, after six in the evening; and if refreshments are to be furnished to a party, it should be either at dinner, at noon, or supper at six o'clock; for no one can eat and drink, especially such trash as is furnished, at midnight with impunity. I can hardly conceive of any instrumentality better calculated to destroy young men and women, both spiritually and physically, than our fashionable parties, as at present conducted. If there is any one passion or faculty of the human soul, which, in the American people, does not require to be cultivated, or stimulated in its perversions, it is love of approbation. Vanity is the form of infernal fire which threatens to consume the very vitals of our Christianity and morality, and it destroys the physical health and lives ot more of our females and, perhaps, even of our males, by the destructive fashions and habits it induces, than the perversions of any other passion. The introduction of young persons, at a tender age, before the rational faculties are fairly developed, into such hot beds of evil, as our fashionable parties, is certainly an abuse of no small magnitude. The young are there taught, practically, that it is right to strive to excel others in the way of expensive suppers, fine furniture, extravagant dresses, and in following destructive habits, such as tight dressing, eating stimulating and late suppers, and gossiping, and even back-biting each other. As the great end and aim of such parties is generally, beyond all question, the gratification of vanity, and not any particular good use, the evils resulting from them can hardly be enumerated. Perhaps more than any other instrumentality they uphold the present destructive habits of dress and indolence among our ladies. They beget an appetite which tends to lead young men to our drinking and eating saloons at midnight, to spend their time and money in worse than useless gratification, and carousing. They beget a love for useless display, and habits of extravagance in the young of both sexes, which tend to discontent, poverty and crime. They beget a love of riches for the sake of selfish sensual gratification. They deter young men from marrying because they feel that they are not able to meet the extravagant mode of life encouraged by such parties. They are so expensive, and cause so much trouble, that no family can afford to give them often, and for the young to have amusements as often as they need social recreation, their circle of acquaintances, or those who give and receive in return invitations, must be large, and consequently these amusements rarely occur at home, immediately within parental influence, even though the young gentlemen and ladies, may attend several evenings during a week; and if they do attend such parties, thus often, late hours and dissipation soon unfit them for the actual duties and uses of life, and destroy health. They are a frequent cause of jealousy, envy, and hatred. They take the place of smaller and less expensive gatherings of friends and neighbors for proper amusements; and, from their glitter and display, they render the latter tame and unsatisfactory, to the young, and the quiet of home, where amusements frequently are not encouraged or practiced, little more satisfactory than the gloom of prison walls. They bring young gentlemen and ladies together amid unnatural glitter, attracted more by gaudy display, than real worth; and afford them little opportunity to become intimately acquainted with each other's disposition, which is so important before any preference, looking towards matrimony, shall have been manifested between the young, after which each is upon the guard, and strives to present the best face possible. As a result of all this artificial state of society, we have the young rushing into the married state with the least possible knowledge of each other's disposition, or fitness; with romantic expectations, which can only result in disappointment and unhappiness. If instead of all this glitter, the young men were in the habit of meeting in the domestic circle, freely, the young ladies, in company with parents, brothers, and sisters, and the young ladies under similar circumstances the gentlemen, and engaging in harmless amusements, and games, which would bring into activity the various faculties of the mind, they would be far better qualified to judge correctly of each others disposition, by the manner in which they treat their parents, brothers, sisters and neighbors, in trifling acts, words, and looks, in unguarded moments, than what they possibly can be in the present artificial state of society, and if they were then to marry they would know what to expect in each other, and be prepared to meet the troubles of married life without disappointment and discontent.

Some of the evils of our present state of society, are well set forth in the following from the New York *Express:*

"Our young men are a painful study. As they lounge about the streets with bold, leering faces, poisoning the air with oaths, or whirl madly along behind lashed horses, or loom up dimly amid the smoky glare of haunts of folly, sin, and shame, it is sickening to think that with them rests the future of the country, and in them lies its hope. It is no wonder that the hearts of fathers and mothers and sisters are filled with dread and grief.

No wonder that the perpetual and earnest advice to the young man is to go into 'ladies' society.' The advice is good. There is positive safety for him in the society of a modest, gentle, kindly, and sensible girl. There is comparative safety for him in the company of a vain, giggling, trifling girl.

"The most empty-headed and empty-hearted of coquettes is a more harmless companion for him than a cursing, tippling fellow, who thinks mainly of all manner of silliness and sin, and will travel fast, although hell yawns at the end of the road. Yes, your young man's salvation is in the sweet smile and voice, the beautiful graces and accomplishments, of some fair creature, attractive alike in mind and body. But your young man dares not go and see a young woman he fancies, and make a friend and companion of her. Will not all the Mrs. Grundies think and say that it means something, and immediately and vigorously set to work to whisper their suspicions loud enough for the world —including the respective families of the young persons—to hear them? Is not your young man a flirt, a desperate fellow, in whom there is danger, if he is known to go to see a half dozen girls at the same time? Has not this propriety which pervades our fine modern life something to do with the terrible outlawry and viciousness of the young men? Has not rigid, ghastly etiquette driven them from the parlor to the rum-shop and worse? In the days when some of us were boys and girls, it was not a proof that two young people were engaged to be married, that they were often together, happy in the interchange of interest and sympathy and all kindly feeling. And somehow there were better boys than there are now; and better girls, too, for that matter."

I am aware that some object to dancing because it has been carried to excess, and because it has, under certain circumstances, led into bad company; but the same objection lies, with even more force, against eating and drinking; yet because multitudes eat and drink to gluttony, and drunkenness, or seek the gratification of their appetite, in the society of the low and vicious, in saloons, groceries and houses of prostitution, is this a reason why we should condemn eating and drinking? certainly not, every one will reply. The first question is, whether eating is essential to our happiness; if it is, it is right to eat. Then it becomes our duty to inquire how much we should eat, how often, what we should eat, when, and where. The same is true in regard to amusements. That they are necessary, for the development and health of body and mind, few will question at this day; and it is manifest that our American people are suffering seriously, both physically and mentally, for the want of suitable amusements, and that this is a fruitful cause of imperfect development, disease, deformity, fanaticism and insanity, in our midst. It is then manifest that our people, young and old, male and female, and especially the ladies in our cities and villages and even in the country, do not have all the amusements they actually need, especially such as will give active exercise to the body. Next, the inquiry legitimately arises how often should we have amusements? Every one will perhaps agree that they should be regular, as far as practicable at stated intervals, and at least daily; and not so long continued as to do harm, or, as to encroach upon time which should be devoted to other duties and uses. Next arises the question, what amusements are the best adapted to answer the end in view? Certainly such as will give active exercise to the faculties of the mind, and muscles of the body, are far more valuable and important than those which simply exercise the mental faculties, such as lectures, concerts, theatrical performances, games of cards, dice, chess, etc., or than those which simply exercise the body, such as gymnastic exercises, walking, riding, or rowing, without any good object in view except exercise. Out door games and sports of an active character, beyond all doubt, are the most valuable and important, as has already been said, for both males and females. But in our cities we often lack play grounds, or yards, for such sports, and are therefore compelled, in a great measure, to depend upon in-door amusements for the exercise of both body and mind at the same time, and such alone can fully satisfy or answer the demands of both soul and body. As I have already said, I know of no in-door amusement that is as proper and useful as dancing, for it exercises both body and mind, and gives health and vigor; and I verily believe that if all of our citizens would spend one hour, every evening, except Sunday evenings, at this exercise, it would be of incalculable benefit to the physical and mental health of our people.

Mr. Peter Bayne, in his "Essays on the Christian life," speaking on the subject of dancing as an amusement, says:

"When you can trustfully grasp the hand extended to yours, when you know the smile on the lip that addresses you to be the speechless voice of the viewless spirit of kindness; when you can be assured that the tongue now tuned to soft geniality and friendliness will not to-morrow slander your name, when mirth flows in its natural channels, and trustful hearts leap in sympathy with trustful hearts, then all is right. And if in such an assemblage the joyous exhilaration will be increased by moving to harmonious sound with gestures of beauty and vivacious grace, let no one object to the dance; the buoyant leaping of the blood is nature's, the laws of beauty in sound and sight are nature's; who can say they are wrong? The rain falls no less cheeringly because the sunbeams painted the clouds with gold and vermilion, industry and action flourish all the better for this sporting in the sunlight of mirth and gladness."

The question is not whether this and other forms of amusements have been, or are abused, and do harm to many as at present practiced, but it is whether in themselves, when rightly used, they are useful and harmless. It is our duty to see that neither ourselves nor our children abuse them, as much as it is to see that we do not make an improper use of good food. We should never resort to amusements which in themselves are wrong, and injurious, any more than we should to food which is injurious. We should certainly use our best judgment in selecting the time and place for amusements, as well as the company, and strive to make them beneficial to both body and mind. We should avoid ostentatious display, and unnecessary expense, and strive to render them simple, attractive and useful.

In almost all amusements we have an opportunity to teach the young lessons of forbearance, kindness, and strict integrity, which we should not fail to improve; for if the young are taught by both precept and example, to be strictly honest in small things, and are led to act accordingly, there will certainly be far less danger of their becoming dishonest in after life. Nothing is hardly more important than "to nip in the bud" any disposition to bet in connexion with amusements. The young should be taught that even the desire to acquire property in any such way, is morally wrong, and that to receive it in this manner without returning a due equivalent, is but little better than stealing. There is a great neglect of correct teachings upon this subject; and, I am sorry to say, even of example. So long as parents will patronize gift concerts, gift stores, purchase chance tickets of any kind, or make bets within the knowledge of their children, they need not be surprised that the latter commence gambling young, and soon become "blacklegs."

It is cheering, at present, to see our churches arousing to a sense of their duty in regard to amusements, to behold their joyous Sabbath School pic-nics; this is a noble beginning towards encouraging cheerful and useful amusements for the young, but in this selfish age of the world, the old need them even more. Let our religious teachers and churches look to this matter, and see if they are discharging their full duty in this respect. Amusements have been given over to the direction of the ungodly long enough, or until they have been terribly perverted; and it remains for Christians to restore them to their true position, and to teach that they have their use, and should never be followed as the chief object of life. Long enough have the ministers of religion battled innocent and necessary amusements, to the neglect of those terrible habits and evils which are destroying the moral and physical stamina of our race. With what just propriety does the Rev. J. L. Corning inquire of his readers:

"Did you ever hear a sermon preached specifically on the sinful excess of ornament and attire connected with large parties?"

He might have included also in his inquiry, if they had ever heard a sermon against tight lacing, low-necked dresses and thin shoes. Again he inquires:

"Did you ever hear a sermon, or read a tract on the wickedness of a system of late hours, on the dreadful sin of thus undermining physical health by depriving the body of rest during the period when God designed it to sleep? Again, did you ever hear a sermon, or read a tract upon the monstrous crime of gormandizing, and that at the most unseasonable hour of the day, universally prevalent at our fashionable entertainments? Again, did you ever hear a sermon or read a tract designed to show the tendency of our parties, as they are constructed, to create and nurture a politeness as hollow and false as the bosom of Judas Iscariot? If you have heard sermons, or read tracts on these crying evils, you have been more thorough in your literary research than I have been. Now, please to remember, that these things can never be right under any circumstances. Late hours, gluttony, extravagant display, hypocritical etiquette, these are never right, and never can be. But here, linked with them is an amusement which, restricted within due limits, and indulged at proper seasons, is not only harmless, but every way beneficial both to body and mind, and lo! this is the great scarecrow of the ecclesiastical conscience. Now let it not be thought that in this we offer the most remotely implied endorsement of dancing as it is practiced at present, with all its sinful appendages and in some of its more fashionable figures. But, take it in its most objectionable form, and I am free to say that, among the evils connected with our fashionable parties, it ranks among the least. Why, I have sat beside a professing Christian woman in one of the beautiful parlors of a fashionable metropolitan avenue, whose jewelled neck, and ears, and fingers, and dazzling brocade, as much as said to the assembled guests, 'none of your dresses cost as much as mine;' and then I have seen her go into the supper-room and eat enough to make a swine have gripes of conscience, and then come out, obese, and panting for breath, made marvelously religious by sandwiches and champagne, and wind up the farce with a pious discourse on the sin of dancing!"

Surely there is hope for the physical and moral regeneration of our race when clergymen are ready to speak thus plainly and boldly of the monster evils of the day, and especially when they have the moral courage to intimate, as does the writer from whom I have just quoted, that a weak stomach instead of Divine grace, ought to have the credit of Paysan's austere melancholy; and that the circulation of the memoirs of pious little children—who invariably, and necessarily die young from a violation of God's laws—as true types of youthful piety, is to be deprecated as conveying to the youthful mind false notions as to the nature and requirements of religion; and that ball playing and skating, with those who need exercise and amusements, may be useful in preparing them for the religious exercises of Wednesday evening.

There is but a single sentiment contained in this work of Rev. Mr. Corning, which does not meet my hearty approval. When he intimates, by quoting St. Paul's rule in regard to the use of meat, that it may be the duty of his readers to shun dancing for fear that some one may be likely to be led into sin by their indulgence, I cannot think he is exactly right, for he admits that the Christian portion of the community are suffering both physically and spiritually for the want of amusements; and he is even compelled to admit that under proper restrictions as to time, place, and company, dancing is one of the most appropriate amusements. If this is true, as it seems to me it certainly is, it would seem to be the duty of the Christian not to shun dancing for fear it may, perchance, offend the morbid consciences of some of his brethren in the church, or because it might be an example in right doing which some evil disposed person might carry out into wrong doing, or abuse, for such a course would sacrifice the general good to individual prejudice. Better, far better, that the Christian should enlighten the consciences of his brethren, teach to all the proper use and abuse of dancing and other innocent amusements, and by heartily engaging in them, set an example in well doing which would at this day if all Christians would follow it, be the means of rescuing multitudes, both within and without the churches, from physical and spiritual destruction.

In finishing what he has to say upon the subject of amusements the writer desires to repeat his sincere conviction that the American people, as a body, are suffering almost to the point of physical and moral destruction for the want of proper amusements. We must have less hard work, both physically and intellectually, among the working portion of the community, and less laziness among the idle, and more active innocent amusement and recreation among both the working and the idle classes.

Amusements can never perform the use for which they were designed, until men are directed and restrained in seeking them by the religious sentiment, and make a good or legitimate use the end and aim. Man will rarely if ever fail to abuse every appetite and passion, when any other motive prompts the gratification.

CHAPTER IX.

IMPROPER USE OF POISONS—NARCOTICS.

We have, in the natural world, two great classes of substances which produce effects on man's body when either taken into the stomach or brought in contact with the living structures so as to be absorbed and taken into the circulation.

The first class comprises all animals, vegetables and minerals, which afford food and drink, and nourish and sustain the body without causing disease or producing any undue excitement or depression of the whole system, or of individual organs. The use of these substances is indispensable to build up the growing organisms of the young, and to supply the waste and sustain the middle aged and the old. But even healthy articles of food and drink may be taken to excess and do injury; here, then, is the legitimate field for temperance, that we may control our appetites and eat and drink only such a quantity as is necessary to sustain the body in health and vigor—"eat and drink to live, and not live to eat and drink." The second class of substances which produces an effect upon the body when taken into the organism, either through the stomach or in any other manner, comprises all the various poisons, animal, vegetable and mineral, which are capable of causing specific diseases, or of producing undue excitement or depression, either general or local. Now, it must be evident to every intelligent individual, that with such substances we have no manner of business as articles of food or drink; and to knowingly use them is a violation of the laws of God as manifested in His creation. But the question arises here, how shall we be able to distinguish between healthy articles and poisons, or improper substances? By their effects we may know them

All healthy articles of food sustain and nourish the body in vigor, but without any unnatural excitement, and the individual has a healthy and natural appetite, which is satisfied by a regular quantity of food, which does not require to be progressively increased in order to satisfy the demands of the appetite. Nor is this all, this healthy appetite will be satisfied by the use of any wholesome article of food, and this is a point to which I desire especially to call the attention of the reader.

A man may live upon potatoes, and a meal of bread will satisfy his appetite, or he may live upon beef, and a meal of mutton or venison will relieve his hunger. So of any proper substance which he may use to nourish his body, even though he may have used it for years, any article which is equally nourishing and easily digested, will satisfy his hunger, or the call of nature for nourishment. In striking contrast with this will be found the appetite for poisonous substances, for such articles, even though used but a short time, beget an appetite which no other substance in nature can satisfy. The craving for alcoholic drinks is never satisfied except by some beverage or substance which contains alcohol. Nor will the appetite for tobacco and opium be satisfied by any other poison except tobacco or opium; even alcohol will not relieve the craving for opium, nor will opium satisfy the appetite for tobacco. Here, then, we have positive evidence that any given article is an improper substance for food or drink, when it excites an unnatural appetite, which no other healthy food will satisfy.

Again; to supply the waste in the adult, or to nourish the growing human body, a regular, constant, and uniform quantity of food is required; and the man at fifty or sixty requires and takes no more than he required at twenty or thirty years of age.

This is not true of poisons, for they seem to beget, as it were, in the human organism, a new life or diseased action, which constantly requires feeding; and by the very law in accordance with which this class of agents usually act—to which I shall presently call the attention of the reader—the amount used requires to be steadily increased, until many times the quantity a healthy man can take with impunity, will be required to satisfy the demands of the appetite. Here, then, we have positive evidence that any substance is not a proper article of diet, which requires to be taken in increased quantities to satisfy the appetite for it. Again; poisons when taken into the stomach, and their use long continued, in quantities which are not inappropriate for healthy articles of food or drink, cause disease; and every poison causes its own specific disease. Opium causes one train of symptoms, alcohol another, antimony still another.

It must be manifest to all that every substance which will cause disease of a specific character, or a disease peculiar to itself, cannot be a suitable article for food or drink and that it should never be used for such a purpose.

Poisons generally act upon the human system as stimulants, or excitants; and, although some of these substances excite in a measure the whole system, yet they generally spend their force more especially upon different organs or parts. Alcohol and opium upon the brain and nervous system; calomel and other mercurials upon the glands about the mouth; antimony and ipecac upon the stomach; jalap and aloes upon the bowels.

When man fell and came to love himself and the gratifications, pleasures, and possessions of earth, more than he loved the Lord and his neighbor, his moral sensibilities became blunted, until at last, he came to be scarcely able to distinguish between good and evil, or between truth and falsehood. Nor did his fall end here, for the nourishing and life giving substances in the natural world correspond to man's good affections and thoughts, for they nourish man's natural body, as heavenly love and wisdom derived from the Lord and His Word, nourish man's spiritual body; but the poisonous substances, and such as became poisonous when perverted from their legitimate use, hold a special relation to man's perverted or evil affections and thoughts; and when used to feed and nourish the natural body, they destroy, more or less rapidly as has already been stated, the natural appetite for simple, plain, food, and the healthy action of the organs of the body, and substitute an unnatural appetite, and a diseased and unnatural action in the organism, which lead to structural diseases and death, in the same manner that their corresponding evils and falses, when harbored, tend to destroy all true or heavenly life in man, and substitute infernal life, or the life of self and worldly love. When man spiritually partook of the tree of knowledge of good and evil, and his affections and understanding became perverted, nothing was more natural than that he should, when he made evils his own by acting them out, desire, or even crave those poisonous substances in the natural world, which corresponded to his own evils and falses, and as far as he could discover their action, use them; for such substances excited and gave new life to the perverted affections, and filled his mental atmosphere with thoughts in harmony with such affections. Thus man began to use various poisonous substances as articles for nourishment, or as luxuries; and as he continued to use them, gradually his perceptions and natural sensibilities became blunted, and his taste perverted, until, at present, he is scarcely able, even with the aid of science, to distinguish between proper and improper food.

We certainly have reason to fear that our race has not yet reached the bottom of the ladder, but that a state of degradation even lower than heretofore reached awaits us, and towards which we are slowly but surely descending. M. J. Michelet, a French writer, in a recent work on "Love," says:

"We cannot conceal from ourselves that in these latter times the Inclinations have undergone profound changes. The causes of this are numerous. I will state two only, mental and physical at the same time, which, going straight to the brain, and deadening it, tend to paralyse all our moral faculties.

"For a century past, the increasing invasion of spirituous liquors and narcotics has been marching irresistibly, with results varying according to the population—here obscuring the mind, hopelessly depraving it—there, penetrating deeper into the physical economy, reaching even the race itself—but everywhere isolating man, giving him, even in his home, a deplorable preference for solitary enjoyment.

"No need to him of society, of love, of family; in their stead the dreary pleasures of a polygamic life, which, imposing no responsibility upon the man, not even protecting the woman (as the polygamy of the East does,) is therefore more destructive, indefinite, limitless, stimulating and enervating continually."

At present, having lost the power of perception, we have no certain means of distinguishing poisons except by carefully watching their effects when they are brought in contact with, or are taken into the living organism.

It would seem then to be a very important preparation for both the spiritual and physical regeneration of individual men, and our race, that we should be able to distinguish poisons from healthy food; and when we possess a knowledge as to what substances are poisons, we can but see that it is all important that we shun their use, as we must the spiritual evils which are stimulated, and, as it were, nourished by them, if we would arrive to a state of health and happiness in this world, and heaven in the next.

Hundreds of physicians, men of science and careful observation, scattered over the world, are engaged in the work of carefully proving the various substances, supposed to be poisonous, upon themselves during health, by cautiously taking them, and carefully watching their effects, or the symptoms which they cause, and writing them down for the benefit of others; so that we now have a knowledge of the effects of a large, and increasing number of poisons, such as man has never had before since the fall.

The reader may perhaps ask, does not the man who is in the constant use of a poison, and has used it for years, understand its effects better than he, who, without a love for it and with an appetite unperverted, takes it simply to watch its effects? He certainly does not, any more than the man who is sunken down in spiritual evils, understands the fearful character and consequences of those evils better than he who shuns them. The evil man makes his evils his delight, and they become his very life, and seem to him as good, and had not the Lord bowed the heavens and come down to man in his lowest estate, in the fullness of time, with the light of His Divine Truth, showing him the evils of his heart, man must have perished spiritually, and by ultimating those evils in external life by the gratification of perverted passions, and sensual appetites, our race would have been swept from the earth. So true is it that man can never, by his own unaided vision, see the evils of his own heart; even conscience becomes seared and it is only by acknowledging the Lord Jesus Christ, who is the way, the truth, and the life, and by receiving into his understanding the truths of the Divine Word, that man can ever see his evils and thereby be enabled to shun them. I met a man one day in the street, who, during conversation, said to me that he was free from sin, that he had no evil desires, and was guilty of no evil acts, and he evidently was sincere, yet this man denied the Lord and His Word; but at the very time of this conversation he was looking at a house which was for sale, and said that he hoped that property would come down to half its value, so that a poor man could get him a house to live in of his own, and that then he would purchase. I said to him that there were two sides to that question; that perhaps a majority of the real estate owners in the city had purchased their homesteads at the present prices, and had paid the hard earnings of years as purchase money, and yet were owing perhaps half, more or less, of the amount they agreed to pay; now if property falls one half, the man who, perchance has purchased the house you are looking at, and has paid but one half the purchase money, say one thousand dollars, will be compelled to sell it, for the value of labor will come down also, and you will be able to purchase it with your one thousand dollars, and he will lose his house and be left penniless; now do you think that would be desirable and right? Well, yes, he seemed to think it would be and, to all appearance, looked on the land with delight, and was anxious to enter in and possess it. How far he came short of coveting his neighbor's house I shall leave the reader to judge.

The more a man strives to shun evils the more distinctly will he be able to see the evils within himself, and it is only after the warfare of a lifetime that the Christian is able to enter into his rest.

As the material body is built up from the natural world, I have assumed that both good and *bad* men require healthy food, to develop and sustain substantial and healthy bodies. Some are disposed to call this in question, and the inquiry has heen made as to what kind of food is required by just such a race of men as we now have, and are, with an intimation that the above position is not correct. But we have only to look and we shall find around us positive evidence, that when men live temperately upon plain, wholesome food, they may become well developed and healthy, even when they are evil, and swayed by the most infernal passions, or by the love of rule, vanity or the love of money; and they may live to old age, provided they do not contract diseases by exposure or other excesses. We have equally good evidence, that neither the good nor the *bad* man, can indulge in the use of poisonous substances as food or drink, without sooner or later, according to his power of resistance or natural constitution, other habits, and the quantity he uses, feeling their effects, or impairing both his spiritual and physical health. The good and bad man will suffer nearly alike, all other things being equal. The child's stomach is "born to expect" nourishment from the maternal breast, in which expectation, I am sorry to say, it is sometimes disappointed in this degenerate age. No child is born drinking whisky, strong beer, coffee, or tea, chewing or smoking tobacco, or opium, or eating mustard, and other spices, or with stomachs, expecting or prepared to receive these substances without being injured by their use; and it is, at least, questionable whether they are ever born with an appetite for them. I do not question but that, owing to hereditary inclination, some children may acquire an appetite for them much more readily than others, especially when their taste is covered by some grateful article, such as sugar, milk, or other wholesome food. I have a strong impression that all careful observation will sustain this position. The goodness and wisdom of the Lord are manifested in a ceaseless effort to preserve the physical integrity of our race, in the new born child. A parent may have lost an eye, arm, or leg, and yet the child be perfect; and, the worst hereditary diseases, with the exception of those which result from the violation of the conjugal relation, and sexual instincts, generally do not manifest themselves during infancy, or even during childhood; so that there is a chance to prevent the development of these diseases by living a true and orderly life, and the future physical regeneration of our race depends, in a great measure, upon this provision. The child inherits a tendency or inclination to evils; but if such evils were active, he would possess no days of freedom, and would not be responsible for his acts, and our race would be speedily destroyed. So if where there is a hereditary tendency to consumption, cancer, gout and insanity, children were generally born already diseased, there would soon be an end to all families contaminated by such diseases. As the days of infancy are passing away the child's stomach expects wholesome nourishing food, and an appetite exists for such food, and, when unperverted, remains during life. Among good and useful articles of food, there is a great difference in the ease with which they are digested and appropriated for the nourishment of the body. All men have not equally strong digestive organs, therefore, while one man may eat almost any proper article of food, another is compelled to select with care from the same articles; one man may live entirely on vegetable diet, another will require some meat; and it certainly is right that we should select such food as is best adapted to nourish the body, and give health and strength. Use should be the end in view, and not sensual gratification.

That poisons are often required, and are useful, as medicines in small doses, for a limited time, I admit; but to my own mind it is equally clear, that there is no hereditary predisposition which either compels or requires their habitual use as articles of food, drink, or as luxuries—that they supply no place which healthy food will not better fill, in the human organism. And it is certain that evil men are not exempt from the pernicious effects which they cause when thus used, and that their use does harm to both body and soul.

But what is to be said in regard to habit? Can men who have been long accustomed to the use of poisons discontinue them suddenly with safety, even though they are being harmed by them? It is certain that they cannot always do it, for diseased excitement and life, caused by the poison used, have taken the place of that which is natural, and the life of the body will sometimes be endangered by this sudden withdrawal. The time required to break up the use of improper substances can only be determined by observation. The man who has been drinking large quantities of alcoholic drinks for a long time, can never discontinue their use at once, without being in danger of having delirium tremens; but he may always do it gradually, so as to cease entirely within a few days, or at most a few weeks, with perfect safety. Dangerous symptoms rarely follow the sudden omission of tobacco, coffee, or tea, or any of the other poisons in common use except perhaps opium, although suffering more or less severe, will follow when the use of either of them is discontinued at once. It is perhaps better in all cases to cease using such substances gradually, if the individual has the strength of purpose to do it thus; and there is no danger in breaking up any such habits in this manner, in a few weeks, I need not say months. And abundant observation establishes the point, that both good and bad men are benefited by the change, so far as health is concerned. It will not do to bring the cravings of appetite to justify the use of improper substances longer than is necessary to safely discontinue them.

No man by his own unaided intellect can ever see that a poison, which he has been using gradually for years, injures him, even although he may be dying from its poisonous effects, and suffering beyond patient endurance; for poisons palliate the symptoms which their habitual use has caused, by feeding or nourishing the perverted or diseased life, which they have caused in the organism; and the man feels in every fibre that they are just what he needs, and he has a realizing sense that their use is good for him, and even necessary to keep him alive; for when he attempts to discontinue using them, suffering follows; the physical organism becomes aroused to the violence which has been done to it, just as man's conscience becomes aroused, when man ceases to do evil, and he thereby comes more clearly to see the extent and consequences of his evils; then mental anguish and regret, or spiritual sufferings follow; but if he again relapses into his evils he fails to see them as evils, to a great extent and conscience gradually ceases to reprove him. A man will never break off from the habitual use of a poison unless he will so far heed the testimony of others, as to the pernicious character of the poison, as to make the attempt to quit it; he may then see its effects for himself, if his understanding has been so far enlightened as to the laws of his organization and the effects of the habitual use of poisons, as to know that the sufferings which he then experiences, are caused by the poison he has been using. If a person who habitually uses a poison, chances to take an unusually large dose, at any time, so as to cause a sudden increase of suffering, he then sees that he has taken too much, just as an evil man perceives he has done wrong, when he has been guilty of an unusually heinous sin.

Many of the poisonous substances in use, are not pleasant to the unperverted taste, but when a man learns from others that their use causes pleasurable excitement, he soon overcomes his repugnance to the taste, and when he finds, by experience, that they excite and give temporary activity to his perverted passions, he is led a willing slave; and is even ready to seek out other poisonous substances which by the excitement they cause, will add to his infernal delights. Thus the glutton seeks those articles which will excite an unnatural appetite; the licentious man selects those substances which are known to excite into unnatural activity his perverted passion; and the man of fight and blood, those which will excite his combativeness and destructiveness. If a man, forsakes the real duties and uses of life, and delights in the revels of a perverted imagination, spending his time in day-dreams, he sips his tea and coffee, and uses opium and tobacco, and other stimulating and narcotic substances, which are known to help in giving activity to his perverted state. Children often acquire a taste for poisons by imitating their parents and guardians, for even a young child will often take and eat the most filthy and ill-flavored substances when it sees older persons use them. Young persons frequently commence the use of poisons to gratify their vanity; the young man struts the street with a cigar in his mouth, or walks up to the bar of a hotel or drinking saloon, and calls for a glass of brandy because he thinks it looks manly; the young lady takes her cup of tea or coffee because she thinks it adds to her importance. But soon, from whatever motives their use has been commenced, they come to use them for the sake of the sensual gratification they experience; and thus a state of unnatural excitement and disease is caused.

Among the pernicious poisonous substances in use at present, not only in our country, but throughout the world, will be found certain narcotic poisons, especially opium and tobacco. The former is not used as extensively as the latter, still its use is on the increase to an alarming extent, and merits special notice. Narcotics are poisons, which, when taken into the system, affect chiefly the functions of the brain and nervous system. When taken in small doses, they generally excite the nervous system to unnatural activity for the time; but, of course, corresponding depression follows. If taken in large doses they act as sedatives, or depress or diminish the natural action; and in very large doses, cause stupor, paralysis, and death. Although narcotics affect chiefly the brain and nervous system, still their action is by no means confined to the brain. It is not improbable but that the symptoms which these agents cause in the functions of the heart and blood-vessels, digestive organs, extremities, and even skin, are principally caused through the deranged action of the nerves which are distributed to such parts. It will be seen then, that these poisons act upon and affect a very important part of the human organism. In fact, the brain and nervous system are the highest and most important, as well as the most delicate, complicated, and beautiful, of all the organs and structures which enter into the formation of the human body. The brain in man is the predominant organ of his whole system, not that it is more important, so far as simple animal life is concerned, for it is even less important to the life of the body, that it should be in a condition to fully perform its functions or office, than that the upper part of the spinal cord or marrow, or than that the great sympathetic nervous system should be, for the latter supply the nervous influence which enables the heart and lungs to act, without which action the body dies. But the brain is the organ through and from which we have manifestations of mind, or of intellect, and will; also, of sensation, and indirectly of voluntary motion. The brain may be compressed so as to destroy consciousness, sensation, and voluntary motion, and yet the body live for days, the action of the heart and lungs still continuing. But, as the brain is the central organ of the mind, of intellect and will, for which the whole body has been formed, it is the highest part of man spiritually, and also naturally, for it is in the head, and even the upper portion of the head, which is the highest part of the body; and phrenology teaches, and that truly I think, that the highest and noblest faculties of the mind such as veneration, conscientiousness, benevolence, hope, and ideality are located in the upper portion of the brain, and that causality, comparison, and the perceptive faculties are in the front portion; whereas the selfish faculties, and passions, occupy the posterior, or back, and the lower portion of the brain. This certainly is beautiful, and apparently as it should be.

OPIUM.

Opium has been used as a medicine from the earliest periods of the medical science, and has, perhaps, been more extensively used than almost any other remedy, and in a greater variety of diseases. Taken in a moderate dose, "it increases the frequency and fullness of the pulse, augments the temperature of the skin, invigorates the muscular system, quickens the senses, animates the spirits, and gives new energy to the intellectual faculties." (U. S. Dispensatory.) This excitement soon subsides and a calmness and placidity of body and mind succeed, all painful impressions, all care and anxiety are banished, and the partaker enters the indolent opium-eater's paradise, and submits to a current of undefined and unconnected, but agreeable fancies, with no other feeling than of quiet and vague enjoyment; which state usually continues from a half hour to an hour, when all consciousness is lost in sleep. After from five to ten hours the subject awakes, and upon attempting to arise from bed, he is usually troubled with more or less headache, dizziness or tremors, also nausea and sometimes vomiting, together with general prostration of the nervous system. In a dose sufficiently large to destroy life, it causes little or no excitement, but almost immediately reduces the frequency but not the force of the pulse, diminishes muscular strength and causes drowsiness, which is soon followed by deep apoplectic sleep; and in six or eight hours or more, if not relieved, the patient dies.

Opium, in any perceptible dose, acts very unpleasantly on some, causing excessive nausea and vomiting, faintness, sometimes spasms of the stomach, and in other instances headache, obstinate wakefulness or even delirium.

The habit of using opium, in this country, is rarely acquired except by using it first as a medicine; for, although the first symptoms are very enticing to many, the secondary effects are so very unpleasant that few persons in health will be found willing to encounter them the second time, simply for the short period of excitement which they experience soon after taking the drug. Opium will generally relieve pain temporarily, and is often given for this purpose, but when used for the relief of pain it is usually but a palliative remedy; yet, in many cases of disease, where the cause is temporary and the disease transient, opium may, and will, if given, relieve the suffering until the disease is overcome; therefore many physicians use this substance extensively, and their patients often think they derive great benefit from its administration, and it is rare that individuals get into the habit of using opium simply from taking it in such transient cases. But there are many diseases which are far more tedious in their duration, and where, if the physician is so unwise as to recommend this remedy, or the patient takes it on his own responsibility, he is almost sure of getting into the habit of using it. This is true in chronic rheumatism, neuralgia, and especially in the various forms of nervous diseases, which are so common among those who pride themselves on looking delicate. This remedy will generally, when its use is first commenced, relieve temporarily the pain in such diseases, although it will not cure them, nor do any permanent good. Not only is this true, but more, it generally seems to fix the disease, as it were, upon the patient, and actually makes it much more obstinate than it otherwise would have been, besides adding to it innumerable symptoms peculiar to this poison.

If a patient, suffering from one of the diseases named above, commences the use of opium, and obtains more relief from pain than he suffers from the effects of this substance, he is almost sure to continue it; for he has entered upon a road which has no end, certainly this side of the grave. It will come, in the language of the late celebrated Dr. Eberlie, "At first like an angel, with its balmy powers, to dispel pain, lowness of spirits, and mental disquietude of every kind; it will bring hilarity and pleasantness of feeling when its aid is invoked; but it will not fail ultimately to insinuate itself into every fibre, and to cause indescribable wretchedness and suffering to the unfortunate victim."

The time will soon come, to the patient, when opium will fail, even in enormous doses, to palliate the symptoms for which it is given; but, unfortunately, before that day arrives, it will have bound its victim over to the judgment of his last day, in chains which few have the resolution ever to break, for the most terrible sufferings follow the attempt to discontinue its use. The poor victim is therefore almost doomed to a life of suffering and wretchedness, a perfect slave; reason controls not, the will is overwhelmed, and he is too frequently a poor helpless wretched sot.

"A total attenuation of body," says Oppenheim, "a withered, yellow countenance, a lame gait, a bending of the spine, and glassy, deep-sunken eyes, betray the opium-eater at the first glance. The digestive organs are in the highest degree disturbed; the sufferer eats scarcely anything; his mental and bodily powers are destroyed—he is impotent."

The use of opium is by far the strongest habit known, and causes the most wretchedness to its victims. Let every one shun this habit, as he values health, life, the use of reason, freedom of will, present and future happiness. Scarcely any one can be so wretched from any chronic malady, as he can be made by the use of this substance alone, and to have added to existing chronic sufferings the torments of the opium-eater, by a voluntary act, is a terrible mistake.

It is wonderful to what extent the human system will accommodate itself to the use of this poison, if it is only gradually taken in steadily increasing doses or quantities. I have known a delicate female to take from eighty to ninety grains a day, whereas a well person, not addicted to its use, cannot take five grains with impunity, and from fifteen to twenty, if retained, will often destroy life.

TOBACCO.

I AM more and more impressed with the conviction that tobacco is doing more towards sapping the physical constitutions of the American people, than even alcoholic drinks. Its effects are more insidious, and comparatively unperceived by the popular eye, and even by the victim himself, therefore destruction is more certain and irresistible. Then, again, the habit is much stronger, and more difficult to break than the habit of using alcoholic drinks, and therefore it makes its votaries more abject slaves. One of the most notorious drunkards I have ever known, who was also in the habit of using tobacco, assured me that he would much sooner be without his whisky than his tobacco; that his sufferings and cravings were less. Such, I think, will generally be found to be the testimony of those who have come fully under the dominion of both habits.

That tobacco is a poison will be questioned by no one who has seen the deadly sickness which a very small dose will cause, in a person not habituated to its use; even smoking a single cigar, or chewing for a few moments a small portion. In fact, tobacco is one of the most virulent poisons in nature. It seems to act, not only upon the brain and spinal cord, but also especially upon the great sympathetic system of nerves, which is the very citadel of organic life. These nerves preside over or supply the nervous influence required by the heart, arteries, lungs and digestive organs, to enable them to perform their functions, and thereby to sustain the life of the whole organism or body.

Few substances in nature are capable of destroying life so suddenly as tobacco. It is said by medical writers, that a single drop of the concentrated oil put upon the tongue of a dog, will destroy life. Dr. Mussey of Cincinnati, rubbed a small drop of the oil of tobacco upon the tongue of a large cat; immediately the animal uttered piteous cries and began to froth at the mouth, followed by various symptoms of distress; seven minutes after applying the first, he rubbed a large drop upon the tongue, in an instant the eyes were closed, the cries were stopped, and the breathing was suffocative and convulsed. In one minute the ears were in rapid convulsive motion, and presently after, tremors and violent convulsions extended over the body and limbs; in three and a half minutes the animal fell upon its side senseless and breathless, and the heart had ceased to beat. In another experiment, three drops of the oil of tobacco were rubbed upon the tongue of a full-sized cat, in an instant the pupils of the eyes were dilated, and breathing convulsed; the animal leaped about as if distracted, and presently took two or three rapid turns in a small circle, then dropped upon the floor in frightful convulsions, and was dead in two minutes and forty-five seconds from the moment the oil, was put upon the tongue.

Dr. Brodie, a celebrated English physician, applied a single drop of this oil to the tongue of a cat, upon which bodily prostration and convulsions ensued. Another drop was applied, and the animal died in two minutes. One drop injected into the rectum of a cat, occasioned death in about five minutes; and two drops administered in the same manner to a dog was followed by the same result. Dr. Franklin applied the oily material which floats on the surface of water, when a current of tobacco smoke is passed into it, to the tongue of a cat, and found it to destroy life in a few minutes; yet the cat is more tenacious of life than almost any other animal.

Tobacco, "when very moderately taken, quiets restlessness calms mental and corporeal inquietude, and produces a state of general languor, or repose, which has great charms for those who are habituated to the impression." But when taken in large quantities, it causes confusion of the head with more or less stupor, great faintness, most distressing nausea and vomiting, great feebleness of the pulse, with death-like paleness of the skin, with coldness of the surface, which is covered with a cold clammy sweat, with great and general debility of the nervous and circulatory functions. Fainting, alarming and fatal prostration, or convulsions and death, soon close the scene, if a very large quantity has been taken. Tobacco is sometimes used as an injection in cases of obstruction of the bowels, but its use requires the utmost care, as death has sometimes occurred from its administration, even in the hands of skillful physicians.

Dr. L. B. Coles, in his excellent work on the "Beauties and Deformities of Tobacco Using," which should be placed in the hands of every young man, says:

"A single leaf, dipped in hot water and laid upon the pit of the stomach, will produce a powerful effect by mere absorption from the surface. By being applied to a spot where the scarf skin, or external surface of the skin is destroyed, fearful results have followed. Professor Mussey, in his essay on Tobacco, gives a case:

"Dr. Long, of New Hampshire, was consulted by a mother, to know whether she might apply tobacco to a ringworm, scarcely three-fourths of an inch in diameter, on the nose of her daughter, then about five years old; he objected to it as an exceedingly hazardous measure, and confirmed his judgment by relating a case which he had seen recorded, in which a father destroyed the life of his son by putting tobacco spittle upon an eruption on the head; immediately after the doctor left, the mother, thinking she knew more than her medical adviser, proceeded to moisten the ringworm from the essence of the grandmother's pipe, remarking that if it should strike to the stomach it must go through the nose; the instant the mother's finger touched the part, the eyes of the patient rolled up in their sockets, she sallied back, and falling, was caught in the arms of the alarmed mother; the part was immediately washed, but to no purpose; the jaws were locked, the patient was senseless, and apparently in a dying state; the doctor was immediately called back, who found the following symptoms:—Coldness of the surface and extremities, no pulsation at the wrist, jaws set, deep insensibility, countenance death-like."

By the application of friction to the surface, and the administration of spirits of ammonia, at the end of about an hour and a half, the patient became able to speak, but did not fully recover from the shock for years. For the first four or five years afterwards she was subject to fainting fits every three or four weeks, which sometimes lasted from twelve to twenty-four hours. The smoking of a single cigar, by a person not long habituated to the use of the weed, will increase the frequency of the pulse from ten to fifteen beats.

I have thus hastily noticed some of the prominent symptoms caused by tobacco when it is taken by persons not previously accustomed to its use; and when it is taken in large quantities even by those who habitually use it; also the alarming and dangerous symptoms which result from an excessive dose. But I desire more particularly to call the attention of the reader to the not less destructive, although more gradual effects which result from its habitual use. These effects are less manifest, for the human organism possesses the capacity to accommodate itself in a wonderful degree, to the use of poisons, if the quantity taken only be gradually increased. We have seen this to be the case with opium, and the same is true of tobacco, and all other poisons. There are many men who use tobacco enough in a single day to kill several who are not accustomed to its use, if they were obliged to take it in the same manner, during the same period.

Among the symptoms and diseases often caused by the habitual use of tobacco, may be named the following:

Depression of spirits, melancholy, and despondency, as a necessary result of over excitement; great fear of death, irritability and peevishness, loss of memory and dullness of perception. One of the most intelligent teachers of Detroit said to me, that those young men under his instruction who used tobacco seemed to be much more dull and stupid, than those who did not use it. He found it far more difficult to make them comprehend or understand subjects taught. Such are a few of the mental symptoms which tobacco causes.

It causes great general weariness, languor, and debility of the extremities, and trembling of the hands and feet, cramps in the muscles, spasms and convulsions, emaciation and even consumption. The late Dr. Twitchel, of New Hampshire, relates a case of consumption saved by giving up tobacco, and also a case of nearly fatal nightmare cured by quitting its use.

"Dr. Twitchel found that nearly all the cases of sudden death, occurring during sleep, which came under his observation, were of men who had indulged largely in tobacco. And the correctness of his statement was confirmed by investigations made by the Boston Society for Medical Observation." I saw a notice of the death of a lady during sleep in a village in the State of Ohio, a few months ago. I immediately wrote to a physician of my acquaintance in the place, and requested him to inquire, and inform me if she was in the habit of using tobacco. I received, as a reply, that she had used it freely for many years.

Dr. Twitchel expressed the opinion that tobacco is doing a worse work to the physical character of the present generation than alcohol. Tobacco causes a great variety of headaches, with dullness and heaviness of the head, heat in the head, congestion of blood to the head, and apoplexy, stoppage of the ears, and deafness; pain and inflammation of the eyes; amaurosis, or paralysis of the optic nerve, and even blindness; various diseases of the tongue, mouth and lips. The celebrated Dr. J. C. Warren, of Boston, reports a case of cancerous tongue, attributable to tobacco, in which the life of the patient could not be saved by an operation.

"Both smoking and chewing produce marked alterations in the most expressive features of the face. The lips are closed by a circular muscle, which completely surrounds them and forms their pulpy fullness. Now, every muscle of the body is developed in precise ratio with its use, as most young men know, they endeavor to develop and increase their muscles in the gymnasium.

In spitting and holding the cigar in the mouth, this muscle is in constant use; hence the coarse appearance and irregular development of the lips, when compared to the rest of the features, in chewers and smokers. The eye loses its natural fire and becomes dull and lurid; it is unspeculative and appreciative, it answers not before the world; its owner gazes vacantly, and often repels conversation by his stupidity."—SCALPEL.

Tobacco is a frequent cause of dyspepsia. It causes spasmodic pressure of the stomach, heartburn, feeling of coldness of the stomach, nausea and frequent eructations; pains in the region of the liver and diseases of this organ; pains in the bowels, with disposition to diarrhœa or costiveness. It causes difficulty of breathing, oppression of the chest, pains in the chest with inability to take in a long breath and violent palpitation of the heart. It causes pain in and stiffness of the back. Tobacco also causes a tendency to paralysis both general and local. It causes drowsiness, unnatural sleep, nightmare, troublesome, anxious and frightful dreams; together with a great variety of symptoms which I have not space to notice. In fact, I have described but a small share of the symptoms and diseases which are noticed by our best medical writers, and most careful observers, as having been caused by the use of this poison. Not that it will cause all of these symptoms in any one person, for it affects different individuals differently, manifesting its action in the weak organs, or upon the parts of the body which are least able to resist its influence. But there is no one who uses tobacco, who will not find himself troubled with more or less of these symptoms the very moment he quits using the poison; but while he is using it freely, it will palliate, as do all poisons, the symptoms its habitual use has caused. In the morning, after having abstained during the night, the tobacco user will get a slight glimpse of his waning vital energies, but his view will soon be covered over by the oblivious leaves of the demon, when he again partakes.

I was never more painfully conscious of the terrible effects of the habitual use of tobacco, than during a recent visit to a locality where reside many of the friends of my childhood and youth.

I found a large number of the gentlemen the sons of robust parents, addicted to its use, and its effects were to be seen in every lineament of their countenances, emaciated, prematurely wrinkled and sallow, looking in fact almost as much like a wilted tobacco leaf, as like human beings in the full pride of manhood. But I found two gentlemen who had used tobacco for many years formerly, and when I last saw them they were suffering excessively from its use, but they had given it up and were looking like new creatures. They were better in flesh, better in spirits, and free from a multitude of aches and pains which had formerly tormented them.

The use of tobacco is a filthy and disgusting habit, as well as destructive to health and life. It causes a constant inclination to spit, which is regarded by all civilized nations, with the exception of Americans and tobacco users, as a filthy and unnecessary practice; and it adds to the character of the saliva the juice of the nauseous weed.

A good anecdote is told by Dr. Coles, in the work to which I have referred, illustrating this point. He says:

"A Professor in a western college related to him the following. He was traveling in company with a clerical brother. They stopped to spend the Sabbath, and the Professor was invited to preach in the evening. His brother in the ministry, who was a practical admirer of tobacco and its fruits, was with him in the desk. The Professor set his hat—a new one—at the end of the pulpit sofa; and while preaching saw his brother, who was near sighted, so that he mistook the hat for a spit-box, delivering the contents of his mouth every moment into his hat. But he was obliged to submit to the process. It would not do to make an apostrophe in his sermon by saying, 'don't spit your vile stuff into my hat!' so he bore it like a saint, and let his brother spit away—casting into his new fashioned spittoon, not only the sirup from his powerful tobacco-mill, but cud after cud of the solid refuse. Think what a hat the Professor had when the meeting was closed."

We are told that he threw it away and went home bare-headed.

So nauseous is even the taste of tobacco that, in all the animal kingdom, but two animals, aside from man, have been discovered which will taste it—the tobacco worm of the South, whose intolerable visage is disgusting, and the rock goat of Africa—the goat is thought by one writer to possess a bodily flavor which prepares it for association with those who create on themselves the tobacco stench. The smell of this goat is so terrible that no other dumb animal will ever associate with it. The very atmosphere for a distance around is tainted with his effluvia, and his whole visage is said to be disgusting. The tobacco user is said to become so pickled with tobacco, that cannibals detect it in the flesh of those who have used it, and throw that flesh away as unfit to use. It is immaterial how tobacco is used, whether it be by smoking, chewing, snuffing or dipping, the effects are similar. As the reader may not understand what is meant by the latter practice I will explain it. Some years ago, while sojourning in a southern state, I frequently noticed ladies with one end of a small stick in the mouth; a lady one day asked me if I thought dipping injured the teeth. Dipping, said I, what do you mean by dipping? She laughed heartily at my ignorance, but very graciously went on to explain the mystery of the small stick, which she exhibited to me. The stick, about as large as a small pipestem, is split or broomed up at one end, this is dipped into a box of snuff, which is then rubbed against the teeth and held in the mouth. I must confess that I was so ungallant as to tell the lady, that I thought if the practice was not very injurious to the teeth, it was at least very filthy.

When tobacco is brought by any of these methods, in contact with the living structures of the body, the poisonous juice is absorbed, enters the circulation, and passes throughout the whole system, even to the delicate structures of the brain and nervous system. It excites directly the various animal propensities beyond their proper balance, and tends to debase the moral character, and to make man more animal and less intellectual and moral. It therefore tends directly to destroy both body and soul. But I fancy I hear some young reader say, my father used tobacco many years, and died an old man; if tobacco killed him it was a very slow poison; let me say to you, young man, that if you were born after your father commenced using tobacco as freely as most young men use it to-day, for that very reason, if not for others, you do not possess your father's strength of constitution, but have to suffer for the folly of your parent, and you cannot follow in his footsteps without going to a premature grave. Nor can you say how much this habit blunted the perceptions of your father in his declining years, clouded his intellect, impaired his health, and shortened his life. The crown upon the head of the old man should be wisdom, and the chief pearl innocence, and in the innocence of wisdom should he go to his fathers free from pain and disease. I am aware that some men of strong constitutions, active life, and of good habits, may use alcohol or tobacco, and even get drunk often, and yet live to a good old age; but they are the exceptions to the general rule; a much greater number will die young. But it will be found that most of those who have lived to old age, did not commence the use of these poisons very young, or else that they either used them moderately, or only occasionally had a spree, and were never what we call hard drinkers or smokers. Whatever impairs the physical energies of individuals, impairs the energies of our race as a whole, and man has no right to entail, through his own folly a tendency to disease, suffering, and premature death to his children. Tobacco is not natural food for man; it will not sustain life; it is a poison, as has abundantly been shown—always injurious during health, and never necessary except in rare cases of disease, and then only for a temporary period. Its use is a bad example to the young, even to innocent children, leading them astray; it is expensive, costing the inhabitants of the United States more than $25,000,000, annually; and even the professed Christians of our country more than $5,000,000. Its use is a direct violation of the Divine command—thou shalt not kill—which includes self-murder, it matters not whether it be done in an hour or more slowly,—the work of years,—therefore more deliberately. I ask all who profess to be Christians or philanthropists, how you can neglect to abstain from this fleshly lust, which not only wars against the soul, but also the body.

How can you spend four times as much to gratify this perverted appetite, as you pay to send abroad the Bible and missionaries, to those whom you acknowledge it to be your duty to feed with the bread of life? Is it not plain that the habitual use of tobacco is a sin against our physical organizations and against our Father in heaven? and that those who are addicted to this habit must shun it as such, or the love of the poison will abide with them.

"A distinguished Doctor of Divinity," says Rev. J. L. Corning in his work on Amusement, "died not long ago, and in the obituary notice which I saw in the newspapers, I observed the remark made by another Doctor of Divinity, that his brother minister died from the effects of hard study. Now I am sorry that a minister of the Gospel should be found uttering such a libel on the Creator. The fact is, the deceased minister had been in the constant practice of chewing tobacco, for more than half a century. And which committed the greatest sin—he, to kill himself in that way, or his brother minister to affirm, in the face of it, that he died of hard study—I will not undertake to say. But that both were great sinners, no man, with any common sense, will deny."

It matters not that good men and even Christians may have used it before our day, or drank brandy, and occasionally, perchance, got drunk; they did it ignorantly and did not violate conscience. But even with them perhaps a certain elderly lady's dream, which is recorded in the spirited work of Dr. Coles to which I have referred, may have been found more than a dream. She is said to have been very pious, "but allowed for many years her devotion to her pipe, like thousands in our churches, to exceed her devotion to her God. She was more sure not to forget her vows to this carnal appetite, than not to forget her closet for prayer. One night she dreamed of an aerial flight to the region of the spirit world, where not only her eyes could feast on the beauties of elysian fields, but where she could converse with perfected spirits. One of these she asked to go and look for her name in the book of life. He complied; but at length returned with a sad countenance, saying it was not there. Again she besought him to go and search more thoroughly. After a more lengthy examination he returned without finding it. She wept bitterly. But she could not rest till a third search should be made. After a long and anxious absence, he returned with a brightened countenance, saying it had, after great labor, been discovered; but that so deep was the covering which years of tobacco smoke had laid over it, that it was with great difficulty that it could be discovered. She awoke and found herself prostrated with weeping. She cast her idol to her feet, and gave unto God, not a divided, but a whole heart; and she no more spent her time, money and vital energies upon its unholy altar."

I have known a man to give up the use of tobacco at the age of ninety years, and as he thought with benefit to his health. It is true he was a man possessing naturally great constitutional vigor, and also unusual mental energy and perseverance; which were manifested not alone in breaking off from the filthy habit of using tobacco, for at the age of ninety-seven he had the misfortune to lose by death his third wife; when he soon commenced looking around among the venerable maidens and widows in search of a suitable candidate to lead to the altar, and to share with him his comfortable homestead, bed and board. He visited one elderly lady and made known his errand, when she inquired his name; he told her his name, when she replied: "Well, I have heard enough of you!" "Well," said he, "I have heard enough of you too!" So on he went. At last, the Lord, he said, sent him a wife exactly to his mind, in the form of a blooming widow of eighty-four years.

I often hear young men of twenty or thirty say that they cannot give up the use of tobacco, and often they have not the energy to even make the attempt. Sad indeed is their fate; poor weak-minded young men, living slaves to their appetite, and dying at their own hands, when a little of the energy and perseverance of the venerable man of ninety, to whom I have referred in the preceding paragraph, would break their chains and save them from disease and a premature death.

Our Heavenly Father has given us reason to guide our footsteps here below, and if he does not intend that we shall be guided by our understanding in our eating and drinking, what mean those denunciations against drunkenness and gluttony, to be found in His Word. I will ask the believers in a divine revelation if a man is not certainly a drunkard or a glutton in the Bible acceptation of these terms when he deliberately uses a poisonous substance, knowing it to be injurious and destructive to health and life, and entirely unnecessary. Loving the sensual gratification, more than he loves his God, or even health, life and the welfare of his neighbor, does he not deliberately make the sensual selfish gratification his ruling love? and must not man's ruling love, when thus deliberately and intelligently formed, govern his destiny to eternity? and will he not almost necessarily seek, as his chief delight, corresponding evils in the next life, when his days of probation here are over?

CHAPTER X.

ALCOHOLIC DRINKS.

THAT such stimulants should never be used by man during health, must, upon careful examination and reflection, be manifest, for it will be found that they are not necessary—yea more, that they are absolutely pernicious.

Dr. Wm. B. Carpenter, the most celebrated English Physiologist living, says:

"The capacity of the human system to sustain so much bodily or mental labor as it can be legitimately called upon to perform, and its power of resisting the extremes of heat and cold, as well as other depressing agencies, are not augmented by the use of alcoholic liquors, but that, on the other hand, their use, under such circumstances tends positively to the impairment of that capacity

"Both the nervous and muscular systems require, for the energetic development and due maintenance of their respective powers that their tissues shall be adequately supplied with the *materials of growth and regeneration;* whereby they shall be able to repair the effects of their loss, which every exercise of their vital endowments involves; and also to develop new tissue to meet increasing demands upon the functional activity.

"Now it may be accepted as an indubitable fact in organic chemistry, that there is not the slightest relation of composition between alcohol and muscular tissue; and all our present knowledge of the subject tends to prove that the albuminous matters of the blood, which constitute the *pabulum* of that tissue, cannot be generated within the body of man, or of any other animal, but are derived immediately from the food. We cannot regard alcoholic liquors then, as contributing to the nutrition of muscular tissue; except in so far as they may contain albuminous matters in addition to the alcohol, which is especially the case with 'malt liquors.' But these matters would have the same nutritive power, if they were taken in the form of solid food."

After quoting a great variety of testimony in regard to the capacity for endurance of iron-workers, furnace-men, sawyers, glass-blowers, harvesters, brick-makers, water-carriers, miners, sailors and soldiers, showing that men can actually perform more physical labor with less fatigue without than with alcoholic drinks in any form, Dr. Carpenter continues:

"Having for several years past been himself performing an amount of steady mental labor, which, to most persons, would appear excessive, the writer may be allowed to refer to his own experience, which is altogether in favor of total abstinence from alcoholic liquors, as a means of sustaining the power of performing it. On determining about four years since, to give up the occasional use of wine, etc., as a social indulgence, he still held himself free to employ it when he might think it likely to increase the general powers of his system; and for some time he continued to have occasional recourse to alcoholic stimulants (never exceeding a single glass of wine, or half a tumbler of bitter ale) when he felt himself suffering under the peculiar depression just referred to. He gradually, however, found reason to doubt the utility of the remedy; and has for the last two years entirely given it up. During these two years, he has gone through a larger amount of mental labor than he ever did before in the same period of time; and he does not hesitate to say, that he has it performed with more ease to himself than on his former system; and that he has been more free than ever from those states of depression of mental energy, which he was accustomed to regard as indicating the need of a temporary support to antagonise the depressing cause. In fact, he now finds that when these do occur, the use of alcoholic stimulants (taken even in very small amount) is decidedly injurious to him: diminishing, rather than increasing his power of mental exertion at the time, and leaving him still less disposed for it after their effects have gone off."

Dr. Carpenter shows by the physiological action of alcohol on the human body, that its use does not enable men to withstand either heat or cold any better than they can without it; and he brings facts, drawn from the observation and experience of travelers and voyagers, in both tropical and arctic regions; and travelers in ascending mountains; also the residence of officers and armies in northern climes, as well as on the burning plains of India, and during great exposure and forced marches, showing conclusively that man can actually stand both heat and cold better without than with any form of alcoholic drinks.

The late General Havelock, after detailing the achievements of the troops during the late war in India, when they had been without alcoholic drinks for some time, has left the following unequivocal testimony upon this subject. He says:

"Since then it has been proved that troops can make forced marches for forty miles and storm a fortress in seventy-five minutes without the aid of rum, behaving after success with a forbearance and humanity unparalleled in history, let it not henceforth be argued that distilled spirits are an indispensable portion of a soldier's rations."

That a man can perform more work or labor both mentally and physically, without than with alcoholic stimulants, will be clearly seen if we bear in mind one of the physiological laws of our being; viz.: all undue or unnatural excitement is followed by corresponding depression. This is a law of the natural and mental organism as fixed as that of the Medes and Persians, which was said to change not. The man who lives upon a plain, wholesome diet, pursues the even tenor of his way, and receives all due or necessary excitement from the use of healthy food, to enable him to perform his daily duties. But how is it with the user of stimulants? Let us take the drinker of alcohol as a representative of this type of humanity, for he stands at the head of the list; and we will commence with his first dram, and confine ourselves to his legitmate history.

A man, entirely unaccustomed to the use of alcohol in all its forms, takes a glass of brandy; this excites and increases both his physical and mental activity above its healthy level, for a few hours, while he is under its direct and stimulating action, and if he repeats the dose once or twice during the day, he may even keep up a state of constant excitement until he retires at night, when nature sinks exhausted into sleep. He awakes in the morning, weak, faint and exhausted, and as both his words and looks will testify, depressed in both body and mind as much below the natural standard as he was excited above it the day before. This may have been very slight, or very great. In either case he manifestly commences his second day of stimulation at a lower point than he did the first; and it follows as a necessary consequence, that the same quantity that he took the day before will not and cannot bring him up to the same degree of excitement that he realized on the preceding day, for he commences in the morning with a lower standard of physical and mental energy.

Here then, there is, as we see, a necessity, resulting from a physiological law, for an increase of the quantity of the stimulant when he once commences using it. It is just as natural for alcoholic drinks to flow with increasing momentum, to supply the waning vital energies of the drinker of stimulants, as it is for water to run down hill.

Steadily the rum drinker continues on, and if he strives to keep up his energies by the use of stimulants, he is necessarily, as we have seen, compelled to increase the quantity, for he gets up in the morning feeling faint and gone, and that nothing but his old friend alcohol can satisfy him. Now if, laying aside his judgment, he follows the full bent of his appetite, and drinks just what is absolutely necessary to make him feel right, he soon begins to reel in the streets and becomes drunk; but if he endeavors to set bounds to his appetite, and in violation of the law to which the attention of the reader has been called, confines himself to moderate drinking, and that only during the day, or hours of labor, and only steadily increases the quantity, to meet the increasing demands of his appetite, drunkenness may never ensue; but, after a time, rum blossoms begin to appear upon his face, and still later, nature either revolts against the use of his accustomed beverages, or an attack of some febrile or acute disease, or mechanical injury, destroys his appetite, and the poor victim begins to tremble with delirium tremens. He does not have this disease so long as he continues to drink; for it is with alcohol as it is with all poisons which are steadily and slowly used, its effects can only be seen and realized when it is discontinued, for all stimulants will palliate the very symptoms which their habitual use has caused. If we would know if a given substance, which we are habitually using, is doing us harm, we have but to discontinue its use for a few days, or weeks, and live upon wholesome food, and if any unusual symptoms of depression follow, any aches, pains or unpleasant feelings, we may know that they are caused by the substance omitted. The headache caused by the habitual use of coffee is far more violent when this beverage is omitted; so the gone feeling, or faintness at the pit of the stomach, and palpitation of the heart, which are caused by tea, are far worse for days after its use is discontinued.

Those who habitually use such beverages, are far more liable to have delirium tremens than those who only occasionally have a spree, even though they may get beastly drunk.

The law to which I have alluded—that all unnatural excitement is surely followed by corresponding depression—produces the siren song which lures the drinker of stimulating drinks on to drunkenness, delirium tremens and death. We have seen that this law absolutely requires a constant and uniform increase in the quantity used, and it therefore follows that drunkenness, delirium tremens, and death, are the legitimate effects of using stimulating drinks, and that no man who habitually uses them has a right to expect to escape this doom.

I am aware that some men have drank brandy and other intoxicating drinks during the active period of a long life, without having become what we call drunkards; but such men have generally taken such beverages because they honestly thought them necessary, and by strong will, sustained by conscience, have, in violation of this law of their being to which I have called the attention of the reader, limited the quantity and frequency of their drams, and have not departed from such limits, even to drink with friends; but men do not generally drink stimulating drinks to-day because they think that they are necessary, or even harmless and safe. Is it not true that they generally partake of them in violation of conscience? and, therefore, that they feel not its restraints to confine them to moderate drinking, as did their fathers, but are left to the guidance of their appetites which we have seen never cease to demand an increased supply to relieve the increasing debility or nervous prostration. If this is so, it is evident that fewer men can now, or will hereafter, drink without becoming drunkards than during any past age of the world.

Here then we have the cause why so many young men are prematurely cut off at this day by the use of alcoholic drinks. It is because they drink more and more constantly; and we certainly need not seek the cause of the increased mortality among rum-drinkers, nor expect to find it in the adulterations to which liquors are subjected at the hands of unscrupulous venders, so long as people continue to die of delirium tremens and drunkenness—the effects of alcohol, and not of the substances added.

Few men ever realize that they drink to excess, they only drink enough to make them feel just right, that is, to bring them up to their ordinary state, and they are generally very indignant if their friends intimate that they drink too much. The reader has doubtless heard the story of the deacon and the drunkard, but as it will illustrate this point, I will repeat it. A church meeting was held for the purpose of considering the propriety of requiring the members to abstain from the use of intoxicating drinks. One of the deacons arose and said that he was opposed to this measure; that it was ultra; that it was carrying the thing too far; he believed in temperate drinking, and thought a little did him good. When he had taken his seat, one of the most notorious drunkards in the country arose and said that he exactly agreed with the good deacon, he despised drunkenness as bad as any one, but he always stopped when he had drank just enough.

But, as we have seen, the just enough of an unnatural stimulant to-day is not enough for to-morrow, for all undue excitement is followed by corresponding depression. This is not the case with natural stimulants, and the natural excitement which follows their use is not so great but that the organism is preserved from debility and exhaustion by rest and sleep, and fully restored to its natural state. Strange as it may seem, there are writers who confound natural and unnatural stimulants, and consider both alike, appropriate and necessary, and on this ground justify the use of alcoholic drinks. J. J. G. Wilkinson, in his work on "The Human Body and its connexion with Man," does this, and thus, as it were, confounds good and evil. Pure water and wholesome nourishing food are natural stimulants to the body, for they supply healthy fluid and substance and meet the demands of the system; we may use these to excess and thus abuse them. Light is a natural stimulant to the eye, at a certain intensity it is exactly what the eye is prepared to receive; but cayenne pepper is not. Sound is a natural stimulant to the ear, but corrosive sublimate is not, although a stimulant. The eye craves light, the ear sound, and the stomach wholesome food. "Poisons," says Dr. Wilkinson, "destroy the structure, or subvert the functions of the body." Surely few poisons more manifestly subvert the functions of the body than alcoholic stimulants. Where can we find a greater perversion of the functions of the body than is to be witnessed in delirium tremens? The healthy structure of the stomach, and other organs, is also impaired by even the temperate use of alcoholic drinks.

Temperate drinking, or using stimulants—substances which excite an unnatural appetite, which no healthy food will appease—drinks which by the very law in accordance with which they act, require to be taken in increased quantities; which are well known to excite disease, and premature death; why! the very word temperance applied to the use of such beverages, is a misnomer; we might as well talk of temperate stealing, temperate lying, or temperate bearing of false witness, for not more surely do the latter violations of the moral law, when continued in, pervert man's spiritual nature, than do stimulants man's natural organism. The one class of violations is poisonous and destructive to the soul when indulgence is permitted, the other to the body, both alike forbidden fruit.

Let no man pride himself in his ability to walk in the road that leads to destruction, without entering the gates of the pit. We have seen that a natural law leads the so-called temperate drinker on to delirium tremens, by requiring him to increase the quantity used. For this reason firmness of will and endurance are no safeguards against drunkenness. An Alexander who had the energy to conquer the world, could not control his appetite, but died an inebriate. Do we not manifest a lack of wisdom when we imagine ourselves possessed of a strength of intellect which will enable us to drink moderately without becoming drunkards? Have we more power of intellect or of will than any of the long list of distinguished statesmen who have died drunkards within the last few years? Nor is even piety a safeguard against drunkenness, if a man permits himself to continue the use of stimulants, for not a few have gone from the sacred desk to fill a drunkard's grave.

There is no safety in living—as the man who uses stimulants does—in open violation of the laws of our being. I well remember—it is as it were but yesterday, so swiftly have the years of my life passed—standing upon my native New England hills, conversing with a young neighbor upon the propriety of resolving to abstain entirely from the use of intoxicating drinks. He said to me that he believed in temperate drinking, and that a little brandy did him good—but that a man was a fool who could not restrain his appetite. In the strong language of assurance he said: "If you ever hear of my drinking to excess, or of my getting drunk, you may tell me, and I will quit drinking." That man was told years ago that he was drinking to excess, and that he had become a drunkard. Did he quit drinking? He spent the fine farm left him by his father, his wife went down to her grave broken-hearted, his children are scattered among strangers, and he is to-day a poor, miserable drunken outcast.

There is no excuse for drinking at all; the well man needs not the stimulating effect of alcohol; and the fact that all undue excitement is necessarily followed by corresponding depression, renders it rarely beneficial for the treatment of the sick; and I can say that, after devoting over eighteen years to the study and the practice of medicine, I have never seen eighteen cases in which the use of alcoholic drinks have done my patients good. I have never seen a patient recover under their use, that I had not good reason to think would have recovered without them. I grant that in cases of temporary prostration, where there is no actual loss of substance, where the organism is capable of taking care of itself when aroused, stimulants may do some good. They may be useful in cases of great prostration from severe mechanical injuries, and in faintness, even sometimes when the latter arises from sudden loss of blood; also for the depression of the vital energies which sometimes occurs during pernicious, or the so-called congestive, intermittent or remittent fevers, when the danger only continues during the paroxysms.

But such cases are very rare in this latitude, therefore stimulants are rarely needed. If given during ordinary chills they do no good, and only increase the reaction, or fever, which follows. They may sometimes check a diarrhœa, or slight attack of dysentery, but if they do not relieve they are sure to aggravate, therefore they are not safe, and I do not use them; nor is their use necessary, as there are a plenty of remedies far more certain as well as more safe. Stimulants are often taken for weakness, to give strength.

I have frequently been called to see feeble persons, especially females, who had been taking wine, beer, brandy and the like for years, to strengthen them, and still they remained weak; and I have found that such patients improved when they were required to live on a proper diet, and discontinue their stimulants. So far from being strengthened they had actually been debilitated by their use. Individuals who have been debilitated by disease frequently take stimulants during the period of recovery, or convalescence, and often think that they derive great benefit, because they continue to improve, when all the strength they gain is the result of the food they eat; and a multitude of physicians, who have carefully watched patients during convalescence under the use of stimulants and without them, can bear testimony to the fact that they generally recover more rapidly and safely without than with them.

It is not my aim to deter any one from taking stimulants when they are prescribed by physicians, for with the physician rests the responsibility, and he is supposed to understand when to give and when to withhold, better than the patient or friends; and while he is in attendance his directions should be followed. But I well know that the importunity of the patient, and his friends to have stimulants used—to say nothing of their adminstration occasionally by friends unknown to the physician—when patients are very weak, is often a great annoyance to the physician, even if it does not induce him to give such remedies, against his better judgment, to the injury of his patient. Every intelligent physician is aware that there is no class of remedies so liable to abuse as the one we are considering; and this is especially true in fevers. That there are conditions or states in typhus fever, or even occasionally in typhoid fever, were stimulants may do good I do not deny; but it requires the judgment of the experienced physician to decide when they are necessary or safe. It is not generally when there is an irritation of the mucous membrane of the stomach and bowels, or when the fluids and solids of the body are gradually wasted, and the loss of strength is not temporary, but gradual and real, for in such cases they rarely fail to do harm; and yet these are the very cases where the attendants, friends and neighbors, are the most anxious to have them given; and I am satisfied, from observation, that many patients die under their use, who would not if they were let alone. How can it be otherwise? Can a man, prostrated to the lowest ebb of life, stand a course of stimulation which all experience shows will prostrate a well man, even to the extent of giving rise to delirium tremens and death? We will take the most critical case, in which the patient is for days in a state where he can barely live without stimulants, as frequently occurs, and what must be the inevitable result of giving them? Bear in mind that this state of depression is the result of the actual condition of the solids and fluids of the body, and is, under the circumstances, as it were a natural condition. Now give such a patient stimulants and an unnatural state of excitement will follow, or a degree of activity above that which the exhausted organism is capable of sustaining; as a necessary consequence, corresponding depression must follow; and, if the patient was barely at the living point before, the prostration, which is sure to follow, must lie below that point.

It may be asked, cannot this state of excitement be kept up for days, until the patient recovers, by the use of stimulants? It cannot be; the over excited organism needs repose, and must and will have it. How is it with the rum-drinker if he attempts to keep up a state of constant excitement day and night? Speedy drunkenness and entire prostration follow, and nature revolts, if he does not omit the stimulus during the night, and if he does omit it he awakes in the morning feeling exhausted and gone. How must it be with the poor typhoid patient, in a most critical case where stimulants are needed if they are needed in any case, when exhausted nature seeks repose under such treatment? Is it not evident that he too must be gone—gone to that last home from whence no traveler returns to his natural body.

Alcohol can give to the body no muscular strength, for physiology teaches, unmistakably, that it gives no substance to supply the waste which always results from all muscular activity, even from the very pulsations of the heart. It therefore excites but to exhaust, as I have shown, by the depression which follows the unnatural excitement, and each step in its use is but a backward step. This may be seen to be true, even in the use of stimulants which have a more local action. Let a healthy man, or one who has slight costiveness, itself perhaps only temporary and of little consequence, commence taking cathartic remedies, which stimulate the bowels and glandular organs which pour their secretions into the bowels; the bowels are excited to an increased motion or peristaltic action, the mucous membrane is excited to increase its secretion, and the bowels become more loose than natural; but if the living forces are able to overcome the diarrhœa thus caused, the bowels become more costive than ever; and the more frequently cathartics are used, the more rapidly does the costiveness increase. I have known a delicate female, from taking cathartics, become so costive as to be under the necessity of taking, every time she desired a passage from her bowels, fifteen cathartic pills, one of which would have acted as a cathartic on a well person. I have often been reminded, by observing the effects of such stimulants, of remarks which I heard Dr. Willard Parker, of the "College of Physicians and Surgeons" of New York, make some fifteen years ago. He said:

"When I see a young man who cannot eat his beef-steak or his mutton-chop, without sprinkling upon it black or Cayenne pepper, or mustard, I expect to see him an old man before he has seen many years. His stomach will be worn out by over excitement, and the whole body will fail with it."

Debility, premature old age and death, are the legitimate effects which result from using stimulants.

Those who actually die from the immediate effects of stimulants—die of drunkenness or delirium tremens—comprise but a small share of the victims who really go down to their graves from the use of alcoholic drinks; for it is a fact well known to all intelligent medical men, that rum-drinkers are far more liable to be attacked with any prevailing disease, and not only is this true, but it is also certain that when they are attacked they are more likely to die from such diseases than those who abstain entirely from such drinks. As a general rule, the first victims to the cholera, the world over, have been drawn from the users of stimulants; and all febrile and inflammatory diseases destroy an undue proportion of this class of the community. We can very readily see why this is so, if we bear in mind the fact that the circulation and nervous energies of the rum-drinker are unduly excited or depressed nearly all the time. The same is true of those who receive severe mechanical injuries, a much larger portion die than of water drinkers.

It is not alone by immediately and directly causing manifest diseases which can readily be traced to this cause, that alcoholic liquors impair health and shorten life. Dr. Carpenter truly says:

"It cannot then, be imagined that even a small habitual excess in diet, induced by the stimulating action of fermented liquors, can be without its remote consequences upon the general system; even though it may be for a time sufficiently compensated by increased activity of the excreting organs. And the disorders of the liver and kidneys, which are so frequent among those who have been accustomed to this mode of living for many years, without, (as they believe,) any injurious consequences, are as surely to be set down to it, as are those congestive and inflammatory diseases of the abdominal viscera, which so much more speedily follow habitual excess in warm climates."

He also points out the effects of alcoholic and fermented liquors, when moderately used, on the stomach, circulation and nervous system; but I have space to do little more than to refer the reader to Dr. Wm. B. Carpenter's "Prize Essay on the use and abuse of Alcoholic Liquors."

Nor does the use of alcoholic drinks, or stimulants of any kind beyond what is contained in wholesome food and pure water, add to the stock of man's enjoyment as a whole. About so much pleasure, or gratification, is to be derived from eating and drinking, and those who live upon the most wholesome plain food actually enjoy the most in eating and drinking. To deny this would be to assert that evil is superior to good, and Hell superior to Heaven. It requires no argument to show the absurdity of such a position.

We find in the Sacred Scriptures the most severe denunciation of drunkenness, and it becomes the believers in Revelation to inquire what is meant by a drunkard, and in what consists the sin of drunkenness, in the Bible acceptation of the term. We know very well that one man may drink a quantity of brandy daily for months, and years, with comparative impunity, which would get another man drunk, and even destroy his life; and the man who drinks habitually has a much stronger appetite for stimulants than he who occasionally gets drunk, and does not drink constantly. Can we say that the latter is morally more guilty than the former? Perhaps so.

So it is not the quantity a man drinks which makes him a drunkard. Two men may drink the same quantity of alcohol from the same strength of appetite, and one may become drunk and the other may not, simply owing to his not being so susceptible to drunkenness. A man may even be a hard drinker for many years and die of delirium tremens, without having been drunk to a state of insensibility; I will not say that he never has been drunk, for really there is no difference between the man who is unduly excited by the use of stimulants, and the one who is called dead drunk, except in degree. One is more drunk than the other, but it would be difficult to draw any distinct line of demarkation between drunkenness, and the excitement which results from what is called temperate drinking. The longer a man has drank, and the more he drinks, the less power he has to control his appetite, and, of course, the less moral responsibility has he for his present acts. Every one will perceive that if he was ever responsible, and ever guilty of wrong doing, it was especially when he took the first glass with the knowledge that it was unnecessary and injurious. The first glass did the greatest violence to the laws of his physical body, and drunkenness, delirium tremens, and death are only the natural consequences, or the legitimate result of an attempt to keep up the state of unnatural excitement, and to prevent the unnatural depression which followed the excitement of the first glass.

The man who violates the laws of his physical being must suffer the consequences, whether he does it knowingly or ignorantly; but spiritually the sin of ignorance, we are told, may be winked at. Is it not plain that the individual who drinks alcoholic drinks moderately, knowing them to be unnecessary and injurious, who is able easily to, but does not restrain his appetite, is actually more guilty, for his present acts, than the one who has gone one step further in the same road, and become what is called a drunkard, when he has not the same control over his appetite? Is it not true that every man who commences using tobacco, opium, or any other poison, for the unnatural excitement it causes, knowing it to be unnecessary and injurious, or who continues its use after coming to the knowledge that it is unnecessary and injurious, is equally guilty of sinning against his physical organization, and of a breach of the moral law, as the drinker of alcohol? How far he comes short of being a drunkard in the Bible acceptation of the term, I shall leave the reader to judge; the latter knowingly uses an injurious substance thereby making it his chief delight, the whisky drinker does no more; the consequences to the community may be more injurious in the one case than in the other, but not, it seems to me, to the man's moral nature.

How often has my heart been made sad to hear individuals, even young persons, say that they would continue the use of certain injurious substances if they knew that it would shorten their lives for years. To such a lamentable degree do these poisons in use blunt the moral nature of man that he becomes but a wreck of a true man.

The greatest slave in the world is he who is a slave to his sensual appetites. I would not have the appetite for, or the love of alcohol, opium or tobacco, for all the gold in California, for all the wealth of the world—for the treasures of earth will pass away, but the effects of these poisons, if their use is continued, will never pass away; even if they are indulged in ignorantly, the appetite for them will but strengthen with time, and eternity cannot eradicate their effects—at best a void will remain in the human soul which should be filled by the development of good and useful affections. Humanity, justice and truth, call upon us to use our utmost efforts to stay the use of these poisons. Every one has more or less influence over his fellow men by precept and example; especially have parents over their children. My father early became a temperance man, and not one of his children to-day uses alcoholic drinks.

The example of a drunken parent, sometimes, by manifesting the disgusting and pernicious consequences of rum-drinking, exercises a restraining influence over children. But the influence of the temperate drinker is much more to be feared. I have seen a man laugh before his children at the idea of a man's joining the temperance society, or resolving never to use alcoholic drinks, thereby signing away his liberty as he said, and I have seen the eyes of such a parent opened by seeing a child become a drunkard, and even when he changed his foolish course for one of total abstinence, I have known a response come back to the already stricken heart of the poor father, as it came to the legitimate successor of Louis Philippe—too late! too late! The grim monster intemperance had fixed his fascinating eyes and soon found other victims beneath the paternal roof. Well may a parent beware what example he sets before his children, and how he attempts by ridicule to prevent being formed, or to overthrow the virtuous, temperate and safe resolutions of the young.

Does the reader question but that to oppose the use of alcoholic drinks, except strictly as medicine, is a right, just and true course? Behold the hundreds of thousands of trembling drunkards in our land, and the sufferings of their worse than widows, and orphan children; look down into the graves of thirty thousand drunkards who die annually in the United States; and if that does not satisfy you, look with the eye of reason, enlightened by revelation, beyond the grave, and read: No drunkard shall inherit the kingdom of God—for he has loved the gratification of his sensual appetite more than he has loved the Lord and his neighbor; yes, even more than the wife of his bosom, and the child of his loins, or his own natural life. Tell me if righteousness, justice and truth, are the causes of all the suffering and wretchedness which flow from the use of alcoholic drinks? When has the most rigid total abstinence ever led to such consequences? Are truth and the laws of God at variance? Judge ye. Does a good and true tree bring forth evil fruits, such as these? These are, as we have seen, the legitimate fruits of temperate drinking, for no man ever became a drunkard who did not commence with temperate drinking; and rarely at this day does a man become a drunkard who has not commenced his career by drinking wine and strong beer.

If this is so—and I ask if it is not true—is it in accordance with truth to justify the use of such wine as we obtain in this country and strong beer during health at all? Do not the claims of humanity require of us, as true men, men who have at heart the welfare of others, and the world around us, to set our faces against the use of all stimulating drinks, and by precept and example do all we can to prevent their use, except strictly as medicine, as we would use arsenic, or any other poison?

The use of beer, especially lager beer, has become very fashionable of late, and it must be evident to every careful observer that it is doing a fearful work for the young men of our cities. It contains alcohol enough to kindle an appetite which will require to be fed by yet stronger drinks, and it is found side by side with such drinks in innumerable saloons in our cities and villages. Does any one suppose for a moment that any form of strong beer is a healthy drink? That a miserable bitter drug, like hops, can be taken into the stomach of a well man daily for months and years, without slowly but surely causing disease; and that even the small quantity of alcohol contained in the weaker varieties is harmless? If there is any one so ignorant, let him take a look at the bloated beer drinker; let him for once behold the terrible tortures which the gout causes for years, and turn to medical writers and learn that the use of beer is one of the chief predisposing causes of this disease. If he should ever chance to feel the twinges of this disease in his own toe joints, before he gets through with it, if he is not well stocked with patience, he will be likely to wish all the brewers and saloon keepers in a hotter place than even the Maine Law men were anxious to place them. In the quotations from Dr. Carpenter it has been shown how such drinks cause chronic diseases of the liver, kidneys, and stomach, by leading to excesses in eating, aside from their own poisonous effects.

"Malt liquors," says a distinguished writer, "though of less alcoholic strength than spirits and most wines, are capable of causing drunkenness, and this is quite a common effect of their use in England. At first apparently more favorable to nutrition than the other classes of alcoholic liquors, by the fullness and corpulency of frame which they induce, they are found to be after a while adverse to a ready and active discharge of the functions. The brain suffers, and the faculties are dull and sodden, or apoplexy strikes down the beer-bibber; the heart suffers, and there is hypertrophy, and retarded and irregular circulation, and danger of sudden death from this cause; the lungs suffer, and there is congestion, pneumonia, and not seldom dropsy of the chest. Other forms of dropsy also succeed to the free use of malt liquors, which kill more speedily, and with preceding symptoms of greater degradation—reduction of man to the mere brute, than even after the habitual use of ardent spirits. Some of the English writers while they admit and deplore these deleterious effects of drinking malt liquors, attribute them to adulteration. They add, however, that the taste of the people generally is so vitiated by the adulterated, in fact poisonous, beer and ale and porter, that even if the brewers were all honest, they would not find customers for their purer liquors. * * * In our climate, even more than in that of England, the habitual use of malt liquors is decidedly injurious. The free acid though partially disguised to the taste is detrimental to digestion, and to all the assimilating functions; it is particularly inimical to the skin and the kidneys."—Bell on Regimen and Longevity.

WINE.

The reader may ask, if the use of wine is not spoken of favorably in the Bible. We are told to give wine and strong drink to those who are ready to perish; and I have endeavored to point out some of the very few cases in which they may be found useful, and even necessary, but such cases are few and far between. But I will call the attention of the reader to a much more important passage, which reads as follows:

"Look not thou upon the wine when it is red, when it giveth its color in the cup, when it moveth itself aright. At the last it biteth like a serpent and stingeth like an adder."

Show me a kind of wine which does not answer this description, or which does not bite like a serpent and sting like an adder, and you will show me a kind of wine not often, if ever, found in our markets. Here, then, we have an express requirement which will condemn the wine to be found in common use in this country. That light wines are to be found in Central and Southern Europe, which are comparatively harmless, and when moderately used, entirely so, I am not disposed to dispute; but that even such are equal to water, as a common drink, is certainly very questionable. If they contain an appreciable quantity of alcohol, they certainly are not. If sugar is added in the manufacture of wine from the juice of the grape, we shall have from the fermentation, or decomposition, of the sugar, an excess of alcohol, which will add materially to the pernicious quality of the wine, and render it unfit for use.

The intoxicating ingredient in all wines is the alcohol which they contain, and in pure wine which is made from the juice of the grape, the alcohol is produced by the decomposition of grape sugar, and the strength of the wine will depend, first, upon the amount of this sugar, or saccharine matter, contained in the juice of the grape, which varies in the different varieties of grapes; and, secondly, upon the extent to which the process of fermentation has proceeded. This process is not completed at once, but continues for many months; and can be increased by the exposure of the wine to the air, and stirring; or lessened by excluding the air when fermentation begins to slacken, and allowing the wine to be at rest. The saccharine matter may all be destroyed and alcohol take its place, or it may not, which will depend, either upon the extent to which the process of fermentation has proceeded, or the relative quantity of other ingredients in the juice of the variety of the grape used.

But in all cases where neither sugar is added to the juice of the grape in the preparation of wine, nor alcohol in any form mixed with the wine, says Dr. Bache:

"The alcohol naturally in wine, is so blended with its other constituents, as to be in a modified state, which renders it less intoxicating and injurious than the same quantity of alcohol separated by distillation and diluted with water."

Still in regard to the use of pure wines he continues:

"The light wines of France are comparatively innocuous; while the habitual use of the stronger ones, such as port, maderia, sherry, etc., even though taken in moderation, is always injurious, as having a tendency to induce gout and apoplexy, and other diseases dependent on plethora and over stimulation. All wines, however, when used habitually in excess, are productive of bad consequences. They weaken the stomach, produce diseases of the liver, and give rise to dropsy, gout, apoplexy, tremors, and not unfrequently mania."

The best then that can be said in regard to the use of wine, when it is pure, is that when it is light and does not contain alcohol enough to intoxicate when drank in ordinary quantities, its occasional use, rather as a luxury than a constant beverage, may be justifiable. But upon strong wine, even when made from the pure juice of the grape, which experience has shown "Biteth like a serpent and stingeth like an adder," we should not even look with a longing eye; and as alcohol is added to, perhaps, all of our imported wines, even when they are otherwise pure, none of them are fit for use as a beverage. It is beyond all question true, that the wine which we generally get in this country contains very little of the juice of the grape, and often none at all, but is manufactured from alcohol, dye-stuff and drugs; and, of course, its use in any quantity can only be injurious to health and destructive to life.

CONCLUSION.

THAT the use of stimulating drinks is entirely unnecessary, during health, will be manifest if we compare the health of that portion of the community who abstain entirely from their use, with the health of those who use them. If we lay aside preconceived opinions, and observe carefully, we shall soon be satisfied that the use of stimulating drinks, during health, in any quantity is only evil, and that continually. All the safety and good are on the side of total abstinence, and truth is always in harmony with good. All the danger and evil lies in the direction of Temperate drinking, and evil and falsehood always make one, or are in harmony. In fact, alcohol, as has been stated above, is a product resulting from the decomposition of sugar, a good and useful article of diet. It is then, from a perversion and destruction of a substance good and true.

I have taken the following remarks from a Boston medical journal, the "*Medical World.*" The writer says:

"Water-drinkers ordinarily outlive spirit-drinkers, we have a remarkable verification of this statement from an old physician of Natchez. After having enumerated the deaths of most of the physicians of that city, who lived there thirty years ago, who were spirit-drinkers, and given the names of those who were not, and who are still living, he says, as it was with the doctors of Natchez and vicinity, so it has been with the lawyers. The lawyers of that city and vicinity, thirty years ago, who were in the habit of using alcoholic beverages in the place of plain water, between meals, are all dead long ago. There is not one left, even to bring the time down to twenty years, there is not one left. While the temperate lawyers of the same locality, from twenty to thirty years ago, are all living at the present time, June, 1853, minus a number less than the natural decrease of mankind, incident to the most healthy countries, as set forth in the Carlisle tables of mortality. The bench and the pulpit have scarcely lost a member, except from accident or old age. The temperate lawyers, with the exceptions just mentioned, are not only all living, but they are all rich, though they began life poor. The contrast arrived at by consulting time and experience, is so great, that it may be said death is in alcohol, and life is in water, when used as a common beverage. That plain, good, pure water is better than alcohol in any form, to enable the human system to endure fatigue and exposure, and to give both body and mind strength and vigor, the history of the above mentioned classes plainly proves."

Such is the testimony of medical writers, which is based upon carefully collected statistics. That the use of stimulants has done much not only to impair the health and to shorten the lives of multitudes of our race, but also to impair by hereditary transmission the physical and even mental constitutions of offspring, must be manifest to every well-informed observer. The gout is a hereditary disease; and the chronic diseases of the stomach, liver and kidneys, as well as the general nervous debility, which are so frequently caused by the moderate use of stimulants, can but result in the transmission of a predisposition to similar diseases to the children of such parents.

Careful inquiry and statistics have shown that congenital idiocy can frequently be traced to drunken parentage; for it has been found that the children of drunkards are much more liable to be idiots, and to become insane than the children of temperate parents. With all the evidence we have of the danger and injury which results from the use of alcoholic drinks, how can any conscientious man justify or countenance their use, knowing them to be entirely unnecessary? How can so many of our ladies, while viewing on every hand drunken parents, children, brothers, and even sisters, and homes made desolate, deliberately place the seductive wine cup before their friends, knowing full well that a fearful retribution so frequently follows such conduct? That even those near and dear to them may become victims, and that they themselves will then have to drink to the very dregs the bitter cup which they have surely aided in preparing for not a few poor wives, mothers, sisters and daughters.

Let not fashion rule us, for she is a relentless tyrant. Let us do our duty and fear not that dark tyranny which would deter us by sneers, innuendoes and sarcasm. Let us have the moral courage to speak the truth upon this subject, and still more, to do in accordance with the truth, and not only not tempt others to their ruin, but also, to say to our friends, neighbors and enemies who may present the poisoned cup to our lips, that we never drink; after which declaration we shall rarely be asked the second time.

I am satisfied from observation, that the ladies of our country, especially in fashionable society, are doing much in the way of encouraging the tendency to dissipation among young men. Few young men have the moral courage to refuse to partake of wine and other stimulants when tendered by ladies whom they esteem. Their use is thus rendered fashionable and enticing; an appetite for them is often acquired, which leads the inexperienced youth to the habits of dissipation.

Reformed drunkards are, in not a few instances, led back to habits of intemperance by first partaking of the social cup with some fair friend; and once they have violated their good resolutions, all barriers are gone, the appetite returns in all its original force, and the drunkard's wretched life returns but to terminate in the grave. Where ladies offer alcoholic drinks to their friends, in not a few instances habits of intemperance will inevitably follow, and they know not who will be the victims, but causes will surely produce their effects; nor are the ladies themselves exempt from danger, for many a woman has thus fallen to rise no more.

He who uses alcoholic, or fermented drinks, at all, can do little or nothing either by precept or example, towards saving his fellow men, or even his own family, from drunkenness, if he can avoid the common fate himself. Alas! too often it is the case that when he claims but to drink temperately, and boasts of his ability to restrain his appetite, his neighbors could tell him that he is a drunkard; which intimation, if made, he, not realizing the fact to which his attention is called, as he feels that he only drinks just enough to give the required cheerfulness and strength, will generally be found as ready to resent, notwithstanding his admission that he uses stimulants, as was a certain sanctimonious man, upon a particular occasion, a somewhat similar intimation. This man had been greatly disturbed by the neglect of a certain skeptical neighbor to attend religious meetings; he often labored with him on account of his neglect of duty. After a time, this neighbor consented to attend a conference meeting with him one evening. During the meeting the professedly pious neighbor arose to tell his experience. He went on to state what a great sinner he had been; how he had violated the laws of God, and that nothing but the mercy of the Lord had saved him from destruction. When he took his seat, his skeptical neighbor arose and said: that he felt it his duty to arise and bear testimony to the truth of all that his neighbor had stated; and, said he: "I have lived by him for many years, and I can assure you that for once he has told the truth, that his statement that he has been a great sinner, and has violated the laws of God and deserves punishment, is true, every word of it." It is false! it is false! exclaimed the confessor; "there is not a word of truth in it."

If we would follow the path of safety which leads to health in this world, and tends to happiness in the next, let total abstinence from all alcoholic drinks ever be our motto. Acting from duty guided by reason, let us ever remember that life in this world is given us for a great and noble end, and that we cannot squander our physical energies and life, by the unlawful gratification of our sensual appetites, and be blameless. We can no more escape the moral consequences which result from our voluntary acts, than we can the physical effects of natural causes.

Let not our reformation, if we have been accustomed to improper indulgences, be a miserable shifting from one bad habit to another; but with "total abstinence," not only from all alcoholic drinks, but also from all known poisonous substances, engraven upon our banner, let us, like the mountain eagle,

"With wing on the wind and eye on the sun,
Swerve not a hair, but bear onward, right on."

CHAPTER XI.

EXCESSIVE LABOR.

It is true both mentally and physically, that "All work and no play makes Jack a dull boy." If all the faculties of the mind and organs of the body could be duly exercised at any one employment, such a result would not follow; but this is impossible. If the entire energies of the mind are devoted to any kind of mental labor, the body suffers, and soon becomes deformed, debilitated, and diseased. Nor are these the only injuries which result, as is shown in the chapter on Amusements, and in other chapters; for the remaining faculties of the mind are sure to suffer, or become debilitated and lose their vitality. The faculty which is constantly exercised becomes unduly developed, out of proportion to the other faculties; and mental deformity, disease, or insanity result as surely as physical deformity and disease result from constantly exercising one set of muscles to the neglect of the rest of the muscular system. We may have very great mental deformity from over exercise of certain faculties and neglect of others, without having actual insanity, just as we may have physical deformity, from undue exercise of one set of muscles to the neglect of others, without having actual disease. In both cases there is no balance—no harmony. Mentally the individual is a one idea man, a fanatic, or an enthusiast, when he escapes monomania. Whatever mental strength is manifested in the favorite direction, as a whole, the mind is feeble and weak; and from the general mental debility, it is impossible for the faculty most exercised, to reach the highest state of activity and power to which it would have been capable of attaining if more attention had been paid toward obtaining a harmonious mental development.

It has been the aim of the writer to impress upon the reader the importance of striving for a symmetrical development of both mind and body; and also the fact that a harmonious development can only be attained, and sustained by the regular exercise of every faculty of the mind, and organ and muscle of the body.

Among the laboring and business men of our country there is generally both mental and physical activity enough, especially after they arrive at adult age, but it is usually partial, and lacks a healthy variety. The gratification of the appetites, acquisitiveness or vanity, is too frequently the motive which prompts to activity, and the prevailing ideas are work! work! work! Intellectual or physical labor, so directed as to secure a return in dollars and cents, in honors or sensual enjoyment, is, apparently, by the great mass of our citizens, alone regarded as a worthy employment for man. As a result of the prevalence of this false sentiment, the nobler faculties of the mind—veneration, benevolence, mirthfulness, and friendship—have languished, until, with multitudes, Christianity has become little better than dead formality, and benevolence a gratification of vanity; until amusements have been perverted so as to minister to unlawful, sensual gratification, by one portion of the community, while by another, their importance is in a great measure overlooked and denied; and until friendship is measured, to a great extent, by dollars and cents, or favors given and received.

How much more important is the cultivation of kindly affections towards our fellow men, or the healthy development of the mind and body, than this incessant labor to make money, or to obtain notoriety, or even to acquire intellectual treasures, which deform and destroy the body, if not all true life in the soul?

It is high time that sedentary men begin to learn that all the faculties of the mind require to be duly exercised; and, especially, that every organ of the body must be properly exercised, in order for strength and health of either mind or body; and that duty to God and man, as well as themselves, and even self interest, require that they should faithfully act accordingly.

Perhaps among no class in the community are the conditions required for a harmonious development, and preservation, of both soul and body, more heedlessly violated than among the Clergy. They often allow their mental faculties to be long bent in one direction, to a particular class of subjects; they neglect needed amusements and recreation, as well as active labor, or other active exercise, almost entirely; as a result, we have among them, many narrow minded men, bigots mentally, and physically sickly and inefficient. There are certainly noble exceptions—men who are mentally and physically worthy.

"A correspondent," says D. H. Jacques, "of one of our religious journals gives his brethren the following timely hints, suggested by the conversion of a noted pugilist:"

"I dislike to see Satan's body-guard—blackguards though they are—six feet high and forty-five inches about the chest; while the servants of God go creeping about—little shad-bellied fellows—scarce able to walk under the Christian armor, much less able to fight in it! * * * * * We want more *muscle*, as well as more *mind*, in our pulpits.

"When Henry Ward Beecher went to be examined by a phrenologist, Fowler walked around him, and eyed him as a jockey would eye a fine horse, and said, 'You're a *splendid animal!*' 'That's just it,' he replied, 'that's the secret of my success.' Truth! When a man's *body* is vigorous, his mind is vigorous, and his thoughts are energetic, searching, and clear. I don't know whether our Christian churches have grown weak because our ministers have grown lean, or whether the ministers have grown lean because the churches have become weak; but of this I am sure, that many of our ministers to-day weigh too little in the pulpit, because they weigh too little on the scales."

That many of our clergy have to perform too much mental labor, for their present physical strength, is beyond question; but, if they would spend a reasonable share of their time in active amusements and labor, or gymnastic exercises, they would be as much better able to perform their present amount of mental labor, as are tailors or shoe-makers better able to perform their daily tasks when they devote two hours to ball-playing, dancing, or active exercises in the gymnasium.

Physicians, I have reason to think from observation, do not generally injure themselves by excessive study, after they have completed the required period of pupilage, but if they are successful in obtaining a large practice, they suffer much from mental anxiety, loss of sleep, and irregular meals and hours, which together with unavoidable exposure to the causes of disease, render them, as a class, short-lived. Physicians in extensive business lack time for domestic and social recreation and amusement, and are more perfect slaves to their calling than any other class of men, for they have not an hour exempt from a liability to interruption by a business call. The community is often too exacting, and seems to forget that a medical man requires rest, regular meals, and recreation, perhaps more than the members of any other profession or calling, in order that he may be prepared to discharge his duties in the best manner. If he has a wife and children, they have claims upon his attention which he cannot neglect, or, at least, should not; yet there are individuals who will censure the physician if he does not answer promptly every call, even to the extent of sacrificing, or seriously risking health and life, and the welfare and happiness of his family; although other physicians, perhaps equally competent, but without his reputation, may be suffering for the want of business. Perhaps in no profession does success in obtaining business depend less on real merit. Often some fortuitous circumstance gives a man notoriety and business, which he retains in spite of want of skill and success; brass, in his case, supplying the place of brains. Pomposity often outsteps modest worth. A young physician of my acquaintance used to say, if he only had a certain doctor's abdomen it would be the making of him in the way of obtaining practice.

Lawyers are generally fond of good cheer, and recreation; and, as a class, suffer less than physicians when they avoid dissipation; still they often destroy health and life by over mental application, and neglect of physical exercise. While earnestly engaged in the examination and preparation for an important trial, if the individual is not careful, the mind becomes so engrossed as to neglect the wants of the body, and health is impaired; but this need not and should not be. Lawyers and Clergymen—and especially the latter—should be, and, when they pay any regard to the laws of God, as manifested in nature, are among the healthiest and longest lived persons in the community.

"It is a shame! It is a burning shame!" that throughout our land the teachers of the young, those who have the care and instruction of children and youth, and whose influence over them for good or evil is next to, and often superior to, parental influence, as a class are perhaps more delicate, sickly, and physically inactive than almost any other portion of the community. If I had to select our teachers, no delicate, pale faced, dyspeptic, or sickly man or woman, who is unavoidably so, or who has not sense, knowledge, and energy enough to preserve health, symmetry of form, beauty, substance, and strength of body, when a healthy organization has been inherited, would ever be employed as teacher. Think you, gentle parent, that no harm is done to the moral and physical well being of your child, by allowing a wrinkled, tobacco-spitting, or pale-faced, thin, lifeless, dyspeptic man, who has barely energy enough to get to the place of meeting, and languidly spend his few hours in teaching the intellect, who cannot set the example of a single active muscular movement, or even play a game of ball, to stand up as a teacher and as a model before him? or by allowing a sickly, nervous, small-waisted, bare-necked, thin-shod woman, who cares more for the gratification of vanity than for health or life, to train up your daughters in the way they should not go—unless you desire to see them travel to a premature grave and perdition?

It is all important that we have a different class of teachers from many of those at present employed—teachers who shall be a moral and physical example to the young, and shall be able to teach them practically the laws of health and life, and lead them by example to obey them. The health and lives of those engaged in this employment are not destroyed by excessive labor as a general rule, for they are only required to teach six hours a day, which is no more than small children are required to sit and study or recite. If such confinement and application destroys the health, and prevents the development of growing children, and youth, as it surely does, it does not follow that it will injure the adult man or woman, especially when they are allowed, to be upon their feet walking around more or less. It is the neglect of physical exercise and amusements, and other bad habits, which destroy the health, strength and energy of so many of our teachers. Turn both teachers and pupils out doors, one-third or one-half of the time they now spend in the school room, and require them to engage in active plays, and gymnastic exercises, and the gain in substance, beauty, strength, health, and life, in the rising generation, within five years, will astonish every one. But there is no need of teachers at present being so delicate and sickly, for they have time enough for exercise out of their school hours, if they would but improve it.

Book-keepers, tailors, and seamstresses, suffer more, perhaps, than any other portion of the community from excessive labor, as many of those engaged at such employments are compelled to work early and late for a bare subsistence for themselves and families; they have very little time for exercise or amusements. Let all such improve every leisure moment in active sports and exercise, and they will thus perform their accustomed task with much greater ease, without impairing health.

Merchants, with few exceptions, suffer from unnatural excitement, over anxiety, want of exercise and recreation; as is manifested in their care-worn features, and hurried gait, and premature old age.

No class in the community is so well situated for development, health, and long life, as farmers. They have, in abundance, pure air, undimmed sunshine, food and raiment, and space for amusements; and they should have time to enjoy the latter, as well as for intellectual culture. How is it with our farmers to-day, with all these natural advantages? Are they progressing physically in manly form, beauty, and symmetry of body? or in domestic and social graces, or in intelligence, towards perfection? They certainly are striving hard to develop into symmetry of form, various domestic animals, and to render them useful; and they are also dilligently cultivating various vegetables, so that they may answer the end for which they were designed, or be useful to man. Would that we could say the same in regard to themselves; but, alas! it is but too evident, that with many of our farmers, even the physical body becomes bowed down, crippled, and diseased from excessive labor, and from an almost total neglect of any systematic training to aid in its development, and preservation. The great ends of life, the cultivation of the religious, domestic, social and intellectual faculties, seem to be almost entirely overlooked, in the strife for material wealth—in a monotonous round of working, sleeping and eating, with no higher end in view than an increase of crops, and acres, and a multiplication of cattle. In connection with this excessive physical labor, there is but little reading, study or thinking; domestic and social amusements, and recreation, are neglected; and thus both body and soul are deformed, and often diseased. This should not be; it need not be; it must not be.

"It is a matter," says an intelligent writer, "of small moment and scarcely a subject for congratulation, that our crops of corn are growing heavier, from year to year, under improved methods of cultivation, while the crops of men and women left without cultivation are rapidly deteriorating."

Proper recreation and amusements to develop and preserve the human body and affections, and the needed relaxation from business necessary for their enjoyment and for intellectual improvement, are far more important to our farmers than myriads of bushels of grain, or hundreds of cattle. Books and periodicals to feed the mind and furnish subjects for thought, are far more important than tobacco, coffee, tea, and the many pernicious condiments so freely used, which but impair health and shorten life.

Not only do our farmers generally over work, but the same is true of our mechanics, and the operatives in our manufactories, they all need more time for amusements and intellectual culture, and for the want of such advantages, many who arrive to middle age become dull and rigid in both mind and body, instead of progressing in intelligence and goodness, and in symmetry and beauty of form, to a noble manhood, and a cheerful old age.

"To lay the foundation for a long life, both body and mind must practice industrious activities. The hod carrier works the body hard, the brain almost none; the power of one is used up, that of the other is not used at all, and he dies of some speedily fatal disease. The mere student exhausts the brain; the body is not worked at all, and he too dies early, with some acute malady. The farmer works his body hard; is in the open air all the time; eats plain food; retires early; rises with the sun; and indulges in no irregular habits; but his mind, beyond a certain routine, which soon becomes mechanical, as to prices, crops and weather, has no waking-up activities, and he too dies before his time, or vegetates in an asylum."—HALL'S JOURNAL OF HEALTH.

There is no state of the human body where it is more essential that excessive labor should be avoided than during pregnancy; yet it is perhaps true that the wives of a majority of the laboring portion of the community, not only harm themselves but also impair the vitality of their offspring by over-work during such periods. Husbands who would not for a moment think of putting a beast during the latter months of pregnancy into a team, or before a plow, do not scruple to see their wives, during the same period, toiling early and late at household labor and sewing, and constantly perplexed by the care of children, in-doors, deprived of out-door exercise, light and air. The essential conditions required for the welfare of a pregnant female, and her offspring, are light employment for the mother and freedom from care, cheerful company, gentle exercise in the open air and sunlight. Idleness and inactivity should be avoided as well as overwork, for both are alike destructive.

DEFORMITY and disease not unfrequently result from permitting the body to assume a bad position in standing, sitting or lying. Individuals who follow avocations which require them to stoop;

while standing, walking, or sitting, or who permit themselves to stoop while walking or sitting, are very sure to become round shouldered; which materially interferes with the action of the lungs, heart and digestive organs, and predisposes to disease of these organs. It is much easier to stand or sit erect, if we but accustom ourselves to it, than it is to assume a bent position, for the head and shoulders then rest upon the spinal column, instead of being sustained by an unnatural position of the muscular system. It is very important that teachers and parents require children and young persons, to sit erect during their studies; and that they do not confine them longer at any one time than they can thus sit without fatigue. It is also important that those whose occupations require them to stoop, should take particular pains to maintain the erect position when not thus occupied, and to exercise the muscles not used during labor.

Deformity frequently results from lying in a bad position; lying with the head too high, or with the head and shoulders elevated higher than the rest of the body, causing curvature of the spine. In lying upon the back a very small pillow only is proper, and in lying upon the side, one should never, during health, be used larger than is sufficient barely to raise the head to a level with the shoulders, or a trifle above. The broad pillows, so much in fashion at present, which not only raise the head, but also the shoulders, are very pernicious, and a fruitful cause of spinal curvatures; and should be banished forthwith.

When spinal curvatures already exist, much can be done towards remedying the deformity by proper care in regard to the position of the body while lying down, and by a persevering effort to sit and stand erect, aided by frequently drawing in a full breath, and swinging by the hands; and if need be by carrying weights upon the head. It is only when the deformity is so great that it is impossible to obtain relief from such measures, that it is best to resort to shoulder straps, and artificial support, for the latter when not absolutely needed, take the place of muscular support, and thereby render the muscles feeble and delicate, and keep up the necessity for constant artificial support, notwithstanding which the deformity is very sure to increase.

It is not my intention to write a work on surgery, or to devote much space to this subject; but as much suffering, and more or less deformity, often result from a want of knowledge on the part of the community, in regard to the proper method of treating wounds, a few suggestions will not be found out of place in this work. It is even more important to say what should not be done, than it is to give directions for the proper treatment of wounds; for more suffering results from the officious meddling of the uninstructed, than from neglect. The services of a surgeon, or physician, should always, when possible, be secured immediately to attend in cases where severe wounds have been received. But in cases of slight wounds or in those more severe where the services of a physician cannot be readily obtained, it is important for the attendants, and the patient, to have some knowledge in regard to the proper treatment; and, especially, in regard to what should not be done.

Incised wounds, are such as are made with a sharp, or cutting instrument. There is more immediate danger of hemorrhage in such than in any other variety of wounds; therefore it is important for all to know how to arrest hemorrhage, temporarily at least, in such cases; and also in all kinds of wounds. If the blood flowing from a wound is dark colored, and does not flow in jets, but in a steady stream, it can generally be checked by applying cold water, and exposing the cut surface to the cold air, if the vessels from which it flows, are small. If these measures do not soon relieve, or if large veins are wounded, they should be compressed by the ends of the fingers, or by a compress, bound to the part by a bandage, or held by the hand. It is never well to heap on a large quantity of rags or cloths, for they only absorb the blood; a few thicknesses with steady compression, are far more efficacious. If the blood is of a bright color, and flows in jets, it shows that an artery has been wounded, and that there is more danger of serious hemorrhage. If the artery is small, by compressing it firmly with the end of a finger for a few moments, the bleeding will often cease. If it is larger, but not very large, and a surgeon is not at hand, it may be compressed by the finger until a small pair of forceps can be obtained, with which the bleeding vessel may be seized, and either twisted around once or twice, or drawn out and tied with a strong thread. If the artery is of any considerable size it will require to be ligatured, or tied, before the hemorrhage can be permanently checked; but the life of the patient often depends upon the prompt application of measures, by the bystanders, or the patient himself, for temporarily restraining the flow of blood, or death results, as it resulted in the following instance: Two men were mowing in a field, when one accidentally struck the other with his scythe, and wounded the artery which passes down behind the inner ankle: they were both frightened at the profuse flow of blood; the well man ran for help, the wounded man, for his house; but the latter fell down exhausted, and bled to death. Had either of these men possessed the requisite knowledge, which every one should possess, he might have checked for the time being, the flow of blood, by the pressure of a finger, either on the end of the wounded vessel, or by pressing the vessel against the bone above the wound. He could then have bound a hard compress so as to press the vessel against the bone, by the means of a handkerchief or suspender, and could have made all secure until he could have obtained the services of a surgeon; or in case no surgeon, forceps or tenaculum, which surgeons use could have been readily obtained, he could have bent the end of a pin into a hook, with which he might have seized the end of the bleeding vessel, drawn it down, and tied it with a thread.

A little presence of mind, and the requisite knowledge, is often all that is necessary to enable any one to save the life of a wounded man, in case of hemorrhage. I have had an intelligent man restrain the flow of blood from a wounded carotid artery, or the large artery which passes up the neck to the head, by pressing the artery below the wound firmly back against the spinal bones of the neck, and by pressure upon the wound, until a messenger could be sent a mile for me, and I had time to dress and go and ligature the vessel.

The blood flows in the arteries from the heart to every part of the body, and pressure, in order to be effectual, must be made at some point in the course of the artery between the heart and the wound, where it can be compressed against a bone, so as to effectually prevent the flow of blood through the vessel at the point. If the large arteries about the neck are wounded, pressure should be made by the thumb on the lower part of the neck, above the collar bone, close to the trachea or windpipe, on the side upon which the hemorrhage occurs. If the end of the bleeding vessel can be seen, it may be directly compressed with the finger, in connection with the compression below. If the wound is low down in the neck, the only chance may be to press into the wound upon the bleeding vessel. If an artery in the arm is wounded, the main artery may be compressed near the arm pit, or lower on the inside of the arm; or a handkerchief may be tied around the arm above the wound, and always above the elbow, even if the wound is below, and, with a stick, the handkerchief may be twisted until it stops the flow of blood. It will the more readily do this if a compress of cloth or of a stick, or stone, half as large as a hen's egg, is placed under the handkerchief, over the course of the artery, on the inner side of the arm. If the main artery in the thigh is wounded high up, or at any point, with the thumb, it can be compressed against the bone as it passes out of the abdomen, high up in the groin, where it can be felt beating, about midway between the front point of the hip bones, and the central point of the bones of the pelvis, in front. If the wound is low down on the thigh, or below the knee in the fleshy part of the leg, the artery can be compressed at the point named above, and a handkerchief can be put around the thigh, with a compress beneath it, and twisted with a stick as directed for the arm. The artery, as it leaves the abdomen, is directly in front of the thigh, but it gradually winds around the inside of the thigh, until it reaches the knee, when it is directly behind; it is necessary to bear this in mind, so as to know at what point to apply the compress in order to have it over the artery; for a compress here is more important than in the arm, and should be nearly or quite as large as a hen's egg. Such measures for checking the flow of blood, of course, are only temporary, and to be used until the bleeding vessel can be ligatured.

Having arrested the hemorrhage the next point is to see that the wound is free from all foreign substances, such as dirt, bits of clothing, and hair; also, as far as practicable, from clots of blood. After the hemorrhage has ceased the wound may be washed out with tepid water, but if there is still some oozing of blood, cold water may be used.

As soon as practicable the wound should be dressed; if it is very large or angular, or about parts where there is much motion, one or more stitches may be required, which can be made with a common needle and coarse linen or silk thread, if a surgeon cannot be obtained within an hour or two. Narrow strips of adhesive plaster should be used to draw the edges of the wound accurately together. The more perfectly the edges are drawn and kept together, the more certainty will there be of a speedy cure. At the end of four days the stitches should be cut on one side close to where they enter the skin, and by taking hold of the knots they should be drawn out. If an artery has been ligatured, one end of the ligature should be left hanging out of the wound when it is first dressed, so that it can be withdrawn when it becomes loose. Over the adhesive plaster may be put a few folds of cotton or linen cloth, and a bandage around the whole, if the parts are adapted to a bandage. The strips of adhesive plaster should not be removed until the wound is well, which will usually require the best part of a week, before it will be safe to remove the dressings entirely, or exercise the part. A cut wound, if it does well, when thus dressed, will heal up, by what surgeons call "first intention," without the discharge of any matter; and when it does so heal it leaves but a very trifling scar, a simple seam; whereas, if it matterates, it will generally require weeks, and often even months, to heal, and will leave a comparatively large scar. All surgeons, at this day, when they have an opportunity to dress them early, aim to have cut, and even lacerated and contused wounds—if the parts are not too much bruised—heal up in this manner. Nature effects the cure; all that art can do, is to furnish favorable conditions. If the parts are not brought together they can not heal, but must suppurate. Excessive inflammation sometimes occurs, although rarely, especially in cut wounds; but when it does, if not soon relieved, it will prevent healing. In such a case cold, and if that does not relieve, warm applications—simple cloths wrung from cold or warm water, or a bread and milk poultice—are all that are necessary, and oiled silk should be placed over the adhesive plasters so as to prevent their getting wet, and being loosened. But where there is not much inflammation, no applications are necessary, more than the first dressings of straps and bandages; and, often, the latter may be dispensed with.

But in order for wounds to thus heal in four or five days, they must not be tampered with before being dressed; they must be dressed within a very few hours—within one or two if possible—after being received, and be let alone after they are dressed until the parts have time to heal.

But a good deal of ignorance prevails with many, which is the cause of much mischief and unnecessary suffering. Every man and woman, almost, has a cure-all for cuts and wounds; one applies soap and sugar, another whisky, another salt, and another some quack plaster, ointment, or liniment. With not a few, tobacco is a sovereign remedy. Not long since I was called to dress a finger, which had been nearly severed, and found the wound stuffed full of this poisonous and filthy weed, the result was the young man lost his finger. All such applications, when applied to the surface of a wound, cause an unnatural irritation, and it is always very difficult to heal a wound, by first intention, after they have been once applied; and it is generally impossible to avoid suppuration, and consequently much unnecessary suffering, loss of time, and deformity. But as wounds generally get well in spite of bad treatment, the nostrum used gains credit, through the ignorance of the user. No application, then, should generally be made, to the kind of wounds we are now considering, except such as are necessary to keep the two surfaces of the wound accurately together; and often all that is needed for this purpose, especially about the extremities, are a bandage, and a small compress, or two, of cloth or cotton. Where these are not sufficient, adhesive plasters, and occasionally stitches, are needed, as directed above. No irritating applications should ever be made to the raw surface of a fresh cut, as it not only causes severe suffering, but it also serves to lessen the chance for a speedy cure. The application of salt, spirits of turpentine, and like stimulating applications, to cut surfaces, in the lower order of animals, is cruel, in the extreme. The oil of turpentine may sometimes be applied to the hair around the wound, when it is difficult to confine dressings to the parts, to keep the flies away, but care should always be taken that it does not enter the wound.

Contused wounds, where the surfaces are badly bruised, so as to impair or destroy their vitality, will not generally heal up by first intention; but even such wounds should be dressed by simple, soothing applications, instead of such as are irritating. To prevent inflammation the applications should be cool, or even cold, but if the wounded surfaces become inflamed, warm applications do better—simply cloths from warm water, or a warm bread and milk poultice. After the imflammation is relieved the more simple the dressings the better, for nature heals the wound, and the danger is that the applications which are made, may do harm, or interfere with her work.

CONCLUSION.

After dwelling upon the evils and consequent diseases of humanity for nearly three hundred and fifty pages, or, including the little work on "Marriage and its Violations," for nearly four hundred pages, it is a relief to the author to feel that his work is done. He does not think that it is faultless, for most of this volume has been written amid the cares and perplexities of an extensive medical practice, but such as it is he permits it to go forth to the public.

As was stated in the Preface, several of the chapters contained in this volume were first written as lectures, and were intended to be somewhat complete separately, which in treating of kindred subjects necessarily required more or less repetition of leading ideas. In two or three instances short quotations from other authors have been repeated verbatim, for the sake of giving point and force to the subject discussed; for the great aim of the author has been to make this volume useful to his countrymen, and not to perfect it beyond the reach of critics.

The little work on "Marriage and its Violations," was intended as a chapter for the present volume when it was written, and comes legitimately within its scope; but as the subjects discussed in it are of a delicate character, and as the simple fact of their being included might lessen the free circulation of this volume, it has been thought best to publish it separately; not that it contains anything which, in the opinion of the author, it is not important that every man and woman, young and old, should understand, or which it would be injurious for a child to read. Every parent might not feel thus in regard to its contents, and that those who have any delicacy upon this subject need not be prevented from placing the present work in the hands of their children, has been a strong argument in favor of a separate volume.

After discussing so freely and sometimes as the reader may think almost disparagingly, the mental and physical evils of humanity the author feels called upon to express his decided conviction that a glorious future is before our race. He does not believe that all the signs of change and progress in science and arts, in morals and religion, are without their significance; and that even the American people are doomed to be destroyed as a race, either in the manner predicted by Miller, or by their own evils. While evil men are growing worse, and multitudes are being destroyed, good men are growing better, at least in intention, and are sincerely striving to act according to their convictions as to what is good and true. But so far as the physical man is concerned darkness prevails over the land; men and women often do not know how they should live in order to avoid disease and premature death. If this volume shall convey to the reader such practical information as will enable him to lead a better life both physically and spiritually, and escape suffering, disease, unhappiness and a premature death, and thus aid in the elevation of our race, it will answer the end for which it has been written.

The world can only become better as individual men and women become better.

www.ingramcontent.com/pod-product-compliance
Lightning Source LLC
LaVergne TN
LVHW010204110826
845151LV00002B/600
* 9 7 8 1 4 2 5 5 3 5 6 7 4 *